Pharmacoresistance in Epilepsy

Luisa Rocha • Esper A. Cavalheiro
Editors

Pharmacoresistance in Epilepsy

From Genes and Molecules to Promising Therapies

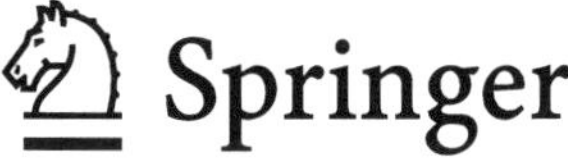

Editors
Luisa Rocha
Department of Pharmacobiology
Center for Research and Advanced Studies
Mexico City, Mexico

Esper A. Cavalheiro
Disciplina de Neurologia Experimental
UNIFESP/EPM, São Paulo, Brazil

ISBN 978-1-4614-6463-1 ISBN 978-1-4614-6464-8 (eBook)
DOI 10.1007/978-1-4614-6464-8
Springer New York Heidelberg Dordrecht London

Library of Congress Control Number: 2013936261

Printed on acid-free paper

Springer is part of Springer Science+Business Media (www.springer.com)

Contents

Contributors

Mario A. Alonso-Vanegas ABC Hospital, Santa Fé, Neurology Center, and National Institute of Neurology and Neurosurgery "Manuel Velasco Suárez", Mexico City, Mexico

Silvana Alvariza Pharmaceutical Sciences Department, Universidad de la República, Montevideo, Uruguay

Rebeca Padrão Amorim Department of Neurology and Neurosurgery, Universidade Federal de São Paulo-UNIFESP, São Paulo, Brazil

Michelle Gasparetti Leão Araújo Department of Neurology and Neurosurgery, Universidade Federal de São Paulo-UNIFESP, São Paulo, Brazil

Ricardo Mario Arida Department of Physiology, Universadade Federal de Sao Paulo, Rua Botucatu, Sao Paulo, Brazil

Carme Auladell Departament de Biologia Cellular, Universitat de Barcelona, Barcelona, Spain

Carlos Beas-Zárate Departamento de Biología Celular y Molecular, Centro Universitario de Ciencias Biologicas y Agropecuarias, Universidad de Guadalajara, Zapopan, Jalisco, México

Marilyn Zaldivar Bermudes Clinical Neurophysiology Service, International Center for Neurological Restoration, Habana, Cuba

Walter G. Besio Department of Electrical, Computer, and Biomedical Engineering, Rhode Island University, Kingston, RI, USA

Luis E. Bruno-Blanch Department of Biological Sciences, Faculty of Exact Sciences, National University of La Plata, La Plata, Argentina

Francisco Velasco Department of Neurology and Neurosurgery, General Hospital of Mexico, Mexico State, Mexico

Ester Verdaguer Cardona Departament de Biologia Cellular, Universitat de Barcelona, Barcelona, Spain

Jose Eduardo Marques Carneiro Department of Neurology and Neurosurgery, Universidade Federal de São Paulo-UNIFESP, São Paulo, Brazil

Esper A. Cavalheiro Disciplina de Neurologia Experimental, UNIFESP/EPM, São Paulo, Brazil

Martha Rivera-Cervantes Departamento de Biologia Celular y Molecular, Centro Universitario de Ciencias Biologicas y Agropecuarias, Universidad de Guadalajara, Zapopan, Jalisco, México

Lilia Maria Morales Chacón Clinical Neurophysiology Service, International Center for Neurological Restoration, Habana, Cuba

Liliana Czornyj Hospital Nacional de Pediatría "Juan P. Garrahan", Combate de los Pozos, Buenos Aires, Argentina

Maria Luisa de Lemos Institute of Biomedicine, Department of Pharmacology and Biomedical Chemistry, University of Barcelona, Barcelona, Spain

Aurelio Vazquez de la Torre Institute of Biomedicine, Department of Pharmacology and Biomedical Chemistry, University of Barcelona, Barcelona, Spain

Maria José da Silva Fernandes Department of Neurology and Neurosurgery, Universidade Federal de São Paulo-UNIFESP, São Paulo, Brazil

Antonio V. Delgado-Escueta West Los Angeles VA Medical Center, Los Angeles, CA, USA

Antoni Camins Espuny Institute of Biomedicine, Department of Pharmacology and Biomedical Chemistry, University of Barcelona, Barcelona, Spain

Pietro Fagiolino Pharmaceutical Sciences Department, Universidad de la República, Montevideo, Uruguay

Alfredo I. Feria-Velasco Departamento de Biología Celular y Molecular, Centro Universitario de Ciencias Biologicas y Agropecuarias, Universidad de Guadalajara, Zapapan, México

Lázaro Gómez Fernández Clinical Neurophysiology Service, International Center for Neurological Restoration, Habana, Cuba

Graciela Gudiño-Cabrera Departamento de Biología Celular y Molecular, Centro Universitario de Ciencias Biologicas y Agropecuarias, Universidad de Guadalajara, Zapopan, Jalisco, México

Laura Elena Hernández-Vanegas Epilepsy Clinic, National Institute of Neurology and Neurosurgery, Mexico City, Mexico

Clinical Epileptology Fellowship, National Autonomous University of Mexico, Mexico City, Mexico

Manuel Ibarra Pharmaceutical Sciences Department, Universidad de la República, Montevideo, Uruguay

Felix Junyent Unitat de Bioquimica, Facultat de Medicina i Ciencies de la Salut, Universitat Rovira i Virgili, Tarragona, Barcelona, Spain

Alberto Lazarowski INFIBIOC-FFyB-UBA-Universidad de Buenos Aires, Buenos Aires, Argentina

Jorge Alfredo León-Aldana Epilepsy Clinic, Hospital General San Juan de Dios, Guatemala City, Guatemala

Cecilia Maldonado Pharmeceutical Sciences Department, Universidad de la República, Montevideo, Uruguay

Iris E. Martínez-Juárez Epilepsy Clinic, National Institute of Neurology and Neurosurgery, Mexico City, Mexico

Clinical Epileptology Fellowship, National Autonomous University of Mexico, Mexico City, Mexico

Ana Luisa Velasco Department of Neurology and Neurosurgery, General Hospital of Mexico, Mexico State, Mexico

Sandra Orozco-Suárez Medical Research Unit in Neurological Diseases, National Medical Center "Siglo XXI", IMSS, Hospital of Specialties, Mexico City, Mexico

Mercè Pallàs Institute of Biomedicine, Department of Pharmacology and Biomedical Chemistry, University of Barcelona, Barcelona, Spain

Lourdes Lorigados Pedre Clinical Neurophysiology Service, International Center for Neurological Restoration, Habana, Cuba

Daniele Suzete Persike Department of Neurology and Neurosurgery, Universidade Federal de São Paulo-UNIFESP, São Paulo, Brazil

Heidrun Potschka Institute of Pharmacology, Toxicology, and Pharmacy, Ludwig-Maximilians-University, Munich, Germany

Otto Trápaga Quincoses Clinical Neurophysiology Service, International Center for Neurological Restoration, Habana, Cuba

Luisa Rocha Department of Pharmacobiology, Center for Research and Advanced Studies, Mexico City, Mexico

Nayelli Rodríguez y Rodríguez Epilepsy Clinic, National Institute of Neurology and Neurosurgery, Mexico City, Mexico

Iris Angélica Feria-Romero Medical Research Unit in Neurological Diseases, National Medical Center "Siglo XXI", IMSS, Hospital of Specialties, Mexico City, Mexico

Francisco Rubio-Donnadieu Programa Nacional de Eplepsia, National Institute of Neurology and Neurosurgery, Mexico City, Mexico

David Escalante-Santiago Medical Research Unit in Neurological Diseases, National Medical Center “Siglo XXI”, IMSS, Hospital of Specialties, Mexico City, Mexico

Carla A. Scorza Department of Neurology and Neurosurgery, Universidade Federal de São Paulo, São Paul, Brazil

Fulvio Alexandre Scorza Department of Neurology/Neurosurgery, Escola Paulista de Medicina/Universidade Federal de Sao Paulo, Rua Botacatu, Sao Paulo, Brazil

Richard J. Staba Department of Neurology, David Geffen School of Medicine at University of California Los Angeles, Los Angeles, CA, USA

Alan Talevi Department of Biological Sciences, Faculty of Exact Sciences, National University of La Plata, La Plata, Argentina

Monica E. Ureña-Guerrero Departamento de Biología Celular y Molecular, Centro Universitario de Ciencias Biológicas y Agropecuarias, Universidad de Guadalajara, Zapopan, Jalisco, Mexico

Marta Vázquez Pharmaceutical Sciences Department, Universidad de la República, Montevideo, Uruguay

Genco Marcio Estrada Vinajera Clinical Neurophysiology Service, International Center for Neurological Restoration, Habana, Cuba

Juana Villeda-Hernandez Pathology Department, National Institute of Neurology and Neurosurgery “Manuel Velasco Suárez”, Mexico City, Mexico

Cecilia Zavala-Tecuapetla Department of Pharmacobiology, Center for Research and Advanced Studies, Mexico City, Mexico

Chapter 1
Pharmacoresistance and Epilepsy

Francisco Rubio-Donnadieu

Abstract Although more than ten new antiepileptic drugs have been developed in the past decade, epilepsy remains resistant to drug therapy in about one-third of patients. Approximately 20 % of patients with primary generalized epilepsy and up to 60 % of patients who have focal epilepsy develop drug resistance during the course of their condition, which for many is lifelong. Managing these patients is a challenge and requires a structured multidisciplinary approach. The present chapter is a general overview of epilepsy as stigma, health and economical problem, and initiatives to change and the conditions of people with epilepsy. Special emphasis is focused to highlight the consequences of pharmacoresistant epilepsy.

Keywords Epilepsy • Pharmacoresistance • Epidemiology • Stigma • Antiepileptic drugs • Burden • Blood brain barrier • International League against Epilepsy • World Health Organization

1.1 Epilepsy

To "take hold of abruptly or to seize" is the meaning of the word Epilepsy, derived from a preposition and an irregular Greek verb *(Epilambanein).* Throughout the last five decades, the definition of epilepsy has been subjected to extensive controversy and debate by different neurological schools. It was not until 1973, that the International League against Epilepsy (ILAE) and the World Health Organization (WHO) published an Epilepsy dictionary in which epilepsy is defined as a chronic affliction of diverse etiology, characterized by recurring seizures due to excessive

F. Rubio-Donnadieu, M.D. (✉)
Programa Nacional de Eplepsia, National Institute of Neurology and Neurosurgery, Insurgentes Sur 3877, Col. La Fama, Mexico City C.P. 14269, Mexico
e-mail: frd@unam.mx

L. Rocha and E.A. Cavalheiro (eds.), *Pharmacoresistance in Epilepsy: From Genes and Molecules to Promising Therapies*, DOI 10.1007/978-1-4614-6464-8_1,

neuronal discharge (epileptic seizures), associated to diverse clinical and paraclinical manifestations. However, one must consider that there are many variables that are not encompassed within this definition, such as genetic aspects, age of onset, and triggering factors, on the one hand. On the other hand, this definition leaves out associated manifestation that have transcended to society, and throughout history led to interpretation of epilepsy as a supernatural phenomenon, as these paroxystic episodes cause fear, surprise and, as a rule, uncertainty.

1.2 Epilepsy as Stigma

The scientific development of medicine has often clashed with religious beliefs, leading to various erroneous concepts that classify epilepsy as the "sacred disease," oblivious to the warning by Hippocrates who tried to convince society that epilepsy was nowise more divine nor more sacred than other diseases, but had a natural cause like other affections. Regardless of Hippocrates wise concepts, absurd beliefs and conceptions multiplied and spread; the epileptic patient has been considered to "be possessed," which, in turn, has resulted in his/her rejection or exclusion not only by society in general, but often by the own family. It is well known that up to this date, the patient with epilepsy is submitted to exorcisms to liberate him/her from "demonic possession" both in highly developed and underdeveloped countries. Few diseases have been associated to such an accumulation of erratic beliefs, based on superstition, prejudice or ignorance, as epilepsy. In fact, in several cases it proves more difficult to control the environment where the epilepsy patient lives, than to obtain good seizure control. The stigma persists and is sustained on mystical bases.

The clinical manifestation of the disease and the different types of epileptic seizures were described since Babylonian times in the earliest handbooks of medicine in a clay tablet called antashubba, which is Sumerian for "falling disease." Regardless of this medical knowledge dating back over 4,000 years, religious beliefs were widely spread through the Bible, the Talmud, and the Koran. Paroxystic episodes are described in the Old Testament and considered as episodes of deep sleep (tardemah) that "took hold of Abra-ham." It is noteworthy that the word "Tardemah" used in Genesis and translated to Greek is understood as ecstasy, episodes that were frequently experienced by the prophets Isaiah, Daniel, Ezekiel and Jeremiah. On the other hand, the Book of Revelations in the New Testament contains a detailed description of what is now called "Saint John's malady," a disease suffered by the apostle himself with clinical features, consistent in auditive manifestations and falls with possible seizures, considered by Dostoyevsky as similar to his own episodes, and that can very likely be considered epileptic seizures.

Furthermore, even in the nineteenth century there were several evidences of erroneous interpretations of the epileptic phenomenon, always related to some famous character in the field of arts or science who exhibited these phenomena. Such is the case of the convulsive seizures presented by Vincent Van Gogh, who according to various reports was assumed to suffer epilepsy. This interpretation has been placed in doubt, considering the clinical history of Van Gogh and the surrounding circumstances of his convulsive episodes, that were most probably non-epileptic seizures associated to alcohol ingestion. The confusion resulting from the interpretation of Van Gogh's convulsive episodes has often led to the association of epileptic disorders with other mental disorders, such as the one suffered by Van Gogh, who, in hindsight, might have suffered from bipolar affective disorder leading to suicide. We can likewise highlight the consequences of the religious beliefs in Christ's miracle when he exorcised the lunatic child to liberate him from the "demonic possession causing epileptic seizures." Unfortunately, there are many examples in the literature that have done nothing more than spread an erroneous understanding of epilepsy, which is ultimately responsible for the persistent stigmatization of the patient with epilepsy.

From the historical point of view, it is a reality that "knowledge" is based on anecdotes, which are translated into facts considered to be incontrovertible, as they are derived from the evolution of culture and, particularly, religion, whether monotheist or polytheist. Thus, throughout the centuries this anecdotic-type beliefs persist and offer resistance to the great advances derived from science, particularly in the last 50 years and the recent knowledge that has resulted from application of the scientific method and led to new theories and continued research related to basic mechanisms; in this case, on the nature of the epileptic discharge. This is why, at the level of society in general, whose behavior is a reflection of cultural beliefs transmitted from generation to generation, it is difficult to obtain a consensus with recent scientific development and advances and modify the concepts that, throughout the centuries, have identified epilepsy as a supernatural phenomenon. Persistence of these erroneous concepts renders epilepsy an even bigger health problem worldwide, and it is why in 1997, the WHO, in conjunction with the ILAE, launched the Global Campaign "Epilepsy out of the shadows."

1.3 Epilepsy and Pharmacoresistance

Epilepsy is a multifactorial disorder from the molecular, genetical, and environmental points of view, which has been the cause of multiple controversies and drawbacks in creating a universal consensus and uniformed criteria that allow determining the magnitude and transcendence of the epileptic phenomenon. Since 1973, according to the WHO and ILAE, epilepsy has been defined as a chronic and recurrent affection of paroxystic seizures (epileptic seizures) resulting from abnormal electrical discharges that have varied clinical manifestations of multifactorial origin and are associated to paraclinical abnormalities (electroencephalographic abnormalities) and present spontaneously. This definition has had the great advantage of being accepted by the different associations and organizations related to the neurosciences, allowing, in the last three decades, a more or less uniformed criterion on what is considered an epileptic phenomenon. This uniformed definition has also contributed largely to the completion of comparative epidemiological studies worldwide, which allow organization of effective and sustainable campaigns against epilepsy to benefit people who suffer epilepsy.

Epilepsy is characterized by abnormal synchronization of neural activity. Pharmacotherapy is the treatment of choice for control of epileptic seizures and the selection of antiepileptic drugs (AEDs) depends on several factors such as the type of epilepsy and drug tolerability (Browne and Holmes 2001).

Though the majority of patients respond to treatment with AEDs adequately, about one third of patients present pharmacologically resistant epilepsy, which is generally defined as the failure of seizures to come under complete control or acceptable control in response to AED therapy (Berg 2009). Clinical characteristics associated to resistance include early onset of epileptic seizures (before 1 year of age), elevated seizure frequency before onset of treatment, history of febrile convulsive seizures, brain lesions, malformations of cortical development and dysembryoplastic neuroepithelial tumors (Rogawski and Johnson 2008; Semah et al. 1998; Regesta and Tanganelli 1999; Sisodiya et al. 2002).

An innate high excitatory neurotransmission could be a neurobiological factor that may underlie augmented susceptibility to develop pharmacoresistance (Arroyo et al. 2002; Rogawski and Johnson 2008; Luna-Munguia et al. 2011). At the cellular level, intractability of epilepsy is associated to factors such as abnormal reorganization of neuronal circuitry, alteration in several neurotransmitter receptors, canalopathies, reactive autoimmunity as well as the abnormal inadequate penetration of AEDs into the epileptic focus due to changes in the blood brain barrier (BBB) (Fig. 1.1) (Kwan and Brodie 2002; Vreugdenhil and Wadman 1994, 1999; Remy et al. 2003; Ellerkmann et al. 2003). Other factors, such as the cell junctions in the vascular endothelium and astrocytes, which undergo important changes as a consequence of repetitive epileptic seizures (Kasantikul et al. 1983; Lamas et al. 2002), also may play a role in pharmacoresistance.

1.4 Epilepsy as Health Problem

Epilepsy is a chronic, recurrent, frequently progressive neurological disorder that affects 1–2 % of the population worldwide. Epilepsy is considered an important public health problem with significant social and economic impact (Engel and Taylor 1997). It is estimated that about 37 million individuals in the world have primary epilepsy, a number that increases to approximately 50 million when epilepsy secondary to other diseases or injuries is considered (World Health Organization 2001). Interestingly, it is calculated that at least 100 million people will have epilepsy at some time in their lives (Reynolds 2002).

In developed countries, the incidence of epilepsy is remarkably consistent across geographical areas, ranging from 24 to 53 per 100,000 person-years (Kurland 1959; Keränen et al. 1989; Olafsson et al. 1996), whereas the prevalence ranges from 3.5 to 10.7 (de Graaf 1974; Haerer et al. 1986). In contrast, epidemiological studies indicate higher prevalence and incidence rates of epilepsy in the general population of developing countries. For example, in Latin America, the median lifetime prevalence in all countries is 17.8 (range 6–43.2) per 1,000 people, and the incidence is

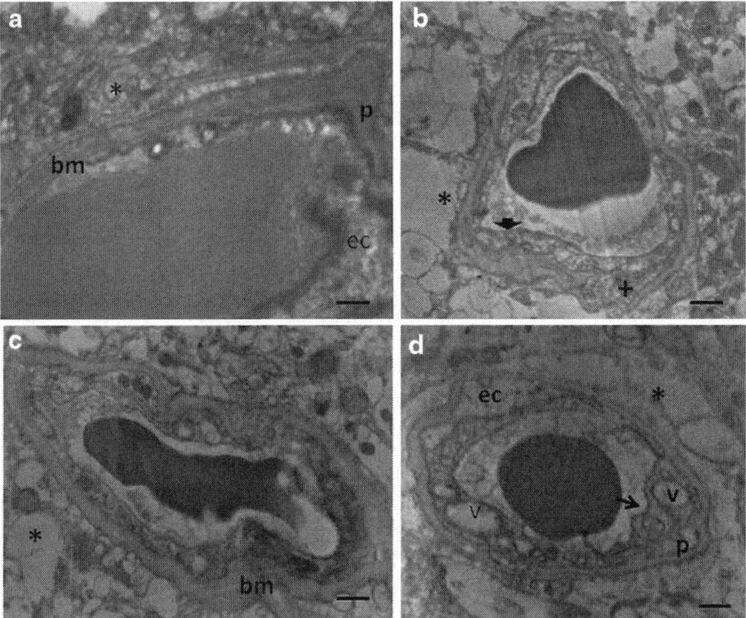

Fig. 1.1 Electron photomicrographs of vessels from epileptic focus of pediatric patients with epilepsy. (**a**) Normal microvessel with normal thickening of the basal membrane. Notice that endothelial cells, pericytes, and the astrocytes feet are preserved. (**b**, **c**) microvessels located in white matter from epileptic focus and (**d**) microvessel in epileptic neocortex. Notice in (**b–d**) degeneration of pericytes, swollen, vacuolation and multivesical bodies (+) inside endothelial cells as well as longitudinal folds and invaginations (*arrows*) on their surface. Abbreviations: *bm*, basal membrane; *ec*, endothelial cells; *p*, pericytes; *v*, vacuolation. Scale bars: (**a**) 0.5 μm, (**b**) 2 μm (**c**, **d**) 1 μm (from Dr. Sandra Orozco-Suárez with permission)

77.7–190 per 100,000 people per year (Burneo et al. 2005). Developing countries concentrate more than 80 % of persons with epilepsy, a situation associated with a lack of appropriate treatment (Carpio and Hauser 2009).

The WHO (2001) highlights that from the 40 million people suffering epilepsy worldwide, only 6 million receive adequate medical treatment. The 34 million people in developing and underdeveloped countries consume 18 % of the antiepileptic medications, whereas 6 million epilepsy patients in the so-called first world consume 82 % of the antiepileptic medications.

1.5 Burden of Pharmacoresistant Epilepsy

The burden of epilepsy is high and, for the year 2000, accounts for approximately 0.5 % of the whole burden of diseases in the world (Leonardi and Ustun 2002; World Health Organization 2001). Patients with epilepsy have significantly higher rates of health-related contacts and medication use as well as a higher socioeconomic cost, lower employment rates and income. Socioeconomic impact of epilepsy has been evaluated in different countries. In the U.K. 400,000 people have active epilepsy and represent a cost of £600 million annually in direct care and £2 billion annually in overall cost to the nation (Bowis 2002). A Danish study indicates that the direct net annual health care and indirect costs are €14,575 for patients in contrast with €1,163 for people without epilepsy, giving a consequent excess cost of €13,412 (Jennum et al. 2011). In the U.S., the direct medical costs for patients with no seizures during the previous year was $US 251, for patients with less-than one-seizure-per-month $US 1,333, and $US 2,439 for patients presenting more than one seizure per month (Annegers et al. 1999; Platt and Sperling 2002). In Mexico, a study published in 2006 revealed that the mean annual healthcare cost per patient with epilepsy was $US 2,646 (García-Contreras et al. 2006). It is important to note that, according to multinational studies, costs of healthcare for patients with pharmacoresistant epilepsy are higher than those for non-refractory epilepsy patients (Begley and Beghi 2002).

In addition to the economical burden, epilepsy may have a substantial social impact because people with this disorder and their families all over the world experience prejudice and discrimination, isolation and exclusion. People with epilepsy are victim of society's stigma and live their life on the margins (Lee 2002). This situation is worsened for patients who experience pharmacoresistant epilepsy (Regesta and Tanganelli 1999).

In carefully selected cases of pharmacoresistant epilepsy, surgical removal of the epileptogenic zone is superior to continued medical treatment in completely controlling seizures and improving health-related quality of life (Wiebe et al. 2001). After epilepsy surgery, total costs for seizure-free patients decline 32 % at a 2-year surgical follow-up due to decreased use of AEDs and inpatient care needs. In the 18–24 months following evaluation, epilepsy-related costs are $US 2,094 in patients with persisting seizures vs. $US 582 in seizure-free patients (Langfitt et al. 2007).

In spite of the high economical burden that pharmacoresistant epilepsy represents, it is important to consider that not all patients with this disorder are candidates for resective epilepsy surgery. Then, there is a great need to develop other therapeutic strategies to control seizure activity for those patients who do not respond to AEDs.

1.6 Epilepsy Care

Given that epilepsy is a public health problem with important social transcendence, affecting the patient's opportunities in the personal, education and employment spheres, extending to the whole family, due to persistent social exclusion, it is the obligation to divulge -across all levels of our communities- that epilepsy is a treatable neurological disorder, which is frequently curable.

In the last few years, several important ILAE initiatives have been taken to change and improve the conditions of people with epilepsy. The main goal of ILAE is to organize successful programs for improving expertise in epileptology in all countries. Under the auspices of the Global Campaign "Epilepsy out of the shadows," knowledge about differences in the pattern of provision of epilepsy care encountered by the ILAE chapters is helpful in the continuing efforts to develop high-quality management of epilepsy all over the world.

For example, the public health sector in Mexico supports and drives assistant programs such as the Epilepsy Priority Program (PPE for its Spanish initials) concerned with prevention, diagnosis, treatment and rehabilitation of patients with epileptic seizures through specialized groups, distributed across the different states and coordinated by neurologist and neuropediatricians, certified by the Mexican Neurology Council. The main objective of the PPE is establishing an efficient reference and contra reference system for patients with epilepsy that works across the three levels of medical health care attention, upon which the National Health System is based. Besides assistant activities, the PPE holds the responsibility to train general and family physicians as well as internists and pediatrician in the diagnosis and treatment of epilepsy, and divulge recent advances in medical and surgical treatment options, and, in many cases, cure of the disease.

Concerted efforts at a global level are needed to improve epilepsy care, and regional surveys concerning the provision of epilepsy care at different levels may be informative and helpful instruments. This is vital because patients identified at early stages may have a proper epilepsy care, avoiding the development or long-term consequences of pharmacoresistant epilepsy.

1.7 Conclusion

Several studies support that in some cases, epilepsy is pharmacoresistant from the onset, even if it appears initially to be benign. At present, there are no biomarkers that allow us to predict confidently whether a newly diagnosed patient will become pharmacoresistant. The knowledge of the mechanisms involved refractoriness, and new strategies in identifying individual genetic variations, might improve our ability to identify patients at risk. In addition, early identification and prompt (and adequate) therapeutic intervention might improve the overall outcome of the disease and maximize quality of life. The future developing of new classes of AEDs with antiepileptogenic properties or focused to block drug transporter effluxes, as well as neuromodulation strategies will change this expectation.

References

Annegers JF, Beghi E, Begley CE. Cost of epilepsy: contrast of methodologies in United States and European studies. Epilepsia. 1999;40 Suppl 8:14–8.

Arroyo S, Brodie MJ, Avanzini G, Baumgartner C, Chiron C, Dulac O, et al. Is refractory epilepsy preventable? Epilepsia. 2002;43:437–44.

Begley CE, Beghi E. The economic cost of epilepsy: a review of the literature. Epilepsia. 2002;43 Suppl 4:3–9.
Berg AT. Identification of pharmacoresistant epilepsy. Neurol Clin. 2009;27:1003–13.
Bowis J. "Out of the shadows": the political view. Epilepsia. 2002;43 Suppl 6:16–7.
Browne TR, Holmes GL. Epilepsy. N Engl J Med. 2001;344:1145–51.
Burneo JG, Tellez-Zenteno J, Wiebe S. Understanding the burden of epilepsy in Latin America: a systematic review of its prevalence and incidence. Epilepsy Res. 2005;66:63–74.
Carpio A, Hauser WA. Epilepsy in the developing world. Curr Neurol Neurosci Rep. 2009;9:319–26.
de Graaf AS. Epidemiological aspects of epilepsy in northern Norway. Epilepsia. 1974;15:291–9.
Ellerkmann RK, Remy S, Chen J, Sochivko D, Elger CE, Urban BW, et al. Molecular and functional changes in voltage-dependent Na+channels following pilocarpine-induced status epilepticus in rat dentate granule cells. Neuroscience. 2003;119:323–33.
Engel JJ, Taylor DC. Neurobiology of behavioral disorders. In: Engel Jr J, Pedley TA, editors. Epilepsy: a comprehensive textbook. Philadelphia: Lippincott-Raven; 1997. p. 2045–52.
García-Contreras F, Constantino-Casas P, Castro-Ríos A, Nevárez-Sida A, Estrada Correa Gdel C, Carlos Rivera F, et al. Direct medical costs for partial refractory epilepsy in Mexico. Arch Med Res. 2006;37:376–83.
Haerer AF, Anderson DW, Schoenberg BS. Prevalence and clinical features of epilepsy in a biracial United States population. Epilepsia. 1986;27:66–75.
Jennum P, Gyllenborg J, Kjellberg J. The social and economic consequences of epilepsy: a controlled national study. Epilepsia. 2011;52:949–56.
Kasantikul V, Brown WJ, Oldendorf WH, Crandall PC. Ultrastructural parameters of limbic microvasculature in human psychomotor epilepsy. Clin Neuropathol. 1983;2:171–8.
Keränen T, Riekkinen PJ, Sillanpää M. Incidence and prevalence of epilepsy in adults in eastern Finland. Epilepsia. 1989;30:413–21.
Kurland LT. The incidence and prevalence of convulsive disorders in a small urban community. Epilepsia. 1959;1:143–61.
Kwan P, Brodie M. Refractory epilepsy: a progressive, intractable but preventable condition? Seizure. 2002;11:77–84.
Lamas M, González-Mariscal L, Gutiérrez R. Presence of claudins mRNA in the brain. Selective modulation of expression by kindling epilepsy. Brain Res Mol Brain Res. 2002;104:250–4.
Langfitt JT, Holloway RG, McDermott MP, Messing S, Sarosky K, Berg AT, et al. Health care costs decline after successful epilepsy surgery. Neurology. 2007;68:1290–8.
Lee P. Epilepsy in the world today: the social point of view. Epilepsia. 2002;43 Suppl 6:14–5.
Leonardi M, Ustun TB. The global burden of epilepsy. Epilepsia. 2002;43 Suppl 6:21–5.
Luna-Munguia H, Orozco-Suarez S, Rocha L. Effects of high frequency electrical stimulation and R-verapamil on seizure susceptibility and glutamate and GABA release in a model of phenytoin-resistant seizures. Neuropharmacology. 2011;61:807–14.
Olafsson E, Hauser WA, Ludvigsson P, Gudmundsson G. Incidence of epilepsy in rural Iceland: a population-based study. Epilepsia. 1996;37:951–5.
Platt M, Sperling MR. A comparison of surgical and medical costs for refractory epilepsy. Epilepsia. 2002;43:25–31.
Regesta G, Tanganelli P. Clinical aspects and biological bases of drug resistant epilepsies. Epilepsy Res. 1999;34:109–22.
Remy S, Gabriel S, Urban BW, Dietrich D, Lehmann TN, Elger CE, et al. A novel mechanism underlying drug resistance in chronic epilepsy. Ann Neurol. 2003;53:469–79.
Reynolds EH. Introduction: epilepsy in the world. Epilepsia. 2002;43 Suppl 6:1–3.
Rogawski MA, Johnson MR. Intrinsic severity as a determinant of antiepileptic drug refractoriness. Epilepsy Curr. 2008;8:127–30.
Semah F, Picot MC, Adam C, Broglin D, Arzimanoglou A, Bazin B, et al. Is the underlying cause of epilepsy a major prognosis factor for recurrence? Neurology. 1998;51:1256–62.

Sisodiya SM, Lin WR, Harding BN, Squier MV, Thom M. Drug resistance in epilepsy: expression of drug resistance proteins in common causes of refractory epilepsy. Brain. 2002;125:22–31.
Vreugdenhil M, Wadman WJ. Kindling-induced long-lasting enhancement of calcium current in hippocampal CA1 area of the rat: relation to calcium-dependent inactivation. Neuroscience. 1994;59:105–14.
Vreugdenhil M, Wadman WJ. Modulation of sodium currents in rat CA1 neurons by carbamazepine and valproate after kindling epileptogenesis. Epilepsia. 1999;40:1512–22.
Wiebe S, Blume WT, Girvin JP, Eliasziw M. A randomized controlled trial of surgery for temporal lobe epilepsy. N Engl J Med. 2001;345:311–8.
World Health Organization. The World Health Report 2001: mental health, new understanding new hope. Geneva: World Health Organization; 2001.

Chapter 2
Genes Involved in Pharmacoresistant Epilepsy

Iris E. Martínez-Juárez, Laura Elena Hernández-Vanegas, Nayelli Rodríguez y Rodríguez, Jorge Alfredo León-Aldana, and Antonio V. Delgado-Escueta

Abstract This chapter is devoted to resistance to antiepileptic drugs (AEDs) and its genetic mechanisms. There are three general hypothesis proposed for pharmacoresistant epilepsy: (1) Target hypothesis, (2) Drug transporter hypothesis, and the (3) Intrinsic Severity Hypothesis (Gorter and Potschka, Jasper's basic mechanisms of the epilepsies, 4th ed. National Center for Biotechnology Information (USA), Bethesda, MD, 2012).

In diagnosing poor response to treatment, it is also important to separate drug resistance from incorrect diagnosis of epilepsy syndrome for example: (a) Epilepsy caused by mutations in Glucose transporter gene 1 (GLUT1) being treated with valproate (VPA) worsens the seizures in this disease whereas replacement of glucose with ketogenic diet alleviates seizures and the glucose deficit in the central

I.E. Martínez-Juárez, M.D. M.Sc. (✉) • L.E. Hernández-Vanegas, M.D.
Epilepsy Clinic, National Institute of Neurology and Neurosurgery, Insurgentes sur 3877, Col. La Fama, Del. Tlalpan, Mexico City, Distrito Federal 14269, Mexico

Clinical Epileptology Fellowship, National Autonomous University of Mexico, Mexico City, Mexico
e-mail: imartinez@innn.edu.mx; hernandez.laura@gmail.com

N. Rodriguez y Rodríguez
Epilepsy Clinic, National Institute of Neurology and Neurosurgery, Insurgentes sur 3877, Col. La Fama, Del. Tlalpan, Mexico City, Distrito Federal 14269, Mexico
e-mail: nayerodri@gmail.com

J.A. León-Aldana, M.D.
Epilepsy Clinic, Hospital General San Juan de Dios, Guatemala city, Guatemala
e-mail: jleonal@yahoo.com.mx

A.V. Delgado-Escueta, M.D.
West Los Angeles VA Medical Center, 11301 Wilshire Blvd, Los Angeles, CA 90073, USA
e-mail: antonio.escueta@med.va.gov

L. Rocha and E.A. Cavalheiro (eds.), *Pharmacoresistance in Epilepsy: From Genes and Molecules to Promising Therapies*, DOI 10.1007/978-1-4614-6464-8_2,

nervous system. (Klepper, Epilepsia 49(Suppl 8):46–49, 2008; Klepper et al., Neuropediatrics 40(5):207–210, 2009) (b) Genetic or idiopathic epilepsies such as Childhood Absence Epilepsy (CAE), Juvenile Myoclonic Epilepsy (JME) and Dravet's Syndrome can be aggravated when treated with Na^+ channel blockers (Genton, Brain Dev 22(2):75–80, 2000; Guerrini et al., Epilepsia 39(5):508–512, 1998; Thomas et al., Brain 129(Pt 5):1281–1292, 2006; Martínez-Juárez et al., Brain 129(Pt 5):1269–1280, 2006) and (c) Mitochondrial disorders can also be aggravated by VPA (Finsterer and Zarrouk Mahjoub, Expert Opin Drug Metab Toxicol 8(1):71–79, 2012).

Herein, we describe the three general hypothesis; we also summarize the "difficult to treat" genetic epilepsies.

Keywords Genes • Drug resistant • Epilepsy • Pharmacoresistant • Target hypothesis • Drug transporter

2.1 Target Hypothesis

A drug must have one or more actions on target sites of the brain to exert its therapeutic action. The resistance to drugs is caused by a structural or functional change at the site of action of drugs causing change in the pharmacodynamics of the drug (Sanchez-Alvarez et al. 2007).

The molecular targets refer to the sites that act as ligands of AEDs by which they exert their mechanism of action. These groups of molecules can be divided into two: voltage-gated channels and neurotransmitter receptors associated with neuronal excitation. These alterations at the site of action may be genetically determined or developed as a result of epigenetic and exogenous environmental factors.

2.1.1 Alterations of Sodium (Na^+) Channels

Sodium channels are the main target of most AEDs, which act by blocking their resting phase (tonic block), preventing channel opening and Na^+ conductance selectively. It has been suggested that mutations in Na^+ channels may affect the clinical response to AEDs (Ragsdale and Avoli 1998).

The Na^+ channels are formed by a pore-forming α subunit and two auxiliary associated subunits β. The modification of any of its subunits may play an important role in drug resistance (Sanchez-Alvarez et al. 2007).

The target theory was based on studies in voltage-regulated Na^+ channel in hippocampal neurons with the use of carbamazepine (CBZ). Most antiepileptic drugs act blocking Na^+ channels in their resting phase (tonic block), which prevents channel opening and ion conductance. It is considered that this alteration may be genetic or acquired. An alteration in the Na^+ channel can modify the sensitivity to one particular drug, but does not necessarily modify all responses to all drugs that share the same mechanism of action in the Na^+ channel.

In genetic drug resistance, it is known that some mutations in genes encoding VGSC subunits may cause refractory or drug-resistant epilepsy (Claes et al. 2001). The *SCN1A* gene is located on chromosome 2q24.3; it has been linked to several diseases, including severe myoclonic epilepsy of infancy or Dravet Syndrome and Generalized Epilepsy with Febrile Seizure Plus (GEFS+). *SCNA1* gene encodes for the α subunit of the VGSC; however, an exact physiological basis of drug resistance related to structural alterations of the subunit of VGSC in Dravet Syndrome has not been demonstrated.

In the *SCN1A* gene, exon 5 encodes for one of the four voltage sensitive channel, the I-S4 domain. This has two versions, one neonatal (N) and another adult (A), which differ in three amino acids. Normally both exons are coexpressed in the adult brain. In studies by Tate et al. (Tate et al. 2005), a G to A polymorphism was identified in the *SCN1A* gene that affects the alternative splicing of exon 5. This polymorphism has been observed in the intron adjacent to exon 5. Apparently this region determines which sequence, either neonatal or adult, is incorporated into each channel. Ancestral allele G allows both exons to be expressed, whereas the mutant allele alters the expression of neonatal exon by interrupting the consensus sequence, reducing the expression of this exon relative to exon 5A. By studying the minimum dose required of two AEDs, namely, CBZ and phenytoin (PHT) prescribed in 706 patients, Tate et al. (2006) found that AA homozygotes had an average dose of CBZ and PHT higher than that of heterozygotes, and the latter also had higher dose than GG homozygotes. A second study by the same authors failed to report this association; therefore, more studies are needed to confirm this (Tate et al. 2006).

An association between polymorphisms of the *SCN2A* gene channel, which codes for the α2 subunit of neuronal Na^+ channel, and resistance to drugs acting on Na^+ channels has also been found (Kwan et al. 2008)

The β subunits function is to modulate the membrane expression of the Na^+ channel. A mutation in the gene encoding for the β1 subunit has been linked with GEFS+. In epilepsy animal models a decreased expression of β1 and β2 subunit has been found. However, this lack of effect of CBZ on Na^+ channels in kindled rats is transient, and the inhibitory effect of CBZ on Na^+ channels is recovered. This effect has not been described in vivo (Gastaldi et al. 1998; Ellerkmann et al. 2003).

In acquired drug resistance, exogenous factors such as the presence of repeated seizures can promote transcriptional or post-transcriptional changes capable of inducing structural changes in VGSC, changes that are enough to induce refractory or drug-resistant epilepsy (Beck 2007). Remy et al. (2003) observed in brain tissue, from patients undergoing surgery for temporal lobe epilepsy with hippocampal sclerosis, a tonic loss of VGSC blockade, in contrast to the CBZ sensitive patient tissue samples.

2.1.2 Alterations of Voltage-Dependent Calcium (Ca^+) Channels

The Ca^+ channels are voltage transmembrane ion channels with an excitatory function. There are at least six types of Ca^+ channels (T, L, N, P/Q, R) classified in two categories on the basis of the voltage necessary for activation: low threshold and high threshold. The T-type channel is the only low-threshold Ca^{2+} channel current described (Shin et al. 2008).

Each VGCC is formed by an $\alpha 1$ subunit which serves as main pore and sensor in potential change, which is encoded by ten distinct genes, and several accessory subunits identified as β, γ, and $\alpha 2\delta$ subunits. The VGCC has a highly functional heterogeneity as a result of its wide distribution.

The T-type calcium channels are involved in generating thalamocortical discharges, involved in the pathophysiology of absence seizures. The $\alpha 1G$ subunit of T-type calcium channels is related to the generation of spike and wave discharges, while the $\alpha 1$ subunit does not have this physiological property. Therefore, it is possible that an imbalance in the proportion of $\alpha 1$ and $\alpha 1G$ subunits in the T Ca^+ channel reduces the response to anti-absence AEDs such as ethosuximide (ESM), lamotrigine (LTG), VPA, and zonisamide (ZNS). However, there is not experimental evidence yet to confirm this hypothesis (Chioza et al. 2001).

2.1.3 Alterations of Gamma Aminobutyric Acid Channels

Gamma Aminobutyric Acid (GABA) is the major inhibitory neurotransmitter in the adult brain. There are two GABA receptors: $GABA_A$ and $GABA_B$. The $GABA_A$ receptor has specific binding sites for benzodiazepines and barbiturates. $GABA_A$ channels mediate most inhibitory neurotransmission in the brain. Most $GABA_A$ channels are assembled by seven different subfamilies, which are defined by similar sequences: α, β, γ, δ, π, θ, and ρ. Most of the $GABA_A$ channels are formed by α, β and γ subunits. The 60 % of $GABA_A$ subunits are assembled by $\alpha_1\beta_2\gamma_2$ subunits. The $GABA_A$ receptor subtypes are distinguished by their affinity for GABA, channel kinetics and the rate of desensitization, distribution and pharmacology. Changes in the composition of the channel may have implications on its role and sensitivity to AEDs, especially of benzodiazepines (Schmidt and Lösher 2005).

In some animal models of chronic epilepsy there has been a progressive decrease in GABA receptor response to benzodiazepines. In these models hippocampal neuronal loss has been observed and has been associated with recurrent seizures with the subsequent development of acquired resistance, secondary to altered $GABA_A$ receptor. Combined molecular and functional studies indicate that the transcriptional change occurs in the α subunit of the $GABA_A$ receptor, consistent with a decrease in the α_1 subunit expression and an increase in the α_4 (Brooks-Kayal et al. 1998).

2.2 Multidrug Transporter Hypothesis (See Fig. 2.1)

The multidrug transporter hypothesis is based on the modification of the drug pharmacokinetics causing an inadequate concentration of antiepileptic drugs in brain tissue. This phenomenon occurs by an increase in cell membrane proteins which expel the endogenous toxins and xenobiotics, thus preventing penetration the blood–brain barrier and a decreased concentration of the medications at the epileptogenic focus or zones.

Drug resistance that occurs as a result of an increase in membrane proteins has become evident in several diseases such as cancer and epilepsy. Now it is considered a major cause of treatment failure. Resistance may be evident from the start of therapy or after an adequate initial response. There may even be cross-resistance to several drugs as a result of overexpression of membrane transport proteins. This phenomenon is called multidrug resistance (MDR).

These proteins are expressed at the luminal surface of cells that form the blood–brain barrier, glial and endothelial cells, and neurons, thus acting as a "second barrier". This would explain why, despite the use of AEDs at maximum doses, these are not effective in patients with refractory or drug-resistant epilepsy (Dombrowski et al. 2001).

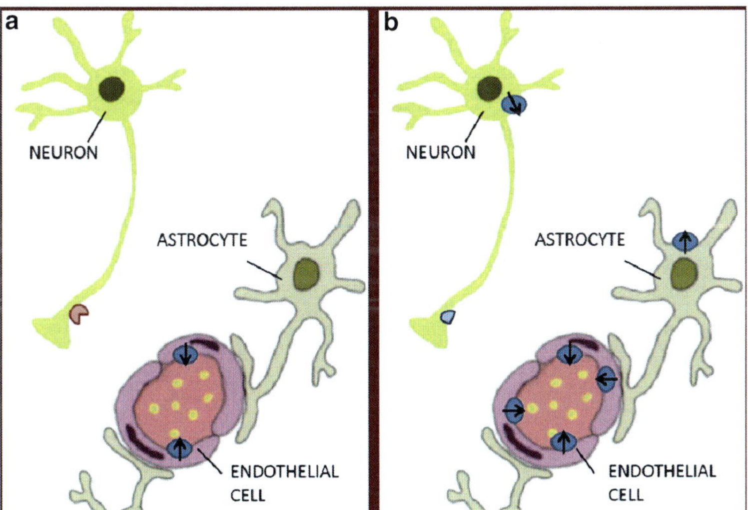

Fig. 2.1 (**a**) Schematic representation of blood brain barrier and normal expression of multidrug transporters. Expression of normal ion channel. (**b**) Epileptogenic-brain tissue with multidrug transporter overexpressed in capillary endothelial cells, astrocytes and neurons. Expression of mutated ion channel

2.2.1 ABC Superfamily (ATP-Binding Cassette Transporters)

The ABC proteins are associated with multiple drug resistance. These are members of an energy-dependent protein superfamily. Several members of the superfamily have been identified and classified into seven subfamilies (ABCA, ABCB, ABCC, ABCD, ABCE, ABCF, and ABCG). Among these, the subfamilies ABCB, ABCC, and ABCG are involved in MDR.

The ABCB1 (*MDR1*) and its protein, P-glycoprotein (P-gp) were the first ones to be described and are the most studied among those associated with resistance to multiple drugs. The *MDR1* gene is located on chromosome 7q21.1. The P-gp is a membrane protein with 1,280 amino acids and sized/weighing 170 kDa. It is found in different tissues with excretory or secretory function, such as liver, pancreas, kidney, intestine, and others. Substances that interact with P-gp are very diverse and have great ability to cross plasma barriers for their characteristics: high molecular weight, positive charge, and high lipophilicity (Kwan and Brodie 2005).

Tishler et al. (1995) suggested that the poor response to AED treatment in patients with refractory epilepsy was secondary to a reduction in the penetration of the drugs to the central nervous system. They observed an increased expression of MDR1 mRNA in 11 of 19 brain tissue of patients undergoing surgery with an increase in P-gp immunostaining. The concentration of PHT in cells was reduced to ¼ in patients expressing MDR1 in contrast to those that did not express it.

The variable expression of P-gp suggests a genetic influence, environmental factors or both. *MDR1* gene is highly polymorphic. More than 50 single nucleotide polymorphism (SNP) along with insertion/deletion polymorphisms have been reported in the *MDR1* (ABCB1) gene that encodes P-gp. Environmental factors could cause the expression of *MDR1* in tissues where it was not previously found; this could explain the fact that symptomatic epilepsies are more resistant to AEDs than idiopathic or genetic epilepsies (Kwan and Brodie 2000, 2005).

An increased expression of multidrug transporters has also been associated with constitutive, genetic or hereditary mechanism. Increased expression of *MDR1* was demonstrated in endothelial cells of the blood–brain barrier up to 130 % in patients with epilepsy, *MRP5* was increased up to 180 % and *MDR2* up to 225 % in comparison to patients without epilepsy (Dombrowski et al. 2001). Siddiqui et al. (2003) reported an association between drug resistance in epilepsy and a polymorphism in the ABCB1 gene. They reported that patients with the CC genotype expressed more P-gp, which was associated with increased drug resistance versus patients with the TT genotype. However, this association has been poorly reproduced and other studies have even documented an inverse association (Tan et al. 2004; Sills et al. 2005).

The association of drug-resistant or refractory epilepsy and some specific etiologies, including mesial temporal sclerosis, cortical dysplasias, and glial tumors has been known now for some time (Semah and Ryvlin 2005). Overexpression of multidrug resistance protein is regionally selective areas, affecting mainly epileptic brain areas. Overexpression of *MRP1* and *MDR1* was demonstrated in perivascular astrocytes of patients with temporal lobe epilepsy due to hippocampal sclerosis.

An aberrant expression in neurons and glial cells was observed as well in patients with dysembryoplastic neuroepithelial tumors and malformation of cortical development (Sisodiya et al. 2002; Sanchez-Alvarez et al. 2007).

It has been proposed that sustained augmentation of glutamate secondary to seizures is the mechanism of acquired increased P-gp expression in cells of the blood–brain barrier. Glutamate acts through NMDA-R, which produces the signal for arachidonic acid, which is then oxidized by the cyclooxygenase 2 (COX-2) producing prostanoids, including prostaglandin E2 (PGE2). PGE2 acts on the Prostaglandin E receptor 1 (EP1-R), which by means of a second messenger system increases transcription of P-gp (Potschka 2012).

Among the drugs transported by P-gp are CBZ, felbamate (FBM), gabapentin (GBP), LTG, phenobarbital (PB), PHT, and topiramate (TPM). Levetiracetam (LVT) and benzodiazepines are not substrates of P-gp in the blood–brain barrier. Kwan et al. (2010) reported a negative relationship between seizure control after epilepsy surgery and P-gp expression on the resected tissue of patients. Various antiepileptic drugs, their mechanisms of action and their corresponding transporters are shown on Table 2.1.

2.3 Intrinsic Severity Hypothesis

A prognostic factor associated with drug-resistant epilepsy is the frequency of seizures at the beginning of the disease, in some cases associated with the number of seizures before the start of treatment (Kwan and Brodie 2000). Even some cases of drug-resistant epilepsies had prolonged episodes of remission in its initial phases. The intrinsic severity hypothesis implies that the frequency of seizures is associated with refractoriness: if seizures are easy to trigger, then seizures will be more difficult to suppress, and the usual dose of the drug will not be enough. There is as yet no evidence that genetic factors directly contribute to the severity of epilepsy in idiopathic (genetic generalized epilepsies, Rogawski and Johnson 2008).

2.4 Genetic Epilepsies "Difficult to Treat"

Pathogenic alterations or mutation in genes and structural abnormalities in chromosomes (deletions, insertions) are responsible of a variety of epilepsies. In some, the possibility of drug-resistant epilepsy is high.

Several mechanisms may be interrelated between genetic disorders and the presence of epilepsy. It is important to distinguish between the susceptibility to generate epilepsy caused by a functional abnormality of a gene, and epilepsy that results from structural or functional abnormalities in a chromosome. Some genetic disorders relate more to certain types of epilepsy but overall any seizure type may be present.

Table 2.2 summarizes some genetic pharmacoresistant epilepsies.

Table 2.1 Antiepileptic drugs, their mechanisms of action and their corresponding transporters

	Mechanism of action							Transporter			
Antiepileptic drug	Blockade of Na^+ channel	Blockade of T-type Ca^+ channel	Blockade of other Ca^+ channels	Blockade of K^+ channel	GABA agonist	Glutamine antagonist	SV2A Action	P-glycoprotein	MRP	MDR	Target
Carbamazepine	+	–	+	–	+	+	–	+	+	+	+
Clobazam/Clonazepam	+	–	+	–	+	–	–	?	?	–	+
Ethosuximide	–	+	–	–	–	–	–	–	?	?	?
Felbatame	+	–	+	–	+	+	–	+	–	+	?
Gabapentin	+	–	+	+	+	+	–	+	?	+	?
Lamotrigine	+	–	+	+	–	+	–	+	–	+	–
Levetiracetam	–	–	+	+	+	–	+	–	–	–	?
Oxcarbazepine	+	–	+	+	–	+	–	+	?	?	?
Phenobarbital/Primidone	+	+	+	–	+	+	–	+	–	–	+
Phenytoin	+	–	+	–	+	–	–	+	+	+	+
Pregabalin	–	–	+	–	–	+	–	?	?	?	?
Topiramate	+	–	+	+	+	+	–	+	?	+	?
Valproate	+	+	+	–	+	+	–	?	+	+	–

+ = effect
– = no effect
? = unknown

Table 2.2 Genetic pharmacoresistant epilepsies

	Disease	Phenotype	Genotype	References
Genes involved in drug resistant epilepsy	Dravet syndrome	Normal development before onset Seizures initially induced by fever. Begin during first year of life Ataxia, mental decline EEG normal initially, generalized spike-wave activity	*SCN1A*, *SCN9A*, *GABRG2*	Dravet (1978), Ohmori, Ouchida, Ohtsuka, Oka and Shimizu (2002), Singh et al. (2001), and Harkin et al. (2007)
	Lafora disease	Insidious onset of progressive neurodegeneration, myoclonic jerks, generalized seizures, and often visual hallucination. Progressive cognitive decline resulting in dementia. Lafora bodies	*NHLRC1*, *EMP2A*	Chan et al. (2003) and Ganesh et al. (2002a, 2002b)
	Unverricht-Lundborg disease	Begin between 6 and 13 years of age. Stimulus sensitive myoclonic jerks, ataxia, incoordination, tremor, dysarthria. The disease stabilizes in early adulthood. No cognitive decline	*CSTB*	Shahwan et al. (2005)
	Pharmacorresistant MTLE with HS[a]	Febrile seizures, complex focal seizures. Epigastric aura, fear and oroalimentary automatisms	*ABCB1*	Kubota et al. (2006)
Genetic alterations associated with drug resistant epilepsies	GLUT1 deficiency syndrome	Infantile-onset epileptic encephalopathy, microcephaly, incoordination and spasticity. Hypoglycorrhachia (<40 mg/dl) and low lactate	*SLC2A1*	Klepper and Voit (2002)
	Tuberous sclerosis	Hamartomas in multiple organ systems, epilepsy, autism, behavioral problems, angiomyolipomas, pulmonary lymphangioleiomyomatosis, melanotic macules, facial angiofibromas	*TSC1*, *TSC2*	Povey et al. (1994)

(continued)

Table 2.2 (continued)

	Disease	Phenotype	Genotype	References
Chromosomal alterations associated with drug resistant epilepsies	Ring chromosome 20 syndrome	Behavioral restlessness and aggression Mental retardation appearing after apparently normal development in a child without dysmorphic features Atypical absence status with diffuse 2–3 Hz slow waves and spikes of possible mesial frontal origin	Ring20	Canevini et al. (1998)
	Fragile X	Learning disorders, hyperactive, autistic child delayed speech, hypotonic, hyperelastic joints, macroorchidism, narrow, long face, large ears with small mandibles and focal epilepsy	Xq27.3	Fu et al. (1991)
	Miller Dieker	Lissencephaly microcephaly, facial dysmorphism, cardiac malformations, growth retardation, mental deficiency, hypotonia and intractable seizures. EEG: focal or multifocal spike-wave discharges, bisynchronous bursts of diffuse paroxysmal activity, and high-voltage diffuse rhythmic theta and beta activity	17p13.3, Deletion or mutation in *LIS 1 gene*	Miller (1963) and Dobyns et al. (1993)
	Angelman syndrome	Mental retardation, microcephaly, movement disorder, abnormal behaviors, and severe alterations in language. Myoclonic jerks, focal and generalised status epilepticus	Maternal deletion on 15q11–q13	Angelman (1965) and Minassian et al. (1998)
	Prader Willi syndrome	Hypotonia, obesity, mental retardation, short stature, hypogonadotropic hypogonadism, and seizures	Paternal deletion *SNRPN gen*	Cassidy et al. (1984)

[a]Mesial temporal lobe epilepsy with hippocampal sclerosis

2.5 Conclusions

2.5.1 Limitations of the Three Hypothesis

To prove a given drug resistance theory, it is important to show that the subgroup of patients with drug resistance has differences in their receptors in comparison to those of responders. However, this is difficult to achieve because patients who respond to drugs are not subjected to epilepsy surgery. Any proposed mechanism for drug resistance must meet the following requirements to be considered valid: be detectable in epileptic brain tissue, have a pathophysiological mechanism, demonstrable in human epilepsy and, when modified, must affect the phenomenon of drug resistance (Sisodiya 2003).

The fact that most patients are resistant to multiple treatments, including several AEDs with different mechanisms of action, suggests that other less specific or unknown mechanisms with some commonality about AED cellular or network actions contribute to drug resistance or that more than one mechanism may be involved (Löscher et al. 2006). Some changes were induced only transiently in animal models of epilepsy which do not necessarily explain chronic pharmacorresistance (Van Vliet et al. 2005; Löscher 2007).

According to Schmidt and Löscher, (2009) the intrinsic hypothesis lacks studies and "a subgroup of patients with a higher seizure frequency at the onset of treatment will become seizure-free but require higher serum concentrations of AEDs to do so than those with a lower seizure frequency".

2.5.2 How to Define Genetic Drug-Resistant Epilepsies?

We have collected over a thousand patients with CAE, JME and CAE evolving to JME, Lafora disease, GEFS+, and Angelman Syndrome. These epilepsies respond variably to AED therapy, depending on their molecular lesion.

This chapter leads us to the question—what is the definition of genetic "drug-resistant" epilepsies. In the end we propose two assertions: (1) epilepsies are drug-resistant because the AED does not have an effect on the specific molecular lesion of the epilepsy syndrome. The epilepsy is supposedly "drug resistant" but seizures do not stop because "the key does not fit the lock in the door" and (2) when the AED has a proven effect on the molecular lesion but seizures persist in spite of AED treatment; this latter, we believe is true genetic pharmacorresistant epilepsy. Therefore, we favor the "intrinsic disease" mechanisms as an explanation for the resistance in genetic epilepsies (Fig. 2.2).

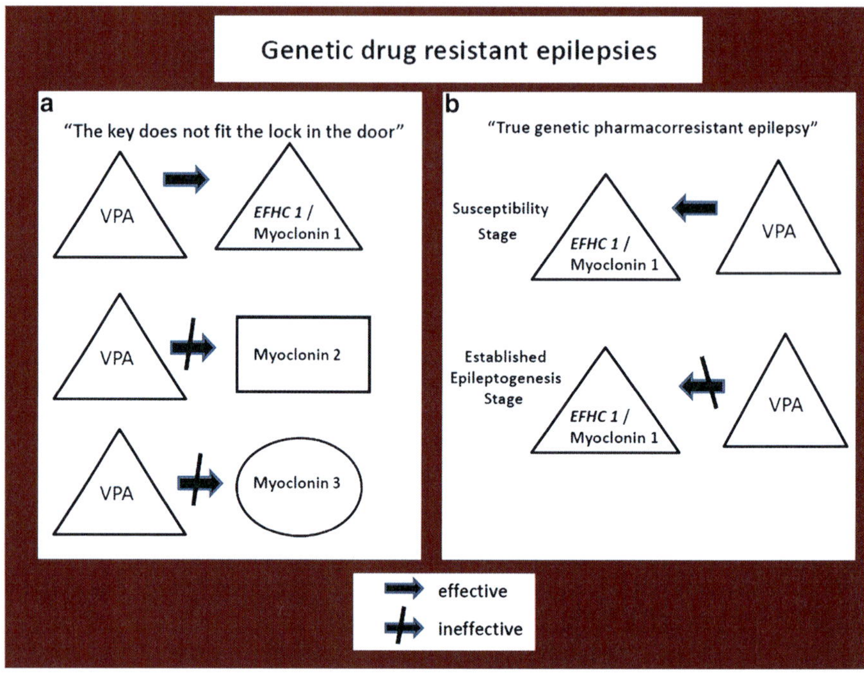

Fig. 2.2 (**a**) *EFHC1*/Myoclonin mutations in Juvenile Myoclonic Epilepsy (JME) frequently respond to treatment with valproate (VPA), however other JME mutations (illustrated as: Myoclonin 2 and Myoclonin 3) might not achieve seizure control due to a different molecular lesion unresponsive to VPA therapy. (**b**) *EFHC1*/Myoclonin mutations in a susceptibility or early stage respond adequately to VPA treatment whereas in established epileptogenesis drug resistance is seen even though the same molecular lesion is present; therefore a true genetic pharmacorresistance is encountered

2.5.3 Future Directions

The question is how to attack the problem in patients. A recommended step now, in assessing AED use, is to genotype epilepsies and use the genotype to guide AED use.

It would be ideal to perform a whole or large scale pharmacogenomic study of how AEDs effects are genetically determined in order to look for responders and non-responders and also for patients that will develop side effects from a specific AED. A large-scale pharmacogenomic studies could also be done in patients who were submitted to surgery for drug-resistant epilepsy. We could study the surgical specimens for their neuropathologic and biochemical abnormalities and correlate the findings with whole genome sequencing.

References

Angelman H. Puppet children: a report on three cases. Dev Med Child Neurol 1965;7:681–8.

Beck H. Plasticity of antiepileptic drug targets. Epilepsia. 2007;48 Suppl 1:14–8.

Brooks-Kayal AR, Shumate MD, Jin H, Rikhter TY, Coulter DA. Selective changes in single cell GABA(A) receptor subunit expression and function in temporal lobe epilepsy. Nat Med. 1998;4(10):1166–72.

Canevini MP, Sgro V, Zuffardi O, Canger R, Carrozzo R, Rossi E, et al. Chromosome 20 ring: a chromosomal disorder associated with a particular electroclinical pattern. Epilepsia. 1998;39(9):942–51.

Cassidy SB, Thuline HC, Holm VA. Deletion of chromosome 15 (q11-13) in a Prader-Labhart-Willi syndrome clinic population. Am J Med Genet. 1984;17(2):485–95.

Chan EM, Young EJ, Ianzano L, Munteanu I, Zhao X, Christopoulos CC, et al. Mutations in NHLRC1 cause progressive myoclonus epilepsy. Nat Genet. 2003;35(2):125–7.

Chioza B, Wilkie H, Nashef L, Blower J, McCormick D, Sham P, et al. Association between the alpha(1a) calcium channel gene CACNA1A and idiopathic generalized epilepsy. Neurology. 2001;56(9):1245–6.

Claes L, Del-Favero J, Ceulemans B, Lagae L, Van Broeckhoven C, De Jonghe P. De novo mutations in the sodium-channel gene SCN1A cause severe myoclonic epilepsy of infancy. Am J Hum Genet. 2001;68(6):1327–32.

Dobyns WB, Reiner O, Carrozzo R, Ledbetter DH. Lissencephaly. A human brain malformation associated with deletion of the LIS1 gene located at chromosome 17p13. JAMA. 1993;270(23):2838–42.

Dombrowski SM, Desai SY, Marroni M, Cucullo L, Goodrich K, Bingaman W, et al. Overexpression of multiple drug resistance genes in endothelial cells from patients with refractory epilepsy. Epilepsia. 2001;42(12):1501–6.

Dravet C. - Vie Med. Les epilepsies graves de l'enfant. 1978. - 543–548: Vol.8.

Ellerkmann RK, Remy S, Chen J, Sochivko D, Elger CE, Urban BW, et al. Molecular and functional changes in voltage-dependent Na(+) channels following pilocarpine-induced status epilepticus in rat dentate granule cells. Neuroscience. 2003;119(2):323–33.

Finsterer J, Zarrouk MS. Mitochondrial toxicity of antiepileptic drugs and their tolerability in mitochondrial disorders. Expert Opin Drug Metab Toxicol. 2012;8(1):71–9.

Fu YH, Kuhl DP, Pizzuti A, Pieretti M, Sutcliffe JS, Richards S, et al. Variation of the CGG repeat at the fragile X site results in genetic instability: resolution of the Sherman paradox. Cell. 1991;67(6):1047–58.

Ganesh S, Delgado-Escueta AV, Sakamoto T, Avila MR, Machado-Salas J, Hoshii Y, et al. Targeted disruption of the Epm2a gene causes formation of Lafora inclusion bodies, neurodegeneration, ataxia, myoclonus epilepsy and impaired behavioral response in mice. Hum Mol Genet. 2002a;11(11):1251–62.

Ganesh S, Delgado-Escueta AV, Suzuki T, Francheschetti S, Riggio C, Avanzini G, et al. Genotype-phenotype correlations for EPM2A mutations in Lafora's progressive myoclonus epilepsy: exon 1 mutations associate with an early-onset cognitive deficit subphenotype. Hum Mol Genet. 2002b;11(11):1263–71.

Gastaldi M, Robaglia-Schlupp A, Massacrier A, Planells R, Cau P. mRNA coding for voltage-gated sodium channel beta2 subunit in rat central nervous system: cellular distribution and changes following kainate-induced seizures. Neurosci Lett. 1998;249(1):53–6.

Genton P. When antiepileptic drugs aggravate epilepsy. Brain Dev. 2000;22(2):75–80.

Gorter JA, Potschka H. Drug Resistance in Noebels JL, Avoli M, Rogawski MA, Olsen RW, Delgado-Escueta AV editors. Jasper's Basic Mechanisms of the Epilepsies. 4th edition. Bethesda (MD): National Center for Biotechnology Information (US); 2012.

Guerrini R, Dravet C, Genton P, Belmonte A, Kaminska A, Dulac O. Lamotrigine and seizure aggravation in severe myoclonic epilepsy. Epilepsia. 1998;39(5):508–12.

Harkin LA, McMahon JM, Iona X, Dibbens L, Pelekanos JT, Zuberi SM, et al. Infantile Epileptic Encephalopathy Referral Consortium, Sutherland G, Berkovic SF, Mulley JC, Scheffer IE. The spectrum of SCN1A-related infantile epileptic encephalopathies. Brain. 2007;130(Pt 3):843–52.
Jq M. Lissencephaly in 2 siblings. Neurology. 1963;13:841–50.
Klepper J. Glucose transporter deficiency syndrome (GLUT1DS) and the ketogenic diet. Epilepsia. 2008;49 Suppl 8:46–9.
Klepper J, Voit T. Facilitated glucose transporter protein type 1 (GLUT1) deficiency syndrome: impaired glucose transport into brain– a review. Eur J Pediatr. 2002;161(6):295–304.
Klepper J, Scheffer H, Elsaid MF, Kamsteeg EJ, Leferink M, Ben-Omran T. Autosomal recessive inheritance of GLUT1 deficiency syndrome. Neuropediatrics. 2009;40(5):207–10.
Kubota H, Ishihara H, Langmann T, Schmitz G, Stieger B, Wieser HG, et al. Distribution and functional activity of P-glycoprotein and multidrug resistance associated proteins in human brain microvascular endothelial cells in hippocampal sclerosis. Epilepsy Res. 2006;68(3):213–28.
Kwan P, Brodie MJ. Early identification of refractory epilepsy. N Engl J Med. 2000;342(5):314–9.
Kwan P, Brodie MJ. Potential role of drug transporters in the pathogenesis of medically intractable epilepsy. Epilepsia. 2005;46(2):224–35.
Kwan P, Poon WS, Ng HK, Kang DE, Wong V, Ng PW, et al. Multidrug resistance in epilepsy and polymorphisms in the voltage-gated sodium channel genes SCN1A, SCN2A, and SCN3A: correlation among phenotype, genotype, and mRNA expression. Pharmacogenet Genomics. 2008;18(11):989–98.
Kwan P, Li HM, Al-Jufairi E, Abdulla R, Gonzales M, Kaye AH, et al. Association between temporal lobe P-glycoprotein expression and seizure recurrence after surgery for pharmacoresistant temporal lobe epilepsy. Neurobiol Dis. 2010;39(2):192–7.
Löscher W. Drug transporters in the epileptic brain. Epilepsia. 2007;48 Suppl 1:8–13.
Löscher W, Poulter MO, Padjen AL. Major targets and mechanisms of antiepileptic drugs and major reasons for failure. Adv Neurol. 2006;97:417–27.
Martínez-Juárez IE, Alonso ME, Medina MT, Durón RM, Bailey JN, López-Ruiz M, et al. Juvenile myoclonic epilepsy subsyndromes: family studies and long-term follow-up. Brain. 2006;129(Pt 5):1269–80.
Minassian BA, DeLorey TM, Olsen RW, Philippart M, Bronstein Y, Zhang Q, et al. Angelmansyndrome: correlations between epilepsy phenotypes and genotypes. Ann Neurol. 1998;43(4):485–93.
Ohmori I, Ouchida M, Ohtsuka Y, Oka E, Shimizu K. Significant correlation of the SCN1A mutations and severe myoclonic epilepsy in infancy. Biochem Biophys Res Commun. 2002;295(1):17–23.
Potschka H. Role of CNS efflux drug transporters in antiepileptic drug delivery: overcoming CNS efflux drug transport. Adv Drug Deliv Rev. 2012;64(10):943–52.
Povey S, Burley MW, Attwood J, Benham F, Hunt D, Jeremiah SJ, et al. Two loci for tuberous sclerosis: one on 9q34 and one on 16p13. Ann Hum Genet. 1994;58(Pt 2):107–27.
Ragsdale DS, Avoli M. Sodium channels as molecular targets for antiepileptic drugs. Brain Res Brain Res Rev. 1998;26(1):16–28.
Remy S, Beck H. Molecular and cellular mechanisms of pharmacoresistance in epilepsy. Brain. 2006;129(Pt 1):18–35.
Remy S, Gabriel S, Urban BW, Dietrich D, Lehmann TN, Elger CE, et al. A novel mechanism underlying drug resistance in chronic epilepsy. Ann Neurol. 2003;53(4):469–79.
Rogawski MA, Johnson MR. Intrinsic severity as a determinant of antiepileptic drug refractoriness. Epilepsy Curr. 2008;8(5):127–30.
Sánchez Alvarez JC, Serrano Castro PJ, Serratosa Fernández JM. Clinical implications of mechanisms of resistance to antiepileptic drugs. Neurologist. 2007;13(6 Suppl 1):S38–46.
Schmidt D, Löscher W. Drug resistance in epilepsy: putative neurobiologic and clinical mechanisms. Epilepsia. 2005;46(6):858–77.
Schmidt D, Löscher W. New developments in antiepileptic drug resistance: an integrative view. Epilepsy Curr. 2009;9(2):47–52.

Semah F, Ryvlin P. Can we predict refractory epilepsy at the time of diagnosis? Epileptic Disord. 2005;7 Suppl 1:S10–3.
Shahwan A, Farrell M, Delanty N. Progressive myoclonic epilepsies: a review of genetic and therapeutic aspects. Lancet Neurol. 2005;4(4):239–48.
Shin HS, Cheong EJ, Choi S, Lee J, Na HS. T-type Ca2+ channels as therapeutic targets in the nervous system. Curr Opin Pharmacol. 2008;8(1):33–41.
Siddiqui A, Kerb R, Weale ME, Brinkmann U, Smith A, Goldstein DB, et al. Association of multidrug resistance in epilepsy with a polymorphism on the drug-transporter GEBE ABCB1. N Engl J Med. 2003;348(15):1442–8.
Sills GJ, Mohanraj R, Butler E, McCrindle S, Collier L, Wilson EA, et al. Lack of association between the C3435T polymorphism in the human multidrug resistance (MDR1) gene and response to antiepileptic drug treatment. Epilepsia. 2005;46(5):643–7.
Singh R, Andermann E, Whitehouse WP, Harvey AS, Keene DL, Seni MH, Crossland KM, Andermann F, Berkovic SF, Scheffer IE. Severe myoclonic epilepsy of infancy: extended spectrum of GEFS+? Epilepsia. 2001;42:837–44.
Sisodiya SM. Mechanisms of antiepileptic drug resistance. Curr Opin Neurol. 2003;16(2):197–201.
Sisodiya SM, Lin WR, Harding BN, Squier MV, Thom M. Drug resistance in epilepsy: expression of drug resistance proteins in common causes of refractory epilepsy. Brain. 2002;125(Pt 1):22–31.
Tan NC, Heron SE, Scheffer IE, Pelekanos JT, McMahon JM, Vears DF, et al. Failure to confirm association of a polymorphism in ABCB1 with multidrug-resistant epilepsy. Neurology. 2004;63(6):1090–2.
Tate SK, Depondt C, Sisodiya SM, Cavalleri GL, Schorge S, Soranzo N, et al. Genetic predictors of the maximum doses patients receive during clinical use of the anti-epileptic drugs carbamazepine and phenytoin. Proc Natl Acad Sci U S A. 2005;102(15):5507–12.
Tate SK, Singh R, Hung CC, Tai JJ, Depondt C, Cavalleri GL, et al. A common polymorphism in the SCN1A gene associates with phenytoin serum levels at maintenance dose. Pharmacogenet Genomics. 2006;16(10):721–6.
Thomas P, Valton L, Genton P. Absence and myoclonic status epilepticus precipitated by antiepileptic drugs in idiopathic generalized epilepsy. Brain. 2006;129(Pt 5):1281–92.
Tishler DM, Weinberg KI, Hinton DR, Barbaro N, Annett GM, Raffel C. MDR1 gene expression in brain of patients with medically intractable epilepsy. Epilepsia. 1995;36(1):1–6.
van Vliet EA, Redeker S, Aronica E, Edelbroek PM, Gorter JA. Expression of multidrug transporters MRP1, MRP2, and BCRP shortly after status epilepticus, during the latent period, and in chronic epileptic rats. Epilepsia. 2005;46(10):1569–80.

Chapter 3
Pathological Oscillations in the Pharmacoresistant Epileptic Brain

Richard J. Staba

Abstract Epilepsy is a serious neurological disorder and in up to one-third of individuals with epilepsy, medication does not adequately control their seizures. Surgery is currently the most effective treatment in patients with pharmacoresistant epilepsy and postsurgical seizure freedom depends on accurately identifying the epileptogenic region. Broad bandwidth direct brain recordings in presurgical patients and chronic models of epilepsy reveal brief spontaneous bursts of electrical activity in the interictal EEG termed high-frequency oscillations (HFOs; 80–600 Hz) that are believed to reflect fundamental neuronal disturbances responsible for epilepsy. In the epileptic brain, pathological HFOs (pHFOs) are strongly linked to brain areas capable of generating spontaneous seizures, and in some cases the occurrence of pHFOs can predict the transition to ictus. Experimental evidence indicates a correlation between postsurgical seizure freedom and removal of tissue generating interictal and ictal pHFOs, thus supporting the view that pathological HFOs could be a biomarker to epileptogenicity.

Keywords Ripples • Fast ripples • Hippocampus • Neocortex • Neuronal mechanism • Synchrony

Abbreviations

EEG	Electroencephalography
HFO	High-frequency oscillation
IPSP	Inhibitory postsynaptic potential

R.J. Staba, Ph.D. (✉)
Department of Neurology, David Geffen School of Medicine at UCLA, 710 Westwood Plaza, Room 2155, Los Angeles 90095, CA, USA
e-mail: rstaba@mednet.ucla.edu

L. Rocha and E.A. Cavalheiro (eds.), *Pharmacoresistance in Epilepsy: From Genes and Molecules to Promising Therapies*, DOI 10.1007/978-1-4614-6464-8_3,

KA	Kainic acid
MRI	Magnetic resonance imaging
MTLE	Mesial temporal lobe epilepsy
non-REM	Non-rapid eye movement sleep
pHFO	Pathological high-frequency oscillation
PIN cluster	Pathologically interconnected neuron cluster
SOZ	Seizure onset zone

3.1 Introduction

3.1.1 Brief History of Electroencephalography

There were many pioneering achievements in the discovery of brain electrical activity and electroencephalography (EEG) that are reviewed in greater detail elsewhere (Brazier 1961; Niedermeyer 1993), but some are highlighted here to place the relatively new domain of high frequency (>80 Hz) activity in the context of EEG. In 1875, Richard Caton first reported spontaneous electrical activity from the brains of rabbits and monkeys (Caton 1875). During this early period of electrophysiological investigation of the brain, there were a number of studies describing spontaneous activity (Beck 1890; Pravdich-Neminsky 1913), evoked brain activity using electrical stimulation (Danilevsky 1891) and studies on abnormal electrical discharges in experimentally induced epilepsy (Kaufman 1912; Cybulski and Jelenska-Maciezyna 1914). Extending the EEG work in animals, groundbreaking studies were carried out by Hans Berger who recorded the first EEG in humans (Berger 1929). Berger's initial study published in 1929 described large amplitude electrical activity occurring at ten waves (cycles) per second (hertz, Hz) in awake subjects with eyes closed that was termed "alpha" rhythm and another faster, smaller amplitude activity (average period of 35 ms) that appeared when subjects opened their eyes that was labeled "beta" waves (Berger 1929). In addition, Berger also observed a 3 Hz rhythm during seizures in patients with epilepsy that was clearly illustrated and thoroughly described by Frederic Gibbs and colleagues as the now typical 3 Hz spike-and-wave ictal rhythm associated with absence epilepsy (Berger 1933; Gibbs et al. 1935, 1936). The number of neurophysiological studies of epilepsy grew rapidly with improvements in EEG instruments and techniques [review by (Collura 1993)], and a clinical role of scalp and intracerebral EEG was established for localizing epileptogenic brain areas in the surgical treatment of epilepsy (Penfield 1939; Bailey and Gibbs 1951; Jasper 1941; Jasper et al. 1951; Talairach et al. 1958; Crandall et al. 1963). Importantly, the increasing practice of intracerebral EEG and the development of wide bandwidth digital recording systems with fast sampling rates revealed ictal and interictal high-frequency oscillations (HFOs) 80 Hz and higher in presurgical patients (Fisher et al. 1992; Allen et al. 1992; Bragin et al. 1999a, b). These more recent developments in the field of EEG have propelled a new line of basic and clinical studies of HFOs associated with normal and abnormal function in the mammalian brain.

3.1.2 EEG Rhythms

In the context of EEG and magnetoencephalography (MEG), the term rhythm or oscillation generally refers to a pattern consisting of a regular variation in the signal around a baseline value repeated over time. Based on a convention of describing electromagnetic oscillations with respect to a dominant period or frequency, the traditional EEG labels and frequency bands consist of delta (1–4 Hz), theta (>4–8), alpha/mu (>8–13 Hz), beta (>13–30 Hz), and gamma (>30–80 Hz). Slow oscillations (<1 Hz) are a relatively new category (Steriade et al. 1993), as is a broad category labeled HFOs that include "ripples" (>80–200 Hz) (O'Keefe and Nadel 1978; Buzsaki et al. 1992), "fast ripples" (>200–600 Hz) (Bragin et al. 1999a, b), and "sigma bursts" (600 Hz and above) (Curio et al. 1994). Gamma could also be considered within the category of HFOs based on similarities in frequency and possibly mechanisms of neuronal synchronization as well as functions (Engel and da Silva 2012). The current discussion, however, concentrates on HFOs defined as oscillations with a central spectral frequency between 80 and 600 Hz that occur in hippocampal formation and neocortex.

In spite of the seemingly distinct EEG frequency bands, oscillation frequency spectra do not always fall within band limits. For example, in the normal mammalian brain, HFOs above 80 Hz and extending up to 200 Hz have been labeled "high" or "fast" gamma (Crone et al. 2006; Sullivan et al. 2011; Belluscio et al. 2012), which overlaps with frequencies associated with ripples generated hippocampus CA1 (Csicsvari et al. 1999a). Evidence suggests gamma proper (i.e., 30–80 Hz) and fast gamma could arise via different mechanisms (Belluscio et al. 2012), while fast gamma in CA3 and ripples in CA1, although spatially distinct patterns, appear to share common mechanistic properties (Sullivan et al. 2011). In addition, fast ripples and fast ripple-frequency HFOs are not always clearly distinguished (e.g., spontaneous vs. sensory evoked, hippocampus or neocortex or both). Furthermore, in the normal dentate gyrus, there is little evidence for ripples, yet the epileptic dentate gyrus can generate ripple-frequency HFOs and fast ripples and both are considered to be pathological (Bragin et al. 2004). These examples illustrate the confusion in the terminology and how labeling oscillations based on frequency alone provides little information on the mechanisms of generation or distinguishing normal from abnormal oscillations (Engel et al. 2009). Recommendations have been made to standardize the description of HFOs not only in terms of (1) frequency range but also indicate (2) whether HFOs arise spontaneously or are evoked, (3) occur during behavior or specific brain state, e.g., non-rapid eye movement (non-REM) or REM sleep, (4) occur transiently (burst) or as a steady state event, and (5) the brain area in which they occur (Jefferys et al. 2012). While additional information will help establish common terminology, identifying different types of HFO in the normal and epileptic brain depends on a better understanding of the mechanism underling their generation.

3.2 High-Frequency Oscillations in Normal Mammalian Brain

3.2.1 Hippocampal Sharp Wave–Ripple Complexes

In order to understand the potential mechanisms and role(s) of abnormal HFOs in the epileptic brain, it would be helpful to first describe the mechanisms generating HFOs in the normal brain. The most well-studied HFO in the normal intact brain are spontaneous ripples (80–200 Hz) in the non-primate hippocampal CA1 and CA3 subfields, subicular and entorhinal cortices (Chrobak and Buzsaki 1996). Ripples are also found in hippocampus and adjacent structures of non-primate human and humans (Skaggs et al. 2007; Bragin et al. 1999a; Le Van Quyen et al. 2008; Staba et al. 2002a). Ripples occur during episodes of waking immobility, feeding and grooming behavior, and non-REM sleep and commonly coincide with large amplitude sharp waves (Fig. 3.1a) (Buzsaki et al. 1992; Buzsaki 1986). The latter EEG events reflect irregular population bursts of CA3 neurons that likely arise when extra-hippocampal inputs (e.g., cholinergic input from septum) that normally suppress burst firing are reduced (Buzsaki et al. 1983). During sharp waves, the CA3 excitatory impulses are projected forward via the Schaffer collateral system onto dendrites of CA1 pyramidal cells and various types of interneurons that increases spike firing (Buzsaki et al. 1992; Csicsvari et al. 1999b; Ylinen et al. 1995; Klausberger et al. 2003). Through local chemical synaptic interactions, and likely gap junction and ephaptic interactions (Draguhn et al. 1998; Schmitz et al. 2001; Traub et al. 1999; Anastassiou et al. 2010; Bikson et al. 2004; Jefferys and Haas 1982), synchronous firing among CA1 pyramidal and some interneurons (e.g., basket cells) triggers a brief (~30–100 ms) ripple oscillation. The extracellular-recorded ripple reflects active inward currents of synchronously discharging neurons, largely pyramidal cells and possibly interneurons, and synchronous fast inhibitory postsynaptic potentials (IPSPs) from basket cells (Ylinen et al. 1995).

3.2.2 Neocortical HFOs

There are several conditions when HFOs occur in normal neocortex, but studies are needed to clarify the mechanisms associated with the different types of HFOs. In cats, neocortical HFOs (80–200 Hz) occur spontaneously during non-REM sleep and ketamine anesthesia (Grenier et al. 2001). In rats, HFOs (400–600 Hz) are associated with high-voltage spindles and can be evoked with electrical stimulation of the thalamus (Kandel and Buzsaki 1997), and mechanical stimulation of the rat's whisker evokes HFOs (200–600 Hz) in somatosensory cortex (Fig. 3.1b) (Jones and Barth 1999). In general, neocortical neuronal firing increases during HFOs and in particular fast-spiking cells (presumably GABAergic interneurons) discharge bursts of spikes time-locked to the negative wave of extracellular spontaneous or sensory-evoked

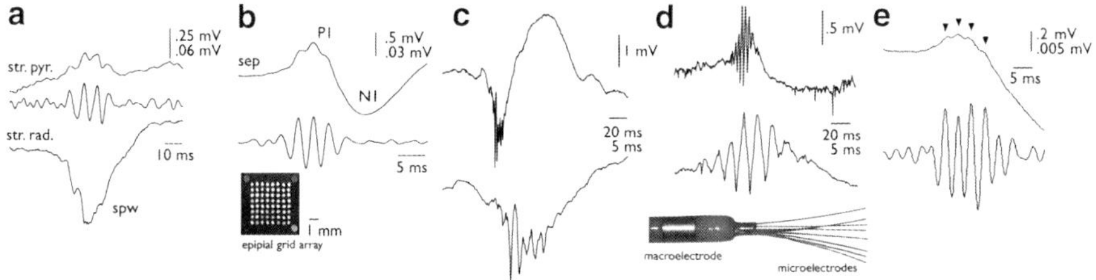

Fig. 3.1 Normal and pathological HFOs. (**a**) *Spontaneous ripple* recorded in CA1 of normal rat during non-REM sleep using tungsten microwires (diameter 40 μm). *Ripple* appears in broad bandwidth (0.1 Hz–1 kHz; *top*) and bandpass filter (80–200 Hz; *middle*) traces recorded above the pyramidal cell layer (str. pyr.). *Sharp wave* (spw) is shown in broad bandwidth trace recorded below pyramidal cell layer within stratum radiatum (str. rad.; *bottom*). (**b**) Averaged somatosensory evoked potential (sep; 1 Hz–2 kHz; *top trace*) recorded in rat barrel cortex during contralateral whisker stimulation. Bandpass filter trace (200–600 Hz; *bottom*) illustrates fast ripple-frequency HFO superimposed the initial component of the biphasic positive–negative (P1–N1) slow wave. Signal recorded on one electrode (diameter 100 μm) of a 64-contact epipial grid electrode array (*bottom*). (**c**) Broad bandwidth (1 Hz–3 kHz; *top trace*) interictal EEG spike associated with pHFO recorded in entorhinal cortex ipsilateral to seizure onset of patient with MTLE. pHFO occurs on descending limb of depth-negative component of interictal spike. *Bottom* trace illustrates pHFO on shorter time scale. Signal recorded on a microelectrode like the one shown at the *bottom of* panel (**d**). (**d**) Spontaneous pHFO in the absence of EEG spike. Interictal pHFO recorded in subiculum ipsilateral to seizure onset of patient with bilateral MTLE on a microelectrode (each 40 μm in diameter) extending beyond the distal tip of a clinical depth electrode (*bottom*). (**e**) Broad bandwidth (1 Hz–3 kHz; *top trace*) EEG illustrating pHFO recording a clinical depth electrode ("macroelectrode" like in panel (**d**)) positioned in anterior hippocampus. Bandpass filtered (200–600 Hz) trace illustrating fast ripple-frequency HFO. Note the small amplitude HFO (denoted by *black triangles*) and difference in amplitude between HFO recorded on clinical depth electrode (~25 μV peak-to-peak) and HFOs captured on microelectrodes in panels (**c**) and (**d**) (>1 mV)

HFO (Grenier et al. 2001; Jones et al. 2000). Some pyramidal cells such as rhythmic bursting cells fire spikes coincident with troughs of the spontaneous HFO (Grenier et al. 2001), while regular-spiking cell responses included a combination of subthreshold potentials, single or less frequently multiple spikes (Jones et al. 2000). Evidence thus far suggests that neocortical HFOs reflect firing of pyramidal cells synchronized through excitatory synaptic transmission (Ikeda et al. 2002) and possibly gap junctions or ephaptic field effects. Interestingly, antagonism of GABA-A receptor-mediated transmission does not suppress sensory-evoked HFOs, but rather significantly increases their duration in rats (Jones and Barth 2002). In this latter study, further antagonism of fast inhibition generated abnormal spontaneous slow waves associated with HFOs similar to the paroxysmal activity observed in cats under ketamine that showed a disruption in time-locked discharges of fast-spiking cells with HFO (Grenier et al. 2003). These data suggest that fast IPSPs do not contribute significantly to extracellular HFO in normal neocortex, but similar to hippocampal ripples, inhibitory processes likely play an important role in regulating principal cell spike firing during spontaneous as well as sensory-evoked neocortical HFOs.

3.2.3 Physiological Significance of HFOs

The synchrony of neuronal activity associated with HFOs has been implicated with physiological processes such as encoding information (Singer 1993), sensorimotor integration (Murthy and Fetz 1992), and memory consolidation (Buzsaki 1996). The former are presumed to be mediated primarily by gamma oscillations, while the latter involve hippocampal ripples. There exists ample neurophysiologic data from non-primate and human studies that supports a role of sharp wave-ripples in memory consolidation during sleep (Kudrimoti et al. 1999; Nadasdy et al. 1999; Clemens et al. 2007; Wierzynski et al. 2009; Siapas and Wilson 1998; Axmacher et al. 2008; Le Van Quyen et al. 2010). Most of the evidence is indirect, however, two studies showed that electrical stimulation timed to disrupt neuronal discharges associated with sharp wave–ripple complexes during slow wave sleep was associated with significant learning and performance impairments during subsequent waking episodes (Girardeau et al. 2009; Ego-Stengel and Wilson 2010). If ripples do play a role in memory consolidation, then hippocampal damage associated with epilepsy such as hippocampal sclerosis in mesial temporal lobe epilepsy (MTLE) might impede ripple generation and produce hippocampal-dependent memory impairments. Indeed, one study found reduced performance on spatial memory tasks in patients with temporal lobe epilepsy (Abrahams et al. 1999). In addition, the generation of spontaneous pathological HFOs could disrupt the normal spatiotemporal sequence of spike firing during endogenous ripples and produce learning or memory deficits (Buzsaki and Silva 2012).

3.3 HFOs in the Epileptic Brain

3.3.1 Pathological HFOs in Epileptic Animals

Spontaneous HFOs termed "fast ripples" (200–600 Hz) were first described in the unilateral intrahippocampal kainic acid (KA) rat model of temporal lobe epilepsy (TLE) (Bragin et al. 1999b, 2000). In these initial studies, fast ripples appeared as brief bursts primarily during interictal episodes while rats were asleep and were considered abnormal because they localized to injected dentate gyrus and hippocampus where seizures began and they could also occur during the onset of some hippocampal seizures. Subsequent studies found fast ripples and ripple-frequency HFOs in the dentate gyrus of epileptic rats and both were considered "pathological HFOs" (pHFOs) because previous studies did not find ripples in the normal dentate gyrus (Bragin et al. 1999b), both were only found in KA-treated rats that subsequently developed spontaneous seizures, and the sooner pHFOs appeared after KA-induced status epilepticus, the sooner spontaneous seizures appeared (Bragin et al. 2004, 2005). Evidence from other chemically induced status epilepticus models (e.g., pilocarpine) supports the strong association between pHFOs and epileptogenicity as well as severity of neuron loss (Foffani et al. 2007; Levesque et al. 2011). However, recent evidence from the intrahippocampal tetanus toxin model of TLE indicates that status epilepticus or extensive neuron loss are not required for the generation of pHFOs (Jiruska et al. 2010b), suggesting there could be different types and mechanisms generating pHFOs.

3.3.2 *Mechanisms Generating pHFOs*

Currently there are no reliable means for separating pHFOs from normal HFOs in the epileptic brain, but understanding the mechanisms generating pathological and normal HFOs could reveal properties unique to each group that could provide the basis for such strategies. Microelectrode recordings in the intact dentate gyrus and hippocampus of post-status epilepticus epileptic rats suggest interictal pHFOs reflect a brief burst of population spikes that arise from clusters of pathologically interconnected neurons (or PIN clusters) that generate abnormally synchronous discharges (Bragin et al. 1999b, 2000, 2007b). It appears principal cells are the primary contributors to pHFOs because in vivo juxta-cellular studies carried out in the dentate gyrus of pilocarpine-treated epileptic rats found an increase in granule cell discharges aligned with the negative waves of the extracellular pHFO (in some cases a single population spike) and reduction in presumed basket cell firing (Bragin et al. 2011) (contrast with normal CA1 ripples described in Sect. 3.2.1). Furthermore, in hippocampal tissue with high concentrations of extracellular K^+, it seems recurrent excitatory connections among CA3 pyramidal cells generate synchronous firing and bursts of population spikes (Dzhala and Staley 2004). These data argue for a limited role of inhibitory processes in the generation of dentate gyrus and hippocampal pHFOs and little contribution of IPSPs to extracellular current sources, which is consistent with persistence of in vitro pHFOs after suppressing GABA-A receptor-mediated transmission (D'Antuono et al. 2005; Foffani et al. 2007).

In spite of results in the preceding paragraph and principal cell's elongated dendritic architecture that can give rise to open fields with strong extracellular current flow, it is possible that some types of interneurons are active during pHFOs and could contribute current flow in the local extracellular environment. While basket cells fire during normal CA1 ripples, other types of interneurons stop firing (Ylinen et al. 1995; Klausberger et al. 2003). It appears Bragin and colleagues were recording from single basket cells during pHFOs in epileptic dentate gyrus (Bragin et al. 2011), but this pattern of activity might not reflect all types of interneurons. Symmetrical depolarization of an interneuron's spherically projecting dendrites would likely generate a close field with current dipoles canceling one another. However, if interneuron dendrites were depolarized in a spatially asymmetrical or temporally asynchronous pattern, then a detectable dipole might be produced (Buzsaki et al. 2012). Morphological alterations in some epileptogenic lesions (e.g., hippocampal sclerosis) might contain axonal sprouting and synaptic reorganization that activate interneurons and produce current sources in a manner not found in normal tissue (Menendez de la Prida and Trevelyan 2011). Studies are needed to determine if this is correct and whether in the epileptic brain there exists unique HFOs that reflect interneuron discharges that might play a role in maintaining the interictal state.

Recordings in the intact rodent epileptic brain explain some but not all of the features associated with pHFOs. For example, the mechanisms that underlie synchronous neuronal spike firing are not known. It is reasonable that gap junctions could play a role and there is evidence from in vitro and network modeling studies for pHFOs in the absence of chemical synaptic transmission (Draguhn et al. 1998; Jiruska et al. 2010a; Roopun et al. 2010). In addition, synchrony of neuronal discharges might be achieved more easily under conditions that promote excitability, e.g., cell type-specific neuron loss, alterations in inhibition, gliosis, axon spouting, synaptic reorganization (Esclapez et al. 1999; Esclapez and Houser 1999; Shao and Dudek 2005; Huberfeld et al. 2007). Indeed, single neuron studies in patients with epilepsy found increased interictal excitability and synchrony of neuronal discharges in the seizure onset zone (SOZ), and more recently evidence for neuronal hyperexcitability associated with gray matter loss in the mesial temporal lobe SOZ (Staba et al. 2002b, 2011).

Evidence for synchronous principal cell bursting appears to explain pHFOs that occur at frequencies up to 300 Hz (Dzhala and Staley 2004; Foffani et al. 2007; Ibarz et al. 2010), but since single neurons rarely fire at frequencies greater than 300 Hz (Colder et al. 1996; Staba et al. 2002b, c), this neuronal mechanism does not adequately explain how pHFOs up to 600 Hz occur. It has been recently proposed that pHFOs such as fast ripples emerge from the out-of-phase firing between small groups of neurons with individual neurons discharging at low frequencies and few neurons firing during consecutive waves of the extracellular pHFO (Foffani et al. 2007; Ibarz et al. 2010; Jiruska et al. 2010a). This hypothesis better explains the precision of spike firing and frequency spectra of individual pHFO, as well as the spectral variability from one pHFO to the next (Dzhala and Staley 2004; Foffani et al. 2007; Ibarz et al. 2010; Menendez de la Prida and Trevelyan 2011). It is less clear how phase differences could arise between groups of neurons, although several possibilities might promote out-of-phase firing, such as weak ephaptic field effects, neuron loss, circuit reorganization, or irregular spread of activity throughout neuronal networks (Menendez de la Prida and Trevelyan 2011; Kohling and Staley 2011).

3.3.3 HFOs in Clinical Epilepsy

3.3.3.1 Recording and Detection of HFOs

The optimal size and configuration of electrodes to capture HFOs is not known. Studies in epileptic rats and presurgical patients using small diameter microelectrodes (40–60 μm) estimate the volume of tissue generating pHFOs could be as small as 1 mm^3 (Bragin et al. 2002a, b). Since a large electrode compared to microelectrode might be positioned at a greater distance from a pHFO-generating site and electrical potential attenuates in direct proportion to the square of distance from the current source(s), a large electrode might record pHFOs less reliably. In addition, the effective surface area of a large electrode would average extracellular current sources within a larger volume of tissue than a microelectrode that might also reduce pHFO signal (e.g., ~6 mm^2 for clinical depth electrode contact versus 0.0013 mm^2 for a microelectrode). A number of studies using electrodes with different diameters and configurations have captured pHFOs with remarkably similar results that suggests the volume of tissue generating pHFOs could be much larger (Bragin et al. 1999a; Staba et al. 2002a; Urrestarazu et al. 2007; Khosravani et al. 2008; Crepon et al. 2010; Schevon et al. 2009). Furthermore, one study compared hippocampal ripples and fast ripples recorded with electrodes of different sizes and found no difference in duration or spectral frequency with respect to electrode diameter (Chatillon et al. 2011). However, in this same study the mean amplitude of ripples and fast ripples was significantly lower and rates of each *higher* compared to the respective amplitudes and rates of these HFOs reported in a previous microelectrode study (compare Fig. 3.1c–e) (Bragin et al. 1999b). By contrast, another study found a significant reduction in the number of fast ripples recorded with standard clinical electrodes compared to microelectrodes (Worrell et al. 2008). Based on current evidence, it is clear that identifying the optimal electrode(s) to reliably capture all types of HFOs and developing uniform HFO criteria and detection strategies will be important for the use of HFOs in clinical studies.

There are no formal criteria for HFOs, but the features typically reported in studies using different types of electrodes include amplitude (10–1,000 μV), frequency (80–600 Hz), and duration (10–100 ms) (Worrell et al. 2012). Detection methods generally fall into categories of manual review, supervised and unsupervised computer-automated detection with strengths and weaknesses associated with all methods (Staba et al. 2002a; Gardner et al. 2007; Crepon et al. 2010; Zelmann et al. 2012). Most strategies include a comparison between the continuous bandpass filtered signal and an energy threshold computed from a baseline period to detect episodes that exceed threshold and selected as putative HFOs. The baseline can be the entire continuous signal that could result in high threshold values for electrodes containing significant HFO activity or computed from epochs that do not contain HFOs, but this requires careful review and no guarantee the chosen epochs is representative of the continuous signal. Scalp and intracranial EEG recordings contain physiological and epileptiform sharp transients (interictal EEG spikes) and artifacts (electrode noise, eye- and muscle-related activity) that contain high frequency power and digital filtering of these events could be incorrectly interpreted as HFOs (Benar et al. 2010; Worrell 2012). Manual post hoc review of putative events in the unfiltered signal can confirm the authenticity of HFOs, although this can be time consuming and subjective. Automated review using other aspects of the signal can also be used (e.g., duration, number of waves, inter-event interval), which imposes restrictions on HFOs features. Based on the potential use of HFOs in the localization of the epileptogenic zone (i.e., brain area(s) necessary and sufficient for generating spontaneous seizures) and surgical planning, it seems prudent that the detection of HFOs should not be based solely on results of signal processing, but include a step of expert review.

3.3.3.2 Interictal HFOs

Initial studies describing spontaneous interictal HFOs (80–600 Hz) were carried out in presurgical patients with MTLE using microelectrodes and found a strong association between fast ripples, but not ripple-frequency HFOs, and the SOZ (Fig. 3.1c–d) (Bragin et al. 1999a, b). Subsequent quantitative studies confirmed the association of fast ripples with SOZ (Staba et al. 2002a), and fast ripples and ripple-frequency HFOs with states of vigilance, finding that the rates of both types of HFOs were highest during episodes of non-REM sleep (Staba et al. 2004). Voltage depth analysis in entorhinal cortex indicated fast ripples and ripple-frequency HFOs were generated within cell lamina of entorhinal cortex, but the fast ripples could arise from smaller cellular areas compared to ripple-frequency HFOs (Bragin et al. 2002b). Moreover, higher rates of fast ripples and lower rates of ripple-frequency HFOs correlated with hippocampal atrophy and reduced neuron densities (Staba et al. 2007; Ogren et al. 2009). These data suggest that morphological alterations associated with hippocampal sclerosis in MTLE could be an anatomical substrate for hippocampal fast ripples and some ripple-frequency HFOs that could also be pathological.

Studies using larger diameter electrodes and commercial clinical electrodes verified and extended microelectrode studies of HFOs. The link between fast ripples, as well as ripple-frequency HFOs, and SOZ was confirmed in MTLE and neocortical epilepsy, although fast ripples appear more specific to the SOZ particularly in MTLE (Jacobs et al. 2008; Crepon et al. 2010). In addition, one study found pHFOs in epileptogenic tissue extending beyond areas pathology in other lesional epilepsies (Jacobs et al. 2009a), and another study found pHFOs in the SOZ of patients with normal MRI (Andrade-Valenca et al. 2012), although histological analysis of resected tissue indicated gliosis and neuron loss in many of these patients. The explanation for association between ripple-frequency HFOs and SOZ is not clear, but these HFOs appear similar to pHFOs described in microelectrode studies and some have suggested a bias of larger diameter electrodes to capture pHFOs versus normal HFO including ripples (Crepon et al. 2010; Engel and da Silva 2012). In contrast to the studies cited above that have focused on pHFOs that occur as brief bursts in the EEG, recent work has identified continuous interictal HFO (>80 Hz, >500 ms in duration) activity in hippocampus of presurgical patients (Mari et al. 2012), although this study did not find evidence for continuous HFO that was unique to epileptogenic tissue.

Several studies have emphasized the spatial and temporal association between pHFOs and interictal EEG spikes. Interictal EEG spikes can be useful for identifying epileptogenic tissue (Lieb et al. 1978), but EEG spikes can also occur outside of the epileptogenic region and their accuracy can dependent on state of vigilance, i.e., wakefulness vs. sleep (Wieser et al. 1979; Lieb et al. 1980; Sammaritano et al. 1991). A large percentage of EEG spikes occur independently of pHFOs and vice versa, although some EEG spikes do contain pHFOs yet the pHFO might not be visible in broad bandwidth recordings unless the signal is filtered or detected using statistical time–frequency analysis (Urrestarazu et al. 2007; Kobayashi et al. 2009). Importantly, studies suggest that EEG spikes with pHFOs as well as pHFOs alone more accurately localize epileptogenic regions than EEG spikes alone (Jacobs et al. 2008, 2010). The mechanisms that give rise to EEG spike–pHFO complexes are not known, but studies have found a dissociation between EEG spikes and pHFOs during medication withdrawal and with respect to seizures (Zijlmans et al. 2009, 2011). In addition, others have proposed that tissue with EEG spikes containing pHFOs reflect hypersynchronous discharges of neurons that actively participate in the generation and propagation of epileptiform activity. By contrast, sites with EEG spikes that do not contain pHFOs receive abnormal input that is not sufficient to generate hypersynchronous neuron activity (Bragin et al. 2010).

As discussed in Sects. 3.3.1 and 3.3.2 ripple-frequency HFOs in dentate gyrus are considered abnormal, but it is not known if ripple-frequency HFOs outside the dentate gyrus are abnormal and, if so, how to distinguish them from normal ripples. In presurgical patients, ripple-frequency HFOs can occur in hippocampus, subicular and entorhinal cortices and share several important features with ripples in the normal rodent hippocampus. Human ripples occur most frequently during the ON-periods (likely the UP-phase) of non-REM sleep and least often during REM sleep (Bragin et al. 1999a; Staba et al. 2002a, 2004; Nir et al. 2011). Single neuron analysis found a significant increase in both putative interneurons and pyramidal cells during spontaneous ripples in entorhinal cortex (Le Van Quyen et al. 2008). In this same study, spike firing was aligned with the negative wave of the extracellular ripple in a cell type-specific, time-dependent manner similar to the firing pattern of pyramidal cells and some interneurons during normal rodent hippocampal ripples (Klausberger et al. 2003). With respect to the hypothesized role of hippocampal ripples in cognitive performance (Sect. 3.2.3), one patient study found that the rate of ripples in rhinal cortex correlated with the number of successfully recalled items learned during a prior waking period (Axmacher et al. 2008). Developing strategies to reliably identify normal HFOs like hippocampal ripples in the epileptic brain will greatly benefit patient studies investigating the functional roles of HFOs in learning, memory, and sleep.

3.3.3.3 Ictal HFOs

Hypotheses for the role of pHFOs in the transition to ictus in clinical epilepsy derive largely from animal studies. In vitro evidence indicates pHFO-generating sites are surrounded by tissue containing strong inhibition and a reduction in inhibition expands the area generating pHFOs (Bragin et al. 2002a). Moreover, in the intact dentate gyrus of epileptic rats showed a progressive increase in pHFO amplitude, power, and duration preceding seizure onset that could reflect the growth and coalescence of PIN clusters (Bragin et al. 2005). Data such as these form the basis of one hypothesis of seizure genesis that proposes pre-ictal pHFOs arising from PIN clusters trigger wide spread feedback inhibition that subsequently evolves into hypersynchronous discharges as a result of rebound from global inhibition (Bragin et al. 2007a). This hypothesis with respect to clinical EEG might appear as a sequence of single or multiple pre-ictal large amplitude spikes associated with slow wave and low voltage fast activity that evolves to slow rhythmic EEG discharges (Spencer et al. 1992a, b; Bragin et al. 2007a). If correct, then analysis of wide bandwidth EEG should detect an increase in spectral power corresponding with pHFO frequencies before or during the onset of seizures. Several patients studies have indeed detected an increase in pHFO power in the SOZ during or preceding ictal onset by several minutes to seconds (Fisher et al. 1992; Allen et al. 1992; Traub et al. 2001; Jirsch et al. 2006; Khosravani et al. 2008; Worrell et al. 2004). In these same studies, changes in pHFO power were chiefly detected in the primary SOZ and rarely in sites of secondarily generalization of patients with focal epilepsy (Jirsch et al. 2006). Similar changes in pHFOs occurred during epileptic spasms and in some cases before the clinical onset (Ochi et al. 2007; Akiyama et al. 2005, 2006; Ramachandran Nair et al. 2008; Nariai et al. 2011a, b). In one of these latter studies (Akiyama et al. 2006), pHFO power could be observed spreading across cortex and increasing in size during the seizure.

Results from the studies cited above contrast with data from other patient studies that found less predictable changes in pHFO during transition ictus (Zijlmans et al. 2011; Jacobs et al. 2009b), suggesting pHFOs could be one of many possible mechanisms involved with seizure genesis. However, in the epileptic brain, if ripple-like HFOs exist that reflect inhibitory processes and regulate neuronal excitability, then the irregular occurrence or progressive reduction of these HFOs might facilitate the transition to ictus (Bragin et al. 2010). An in vitro study found beta-frequency oscillatory activity largely driven by interneuron firing during seizure onset, but IPSPs progressively declined and principal cell firing increased along with the evolution of the seizure (Gnatkovsky et al. 2008). One interpretation of these data is that some HFOs in the intact epileptic brain are associated with inhibitory processes that could *prevent* the transition to ictus.

3.3.3.4 Role of pHFOs in Epilepsy

Since pHFOs appear to reflect unique epileptic neuronal disturbances, pHFOs provide a novel approach to investigate basic neuronal mechanisms of epileptogenicity, seizure generation and epileptogenesis, the development and progression of tissue capable of generating spontaneous seizures (Bragin et al. 2004; Engel and da Silva 2012). Experimental studies in animals and presurgical patients with epilepsy described in the preceding sections indicate pHFOs could be used to identify epileptogenic tissue and thus serve as a biomarker of epileptogenicity (Bragin et al. 2008). Additional evidence in support of this role derive from retrospective studies that show a strong correlation between postsurgical seizure freedom and removal of tissue generating interictal or ictal pHFOs (Jacobs et al. 2010; Wu et al. 2010; Akiyama et al. 2011; Ochi et al. 2007; Nariai et al. 2011b; Fujiwara et al. 2012). As a biomarker of epileptogenicity pHFOs could also identify the presence and severity of the epileptic condition (Ogren et al. 2009; Staba 2012). Scalp EEG or other non-invasive modalities such as MEG or EEG with functional MRI that might detect pHFOs could be used in differential diagnosis of epilepsy versus acute symptomatic seizures and administer appropriate treatment immediately (Engel and da Silva 2012). Towards these goals a recent study recording EEG from scalp electrodes found gamma (40–80 Hz) and HFOs (>80 Hz) that were associated with the SOZ in patients with focal seizures (Andrade-Valenca et al. 2011). Pathological HFOs might be used as a biomarker to evaluate the efficacy of therapy more quickly without having to wait for the occurrence of seizures. Finally, pHFOs could be used to identify individuals at risk for epilepsy after potential epileptogenic insults and evaluating antiepileptogenic therapy or possibly provide an indication for surgical referral in cases of pharmacoresistant epilepsy (Engel and da Silva 2012).

3.4 Conclusions

Results from chronic animal models of epilepsy and presurgical patients with focal epilepsy suggest pHFOs can accurately identify the epileptogenic region and possibly the development of epilepsy after an epileptogenic injury. Currently it is not yet possible to unequivocally distinguish pathological from normal HFOs, although in the normal brain HFOs reflect strong inhibitory processes that regulate principal cell firing, whereas in the epileptic brain pHFOs arise from abnormally synchronous principal cell discharges. It appears morphological alterations associated with epileptogenic lesions contribute to the generation of some pHFOs, but not others that primarily arise from functional disturbances in principal and inhibitory circuits. It is anticipated that optimizing electrodes and methods for capturing and analyzing HFOs will provide insight into the mechanisms that synchronize neuronal activity and a basis for separating normal HFOs from pHFOs, and likely identify unique pHFOs in different types of epilepsy. Interictal pHFOs, thus far, are one of few potential biomarkers of epileptogenicity that could be used to localize the epileptogenic zone and assist in the surgical treatment of pharmacoresistant epilepsy, identify the presence and severity of the epileptic condition, and possibly serve as a biomarker to evaluate the efficacy of new antiseizure and anti-epileptogenic therapies.

Acknowledgments The author would like to thank Dr. Jerome Engel, Jr. for his helpful comments in reviewing this manuscript. The author is supported by NINDS RO1 071048 & 33310.

References

Abrahams S, Morris RG, Polkey CE, Jarosz JM, Cox TC, Graves M, et al. Hippocampal involvement in spatial and working memory: a structural MRI analysis of patients with unilateral mesial temporal lobe sclerosis. Brain Cogn. 1999;41(1):39–65. doi:10.1006/brcg.1999.1095.

Akiyama T, Otsubo H, Ochi A, Ishiguro T, Kadokura G, RamachandranNair R, et al. Focal cortical high-frequency oscillations trigger epileptic spasms: confirmation by digital video subdural EEG. Clin Neurophysiol. 2005;116(12):2819–25.
Akiyama T, Otsubo H, Ochi A, Galicia EZ, Weiss SK, Donner EJ, et al. Topographic movie of ictal high-frequency oscillations on the brain surface using subdural EEG in neocortical epilepsy. Epilepsia. 2006;47(11):1953–7.
Akiyama T, McCoy B, Go CY, Ochi A, Elliott IM, Akiyama M, et al. Focal resection of fast ripples on extraoperative intracranial EEG improves seizure outcome in pediatric epilepsy. Epilepsia. 2011;52(10):1802–11. doi:10.1111/j.1528-1167.2011.03199.x.
Allen PJ, Fish DR, Smith SJ. Very high-frequency rhythmic activity during SEEG suppression in frontal lobe epilepsy. Electroencephalogr Clin Neurophysiol. 1992;82(2):155–9.
Anastassiou CA, Montgomery SM, Barahona M, Buzsaki G, Koch C. The effect of spatially inhomogeneous extracellular electric fields on neurons. J Neurosci. 2010;30(5):1925–36. doi:10.1523/JNEUROSCI.3635-09.2010.
Andrade-Valenca LP, Dubeau F, Mari F, Zelmann R, Gotman J. Interictal scalp fast oscillations as a marker of the seizure onset zone. Neurology. 2011;77(6):524–31. doi:10.1212/WNL.0b013e318228bee2.
Andrade-Valenca L, Mari F, Jacobs J, Zijlmans M, Olivier A, Gotman J, et al. Interictal high frequency oscillations (HFOs) in patients with focal epilepsy and normal MRI. Clin Neurophysiol. 2012;123(1):100–5. doi:10.1016/j.clinph.2011.06.004.
Axmacher N, Elger CE, Fell J. Ripples in the medial temporal lobe are relevant for human memory consolidation. Brain. 2008;131(7):1806–17. doi:10.1093/brain/awn103.
Bailey P, Gibbs FA. The surgical treatment of psychomotor epilepsy. J Am Med Assoc. 1951;145(6):365–70.
Beck A. Die Bestimmung der Localisation der Gehirn- und Ruckenmarksfunctionen vermittelst der elektrischen Erscheinungen. Zbl Physiol. 1890;4:473–6.
Belluscio MA, Mizuseki K, Schmidt R, Kempter R, Buzsaki G. Cross-frequency phase-phase coupling between theta and gamma oscillations in the hippocampus. J Neurosci. 2012;32(2):423–35. doi:10.1523/JNEUROSCI.4122-11.2012.
Benar CG, Chauviere L, Bartolomei F, Wendling F. Pitfalls of high-pass filtering for detecting epileptic oscillations: a technical note on "false" ripples. Clin Neurophysiol. 2010;121(3):301–10.
Berger H. Uber das Electrenkephalogram des Menschen. Arch Psychiatr Nervenkr. 1929;87:527.
Berger H. Uber das elektrenkephalogramm des menschen. Arch Psychiatr Nervenkr. 1933;100:301–20.
Bikson M, Inoue M, Akiyama H, Deans JK, Fox JE, Miyakawa H, et al. Effects of uniform extracellular DC electric fields on excitability in rat hippocampal slices in vitro. J Physiol. 2004;557(Pt 1):175–90. doi:10.1113/jphysiol.2003.055772.
Bragin A, Engel Jr J, Wilson CL, Fried I, Buzsaki G. High-frequency oscillations in human brain. Hippocampus. 1999a;9:137–42.
Bragin A, Engel Jr J, Wilson CL, Fried I, Mathern GW. Hippocampal and entorhinal cortex high-frequency oscillations (100–500 Hz) in human epileptic brain and in kainic acid–treated rats with chronic seizures. Epilepsia. 1999b;40(2):127–37.
Bragin A, Wilson CL, Engel Jr J. Chronic epileptogenesis requires development of a network of pathologically interconnected neuron clusters: a hypothesis. Epilepsia. 2000;41 Suppl 6:S144–52.
Bragin A, Mody I, Wilson CL, Engel Jr J. Local generation of fast ripples in epileptic brain. J Neurosci. 2002a;22(5):2012–21.
Bragin A, Wilson CL, Staba RJ, Reddick M, Fried I, Engel Jr J. Interictal high-frequency oscillations (80–500 Hz) in the human epileptic brain: entorhinal cortex. Ann Neurol. 2002b;52(4):407–15. doi:10.1002/ana.10291.
Bragin A, Wilson CL, Almajano J, Mody I, Engel Jr J. High-frequency oscillations after status epilepticus: epileptogenesis and seizure genesis. Epilepsia. 2004;45(9):1017–23.

Bragin A, Azizyan A, Almajano J, Wilson CL, Engel JJ. Analysis of chronic seizure onsets after intrahippocampal kainic acid injection in freely moving rats. Epilepsia. 2005;46(10):1592–8.
Bragin A, Claeys P, Vonck K, Van Roost D, Wilson C, Boon P, et al. Analysis of initial slow waves (ISWs) at the seizure onset in patients with drug resistant temporal lobe epilepsy. Epilepsia. 2007a;48(10):1883–94.
Bragin A, Wilson CL, Engel Jr J. Voltage depth profiles of high-frequency oscillations after kainic acid-induced status epilepticus. Epilepsia. 2007b;48(s5):35–40.
Bragin A, Staba RJ, Engel Jr J. The significance of fast ripples in the evaluation of the epileptogenic zone. In: Luders HO, editor. Textbook of Epilepsy Surgery. Abingdon: Taylor & Francis; 2008. p. 530–6.
Bragin A, Engel Jr J, Staba RJ. High-frequency oscillations in epileptic brain. Curr Opin Neurol. 2010;23(2):151–6.
Bragin A, Benassi SK, Kheiri F, Engel Jr J. Further evidence that pathologic high-frequency oscillations are bursts of population spikes derived from recordings of identified cells in dentate gyrus. Epilepsia. 2011;52(1):45–52. doi:10.1111/j.1528-1167.2010.02896.x.
Brazier MAB. A history of the electrical activity of the brain: the first half-century. London: Pitman; 1961.
Buzsaki G. Hippocampal sharp waves: their origin and significance. Brain Res. 1986;398: 242–52.
Buzsaki G. The hippocampo-neortical dialogue. Cereb Cortex. 1996;6:81–92.
Buzsaki G, Silva FL. High frequency oscillations in the intact brain. Prog Neurobiol. 2012;98(3):241–9. doi:10.1016/j.pneurobio.2012.02.004.
Buzsaki G, Leung LW, Vanderwolf CH. Cellular bases of hippocampal EEG in the behaving rat. Brain Res. 1983;287(2):139–71.
Buzsaki G, Horvath Z, Urioste R, Hetke J, Wise K. High-frequency network oscillation in the hippocampus. Science. 1992;256:1025–7.
Buzsaki G, Anastassiou CA, Koch C. The origin of extracellular fields and currents–EEG, ECoG, LFP and spikes. Nat Rev Neurosci. 2012;13(6):407–20. doi:10.1038/nrn3241.
Caton R. The electrical currents of the brain. Br Med J. 1875;2:278.
Chatillon CE, Zelmann R, Bortel A, Avoli M, Gotman J. Contact size does not affect high frequency oscillation detection in intracerebral EEG recordings in a rat epilepsy model. Clin Neurophysiol. 2011;122(9):1701–5. doi:10.1016/j.clinph.2011.02.022.
Chrobak JJ, Buzsaki G. High-frequency oscillations in the output of the hippocampal-entorhinal axis of the freely behaving rat. J Neurosci. 1996;16(9):3056–66.
Clemens Z, Molle M, Eross L, Barsi P, Halasz P, Born J. Temporal coupling of parahippocampal ripples, sleep spindles and slow oscillations in humans. Brain. 2007;11:2868–78. doi:10.1093/brain/awm146.
Colder BW, Wilson CL, Frysinger RC, Harper RM, Engel Jr J. Interspike intervals during interictal periods in human temporal lobe epilepsy. Brain Res. 1996;719(1–2):96–103.
Collura TF. History and evolution of electroencephalographic instruments and techniques. J Clin Neurophysiol. 1993;10(4):476–504.
Crandall PH, Walter RD, Rand RW. Clinical applications of studies on stereotactically implanted electrodes in temporal lobe epilepsy. J Neurosurg. 1963;20:827–40.
Crepon B, Navarro V, Hasboun D, Clemenceau S, Martinerie J, Baulac M, et al. Mapping interictal oscillations greater than 200 Hz recorded with intracranial macroelectrodes in human epilepsy. Brain. 2010;133:33–45. doi:10.1093/brain/awp277.
Crone NE, Sinai A, Korzeniewska A. High-frequency gamma oscillations and human brain mapping with electrocorticography. Prog Brain Res. 2006;159:275–95. doi:10.1016/S0079-6123(06)59019-3.
Csicsvari J, Hirase H, Czurko A, Mamiya A, Buzsaki G. Fast network oscillations in the hippocampal CA1 region of the behaving rat. J Neurosci. 1999a;19(RC20):1–4.
Csicsvari J, Hirase H, Czurko A, Mamiya A, Buzsaki G. Oscillatory coupling of hippocampal pyramidal cells and interneurons in the behaving rat. J Neurosci. 1999b;19(1):274–87.

Curio G, Mackert BM, Burghoff M, Koetitz R, Abraham-Fuchs K, Harer W. Localization of evoked neuromagnetic 600 Hz activity in the cerebral somatosensory system. Electroencephalogr Clin Neurophysiol. 1994;91(6):483–7.
Cybulski N, Jelenska-Maciezyna X. Action currents of the cerebral cortex (in Polish). Bull Acad Sci Krakow. 1914;Ser B:776–81.
Danilevsky VY. Electrical phenomena of the brain. Fiziol Sbornik. 1891;2:77–88.
D'Antuono M, de Guzman P, Kano T, Avoli M. Ripple activity in the dentate gyrus of disinhibited hippocampus-entorhinal cortex slices. J Neurosci Res. 2005;80:92–103.
Draguhn A, Traub RD, Schmitz D, Jefferys JGR. Electrical coupling underlies high-frequency oscillations in the hippocampus in vitro. Nature. 1998;394:189–92.
Dzhala VI, Staley KJ. Mechanisms of fast ripples in the hippocampus. J Neurosci. 2004;24(40):8896–906.
Ego-Stengel V, Wilson MA. Disruption of ripple-associated hippocampal activity during rest impairs spatial learning in the rat. Hippocampus. 2010;20(1):1–10. doi:10.1002/hipo.20707.
Engel Jr J, da Silva FL. High-frequency oscillations: where we are and where we need to go. Prog Neurobiol. 2012;98(3):316–8. doi:10.1016/j.pneurobio.2012.02.001.
Engel Jr J, Bragin A, Staba RJ, Mody I. High-frequency oscillations: what is normal and what is not? Epilepsia. 2009;50(4):598–604.
Esclapez M, Houser CR. Up-regulation of GAD65 and GAD67 in remaining hippocampal GABA neurons in a model of temporal lobe epilepsy. J Comp Neurol. 1999;412(3):488–505.
Esclapez M, Hirsch JC, Ben-Ari Y, Bernard C. Newly formed excitatory pathways provide a substrate for hyperexcitability in experimental temporal lobe epilepsy. J Comp Neurol. 1999;408:449–60.
Fisher RS, Webber WR, Lesser RP, Arroyo S, Uematsu S. High-frequency EEG activity at the start of seizures. J Clin Neurophysiol. 1992;9(3):441–8.
Foffani G, Uzcategui YG, Gal B, Menendez de la Prida L. Reduced spike-timing reliability correlates with the emergence of fast ripples in the rat epileptic hippocampus. Neuron. 2007;55(6):930–41.
Fujiwara H, Greiner HM, Lee KH, Holland-Bouley KD, Seo JH, Arthur T, et al. Resection of ictal high-frequency oscillations leads to favorable surgical outcome in pediatric epilepsy. Epilepsia. 2012;53(9):1607–17. doi:10.1111/j.1528-1167.2012.03629.x.
Gardner AB, Worrell GA, Marsh E, Dlugos D, Litt B. Human and automated detection of high-frequency oscillations in clinical intracranial EEG recordings. Clin Neurophysiol. 2007;118(5):1134–43.
Gibbs FA, Davis H, Lennox WG. The electroencephalogram in epilepsy and in conditions of impaired conciousness. Arch Neurol Psychiatry. 1935;34:1133–48.
Gibbs FA, Lennox WG, Gibbs EL. The electro-encephalogram in diagnosis and in localization of epileptic seizures. Arch Neurol Psychiatry. 1936;36:1225–35.
Girardeau G, Benchenane K, Wiener SI, Buzsaki G, Zugaro MB. Selective suppression of hippocampal ripples impairs spatial memory. Nat Neurosci. 2009;12(10):1222–3. doi:10.1038/nn.2384.
Gnatkovsky V, Librizzi L, Trombin F, de Curtis M. Fast activity at seizure onset is mediated by inhibitory circuits in the entorhinal cortex in vitro. Ann Neurol. 2008;64(6):674–86. doi:10.1002/ana.21519.
Grenier F, Timofeev I, Steriade M. Focal synchronization of ripples (80–200 Hz) in neocortex and their neuronal correlates. J Neurophysiol. 2001;86(4):1884–98.
Grenier F, Timofeev I, Steriade M. Neocortical very fast oscillations (ripples, 80–200 Hz) during seizures: intracellular correlates. J Neurophysiol. 2003;89(2):841–52.
Huberfeld G, Wittner L, Clemenceau S, Baulac M, Kaila K, Miles R, et al. Perturbed chloride homeostasis and GABAergic signaling in human temporal lobe epilepsy. J Neurosci. 2007;27(37):9866–73. doi:10.1523/JNEUROSCI.2761-07.2007.
Ibarz JM, Foffani G, Cid E, Inostroza M, Menendez de la Prida L. Emergent dynamics of fast ripples in the epileptic hippocampus. J Neurosci. 2010;30(48):16249–61. doi:30/48/16249 [pii] 10.1523/JNEUROSCI.3357-10.2010.

Ikeda H, Leyba L, Bartolo A, Wang Y, Okada YC. Synchronized spikes of thalamocortical axonal terminals and cortical neurons are detectable outside the pig brain with MEG. J Neurophysiol. 2002;87(1):626–30.
Jacobs J, LeVan P, Chander R, Hall J, Dubeau F, Gotman J. Interictal high-frequency oscillations (80–500 Hz) are an indicator of seizure onset areas independent of spikes in the human epileptic brain. Epilepsia. 2008;49(11):1893–907.
Jacobs J, Levan P, Chatillon CE, Olivier A, Dubeau F, Gotman J. High frequency oscillations in intracranial EEGs mark epileptogenicity rather than lesion type. Brain. 2009a;132(Pt 4):1022–37.
Jacobs J, Zelmann R, Jirsch J, Chander R, Châtillon CE, Dubeau F, et al. High frequency oscillations (80-500Hz) in the preictal period in patients with focal seizures. Epilepsia. 2009b;50(7):1780–92.
Jacobs J, Zijlmans M, Zelmann R, Chatillon CE, Hall J, Olivier A, et al. High-frequency electroencephalographic oscillations correlate with outcome of epilepsy surgery. Ann Neurol. 2010;67(2):209–20.
Jasper HH. Electroencephalography. In: Penfield W, Erickson TC, editors. Epilepsy and cerebral localization. Springfield, IL: Charles C. Thomas; 1941. p. 380–454.
Jasper H, Pertuisset B, Flanigin H. EEG and cortical electrograms in patients with temporal lobe seizures. AMA Arch Neurol Psychiatry. 1951;65(3):272–90.
Jefferys JG, Haas HL. Synchronized bursting of CA1 hippocampal pyramidal cells in the absence of synaptic transmission. Nature. 1982;300(5891):448–50.
Jefferys JG, de la Prida LM, Wendling F, Bragin A, Avoli M, Timofeev I, et al. Mechanisms of physiological and epileptic HFO generation. Prog Neurobiol. 2012;98(3):250–64. doi:10.1016/j.pneurobio.2012.02.005.
Jirsch JD, Urrestarazu E, LeVan P, Olivier A, Dubeau F, Gotman J. High-frequency oscillations during human focal seizures. Brain. 2006;129(6):1593–608.
Jiruska P, Csicsvari J, Powell AD, Fox JE, Chang W-C, Vreugdenhil M, et al. High-frequency network activity, global increase in neuronal activity, and synchrony expansion precede epileptic seizures in vitro. J Neurosci. 2010a;30(16):5690–701. doi:10.1523/jneurosci.0535-10.2010.
Jiruska P, Finnerty GT, Powell AD, Lofti N, Cmejla R, Jefferys JG. Epileptic high-frequency network activity in a model of non-lesional temporal lobe epilepsy. Brain. 2010b;133:1380–90.
Jones MS, Barth DS. Spatiotemporal organization of fast (>200 Hz) electrical oscillations in rat Vibrissa/Barrel cortex. J Neurophysiol. 1999;82(3):1599–609.
Jones MS, Barth DS. Effects of bicuculline methiodide on fast (>200Hz) electrical oscillations in rat somatosensory cortex. J Neurophysiol. 2002;88(2):1016–25.
Jones MS, MacDonald KD, Choi B, Dudek FE, Barth DS. Intracellular correlates of fast (>200 Hz) electrical oscillations in rat somatosensory cortex. J Neurophysiol. 2000;84:1505–18.
Kandel A, Buzsaki G. Cellular-synaptic generation of sleep spindles, spike-and-wave discharges, and evoked thalamocortical responses in the neocortex of the rat. J Neurosci. 1997;17(17):6783–97.
Kaufman PY. Electrical phenomena in the cerebral cortex (in Russian). Oborz Psikhiat Nevrol eksper Psikol. 1912;7–8(403–424):513–35.
Khosravani H, Mehrotra N, Rigby M, Hader WJ, Pinnegar CR, Pillay N, et al. Spatial localization and time-dependant changes of electrographic high frequency oscillations in human temporal lobe epilepsy. Epilepsia. 2008;50(4):605–16.
Klausberger T, Magill PJ, Marton LF, Roberts JDB, Cobden PM, Buzsaki G, et al. Brain-state and cell-type specific firing of hippocampal interneurons in vivo. Nature. 2003;42:844–8.
Kobayashi K, Jacobs J, Gotman J. Detection of changes of high-frequency activity by statistical time-frequency analysis in epileptic spikes. Clin Neurophysiol. 2009;120(6):1070–7.
Kohling R, Staley K. Network mechanisms for fast ripple activity in epileptic tissue. Epilepsy Res. 2011;97(3):318–23. doi:10.1016/j.eplepsyres.2011.03.006.
Kudrimoti HS, Barnes CA, McNaughton BL. Reactivation of hippocampal cell assemblies: effects of behavioral state, experience, and EEG dynamics. J Neurosci. 1999;19(10):4090–101.

Le Van Quyen M, Bragin A, Staba R, Crepon B, Wilson CL, Engel Jr J. Cell type-specific firing during ripple oscillations in the hippocampal formation of humans. J Neurosci. 2008;28(24):6104–10.

Le Van Quyen M, Staba R, Bragin A, Dickson C, Valderrama M, Fried I, et al. Large-scale microelectrode recordings of high-frequency gamma oscillations in human cortex during sleep. J Neurosci. 2010;30(23):7770–82. doi:10.1523/JNEUROSCI.5049-09.2010.

Levesque M, Bortel A, Gotman J, Avoli M. High-frequency (80–500 Hz) oscillations and epileptogenesis in temporal lobe epilepsy. Neurobiol Dis. 2011;42(3):231–41. doi:S0969-9961(11)00008-8 [pii] 10.1016/j.nbd.2011.01.007.

Lieb JP, Woods SC, Siccardi A, Crandall PH, Walter DO, Leake B. Quantitative analysis of depth spiking in relation to seizure foci in patients with temporal lobe epilepsy. Electroencephalogr Clin Neurophysiol. 1978;44:641–63.

Lieb JP, Joseph JP, Engel Jr J, Walker J, Crandall PH. Sleep state and seizure foci related to depth spike activity in patients with temporal lobe epilepsy. Electroencephalogr Clin Neurophysiol. 1980;49(5–6):538–57.

Mari F, Zelmann R, Andrade-Valenca L, Dubeau F, Gotman J. Continuous high-frequency activity in mesial temporal lobe structures. Epilepsia. 2012;53(5):797–806. doi:10.1111/j.1528-1167.2012.03428.x.

Menendez de la Prida L, Trevelyan AJ. Cellular mechanisms of high frequency oscillations in epilepsy: on the diverse sources of pathological activities. Epilepsy Res. 2011;97(3):308–17. doi:10.1016/j.eplepsyres.2011.02.009.

Murthy VN, Fetz EE. Coherent 25- to 35-Hz oscillations in the sensorimotor cortex of awake behaving monkeys. Proc Natl Acad Sci U S A. 1992;89(12):5670–4.

Nadasdy Z, Hirase H, Czurko A, Csicsvari J, Buzsaki G. Replay and time compression of recurring spike sequences in the hippocampus. J Neurosci. 1999;19(21):9497–507.

Nariai H, Matsuzaki N, Juhasz C, Nagasawa T, Sood S, Chugani HT, et al. Ictal high-frequency oscillations at 80–200 Hz coupled with delta phase in epileptic spasms. Epilepsia. 2011a;52(10):e130–4. doi:10.1111/j.1528-1167.2011.03263.x.

Nariai H, Nagasawa T, Juhasz C, Sood S, Chugani HT, Asano E. Statistical mapping of ictal high-frequency oscillations in epileptic spasms. Epilepsia. 2011b;52(1):63–74. doi:10.1111/j.1528-1167.2010.02786.x.

Niedermeyer E. Historical aspects. In: Niedermeyer E, Lopes da Silva F, editors. Electroencephalography: basic principles, clinical applications, and related field. Baltimore: Williams & Wilkins; 1993. p. 1–14.

Nir Y, Staba RJ, Andrillon T, Vyazovskiy VV, Cirelli C, Fried I, et al. Regional slow waves and spindles in human sleep. Neuron. 2011;70(1):153–69. doi:10.1016/j.neuron.2011.02.043.

Ochi A, Otsubo H, Donner EJ, Elliott I, Iwata R, Funaki T, et al. Dynamic changes of ictal high-frequency oscillations in neocortical epilepsy: using multiple band frequency analysis. Epilepsia. 2007;48(2):286–96.

Ogren JA, Wilson CL, Bragin A, Lin JJ, Salamon N, Dutton RA, et al. Three dimensional surface maps link local atrophy and fast ripples in human epileptic hippocampus. Ann Neurol. 2009;66(6):783–91.

O'Keefe J, Nadel J. The Hippocampus as a Cognitive Map. Oxford: Clarendon Press; 1978.

Penfield W. The epilepsies: with a note on radical therapy. N Engl J Med. 1939;221(6):209–18.

Pravdich-Neminsky WW. An experiment in the recording of electrical phenomena in the brain of mammals. Zbl Physiol. 1913;27:957–60.

RamachandranNair R, Ochi A, Imai K, Benifla M, Akiyama T, Holowka S, et al. Epileptic spasms in older pediatric patients: MEG and ictal high-frequency oscillations suggest focal-onset seizures in a subset of epileptic spasms. Epilepsy Res. 2008;78(2–3):216–24.

Roopun AK, Simonotto JD, Pierce ML, Jenkins A, Nicholson C, Schofield IS, et al. A nonsynaptic mechanism underlying interictal discharges in human epileptic neocortex. Proc Natl Acad Sci U S A. 2010;107(1):338–43.

Sammaritano M, Gigli GL, Gotman J. Interictal spiking during wakefulness and sleep and the localization of foci in temporal lobe epilepsy. Neurology. 1991;41:290–7.

Schevon CA, Trevelyan AJ, Schroeder CE, Goodman RR, McKhann Jr G, Emerson RG. Spatial characterization of interictal high frequency oscillations in epileptic neocortex. Brain. 2009;132(11):3047–59. doi:10.1093/brain/awp222.

Schmitz D, Schuchmann S, Fisahn A, Draguhn A, Buhl EH, Petrasch-Parwez E, et al. Axo-axonal coupling. a novel mechanism for ultrafast neuronal communication. Neuron. 2001;31(5): 831–40.

Shao LR, Dudek FE. Changes in mIPSCs and sIPSCs after kainate treatment: evidence for loss of inhibitory input to dentate granule cells and possible compensatory responses. J Neurophysiol. 2005;94(2):952–60. doi:10.1152/jn.01342.2004.

Siapas AG, Wilson MA. Coordinated interactions between hippocampal ripples and cortical spindles during slow-wave sleep. Neuron. 1998;21:1123–8.

Singer W. Synchronization of cortical activity and its putative role in information processing and learning. Annu Rev Physiol. 1993;55:349–74.

Skaggs WE, McNaughton BL, Permenter M, Archibeque M, Vogt J, Amaral D, et al. EEG sharp wave and sparse ensemble unit activity in the macaque hippocampus. J Neurophysiol. 2007;98:898–910.

Spencer SS, Guimaraes P, Katz A, Kim J, Spencer DD. Morphological patterns of seizures recorded intracranially. Epilepsia. 1992a;33(3):537–45.

Spencer SS, Kim J, Spencer DD. Ictal spikes: a marker of specific hippocampal cell loss. Electroencephalogr Clin Neurophysiol. 1992b;83(2):104–11.

Staba RJ. Normal and pathologic high-frequency oscillations. In: Noebels JL, Avoli M, Rogawski MA, Olsen RW, Delgado-Escueta AV, editors. Jasper's basic mechanisms of the epilepsies. 4th ed. Bethesda, MD: National Center for Biotechnology Information (USA); 2012.

Staba RJ, Wilson CL, Bragin A, Fried I, Engel Jr J. Quantitative analysis of high-frequency oscillations (80–500 Hz) recorded in human epileptic hippocampus and entorhinal cortex. J Neurophysiol. 2002a;88(4):1743–52.

Staba RJ, Wilson CL, Bragin A, Fried I, Engel Jr J. Sleep states differentiate single neuron activity recorded from human epileptic hippocampus, entorhinal cortex, and subiculum. J Neurosci. 2002b;22(13):5694–704. doi:20026532.

Staba RJ, Wilson CL, Fried I, Engel Jr J. Single neuron burst firing in the human hippocampus during sleep. Hippocampus. 2002c;12(6):724–34. doi:10.1002/hipo.10026.

Staba RJ, Wilson CL, Bragin A, Jhung D, Fried I, Engel J. High-frequency oscillations recorded in human medial temporal lobe during sleep. Ann Neurol. 2004;56:108–15.

Staba RJ, Frighetto L, Behnke EJ, Mathern GW, Fields TA, Bragin A, et al. Increased fast ripple to ripple ratios correlate with reduced hippocampal volumes and neuron loss in temporal lobe epilepsy patients. Epilepsia. 2007;48(11):2130–8.

Staba RJ, Ekstrom AD, Suthana NA, Burggren A, Fried I, Engel Jr J, et al. Gray matter loss correlates with mesial temporal lobe neuronal hyperexcitability inside the human seizure-onset zone. Epilepsia. 2011;53(1):25–34. doi:10.1111/j.1528-1167.2011.03333.x.

Steriade M, Nunez A, Amzica F. A novel slow (<1 Hz) oscillation of neocortical neurons in vivo: depolarizing and hyperpolarizing components. J Neurosci. 1993;13(8):3252–65.

Sullivan D, Csicsvari J, Mizuseki K, Montgomery S, Diba K, Buzsaki G. Relationships between hippocampal sharp waves, ripples, and fast gamma oscillation: influence of dentate and entorhinal cortical activity. J Neurosci. 2011;31(23):8605–16. doi:10.1523/JNEUROSCI.0294-11.2011.

Talairach J, David M, Tournoux P. L'exploration chirurgicale stereotaxique du lobe temporal dans l'epilepsie temporale. Paris: Mason; 1958.

Traub RD, Schmitz D, Jefferys JG, Draguhn A. High-frequency population oscillations are predicted to occur in hippocampal pyramidal neuronal networks interconnected by axoaxonal gap junctions. Neuroscience. 1999;92(2):407–26.

Traub RD, Whittington MA, Buhl EH, LeBeau FE, Bibbig A, Boyd S, et al. A possible role for gap junctions in generation of very fast EEG oscillations preceding the onset of, and perhaps initiating, seizures. Epilepsia. 2001;42(2):153–70.

Urrestarazu E, Chander R, Dubeau F, Gotman J. Interictal high-frequency oscillations (100–500 Hz) in the intracerebral EEG of epileptic patients. Brain. 2007;130(9):2354–66.

Wierzynski CM, Lubenov EV, Gu M, Siapas AG. State-dependent spike-timing relationships between hippocampal and prefrontal circuits during sleep. Neuron. 2009;61(4):587–96.

Wieser HG, Bancaud J, Talairach J, Bonis A, Szikla G. Comparative value of spontaneous and chemically and electrically induced seizures in establishing the lateralization of temporal lobe seizures. Epilepsia. 1979;20(1):47–59.

Worrell G. High-frequency oscillations recorded on scalp EEG. Epilepsy Curr. 2012;12(2):57–8. doi:10.5698/1535-7511-12.2.57.

Worrell GA, Parish L, Cranstoun SD, Jonas R, Baltuch G, Litt B. High-frequency oscillations and seizure generation in neocortical epilepsy. Brain. 2004;127(Pt 7):1496–506.

Worrell GA, Gardner AB, Stead SM, Hu S, Goerss S, Cascino GJ, et al. High-frequency oscillations in human temporal lobe: simultaneous microwire and clinical macroelectrode recordings. Brain. 2008;131(4):928–37.

Worrell GA, Jerbi K, Kobayashi K, Lina JM, Zelmann R, Le Van Quyen M. Recording and analysis techniques for high-frequency oscillations. Prog Neurobiol. 2012;98(3):265–78. doi:10.1016/j.pneurobio.2012.02.006.

Wu JY, Sankar R, Lerner JT, Matsumoto JH, Vinters HV, Mathern GW. Removing interictal fast ripples on electrocorticography linked with seizure freedom in children. Neurology. 2010;75(19):1686–94. doi:10.1212/WNL.0b013e3181fc27d0.

Ylinen A, Bragin A, Nadasdy Z, Jando G, Szabo I, Sik A, et al. Sharp wave-associated high-frequency oscillation (200Hz) in the intact hippocampus: network and intracellular mechanisms. J Neurosci. 1995;15(1):30–46.

Zelmann R, Mari F, Jacobs J, Zijlmans M, Dubeau F, Gotman J. A comparison between detectors of high frequency oscillations. Clin Neurophysiol. 2012;123(1):106–16. doi:10.1016/j.clinph.2011.06.006.

Zijlmans MM, Jacobs JM, Zelmann RM, Dubeau FM, Gotman JP. High-frequency oscillations mirror disease activity in patients with epilepsy. Neurology. 2009;72(11):979–86.

Zijlmans M, Jacobs J, Kahn YU, Zelmann R, Dubeau F, Gotman J. Ictal and interictal high frequency oscillations in patients with focal epilepsy. Clin Neurophysiol. 2011;122(4):664–71. doi:10.1016/j.clinph.2010.09.021.

Chapter 4
Molecular Mechanisms of Pharmacoresistant Epilepsy

Alberto Lazarowski and Liliana Czornyj

Abstract Epilepsy is a common neurological disorder and despite significant advances in therapy over recent decades, about 30–40 % of epileptic patients will remain refractory to pharmacological therapies despite optimized drug treatment. Taking a carefully reviewed definition of "drug-resistance" into account, two main concepts were proposed to explain the development of pharmacoresistance in epilepsy. The "target" hypothesis indicates that changes in the properties of the drug targets themselves may result in reduced sensitivity to antiepileptic drugs (AEDs). This hypothesis is supported by several pharmacodynamic modifications leading to loss of drugs' effects in refractory epilepsy. However, it cannot explain the refractoriness observed after polytherapeutic trials using several recommended AEDs at appropriate doses. Consequently, a mechanism of multidrug resistance (MDR) as previously described in cancer could also explain—at least in part—the reason for this particular phenotype. The so-called "transporters" hypothesis suggests that functional over-expression of multidrug transporters in brain could reduce AEDs access to the central nervous system. Both mechanisms could be active simultaneously in refractory epilepsy and possibly also, not represent the only mechanisms involved.

Keywords Refractory epilepsy • Target hypotheses • Pharmacodynamic • Antiepileptic drugs • Multidrug resistance • P-glycoprotein • ABC-transporters • Pharmacokinetics • Depolarized membrane

---

A. Lazarowski, M.S., Ph.D. (✉)
INFIBIOC-FFyB-UBA-Universidad de Buenos Aires,
Junín 856 (1113 AAD), Buenos Aires, Argentina
e-mail: alazarowski@gmail.com

L. Czornyj, M.D.
Hospital Nacional de Pediatría "Juan P. Garrahan",
Combate de los Pozos 1245 (1245 AAM), Buenos Aires, Argentina
e-mail: tominadia@hotmail.com

L. Rocha and E.A. Cavalheiro (eds.), *Pharmacoresistance in Epilepsy: From Genes and Molecules to Promising Therapies*, DOI 10.1007/978-1-4614-6464-8_4,

4.1 Introduction

Epilepsy is one of the most common neurological problems and close to 3 % of individuals within the general population will have epilepsy during their lives. Both primary and secondary mechanisms are involved in the development of epileptic syndromes falling into two broad categories: generalized epilepsy (seizures begins simultaneously in both cerebral hemispheres) and partial epilepsy, characterized by localization-related seizures, originated in one or more foci, although they can spread to involve the entire brain (Benbadis 2001).

Despite considerable advances in pharmacotherapy, about 30 % of patients with epilepsy are refractory to pharmacotherapy (Temkin 2001). Seizures are not controlled in these patients in spite of several antiepileptic drugs (AEDs), even at maximum tolerated doses. This multidrug resistance phenotype (Fig. 4.1) may be present in the early stage of the disease (Elger 2003). Why does a subgroup of patients repeatedly fail to obtain seizure control with one AED after another? (Kwan and Brodie 2000). One explanation is that patients with epilepsy do not receive the correct treatment (Sisodiya 2005). Clinically, refractory epilepsy (RE) should be defined as the failure to achieve seizure freedom after a 9- or 18-month period of continued appropriate AEDs therapy in adults and children, respectively (Berg et al. 2001).

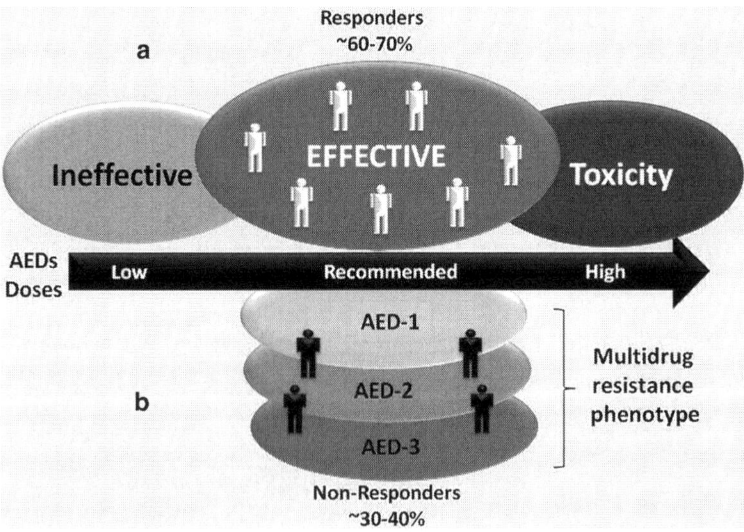

Fig. 4.1 Distribution of responder vs. nonresponder patients with multidrug resistance phenotypes. The *arrow* marks the administered escalating doses of AEDs. The *silhouettes* represent percentage of cases with each phenotype. (**a**) The typical distribution of the therapeutic response after the administration of appropriate AED (monotherapy): *Left*: insufficient dose (ineffective), *Center*: recommended dose (effective), and *Right*: high dose (toxicity). (**b**) The *lower part* represents the typical phenotype of patients refractory to treatment with three different AEDs, which all together are ineffective, even at doses inducing toxic effects

The following risk factors are considered important for the development of the RE phenotype.

- Age of the patient at the time of epilepsy onset
- Type and etiology of seizures
- Number and severity of seizures before the start of the treatment

In the presence of adequate doses and carefully monitored serum AEDs levels, drugs have to traverse the blood–brain barrier (BBB), achieve a sufficient minimum therapeutic concentration in the brain and activate specific target sites. According to this situation, two nonexclusive hypotheses have been postulated to explain refractoriness in epilepsy: the functional/structural modification of targets and/or the over-expression of drug-transporters in the brain (Remy and Beck 2006).

4.2 The Target Hypothesis or Pharmacodynamic Changes in Pharmacoresistance

After AEDs permeation into the central nervous system (CNS) parenchyma, drugs have to bind to one or more targets to exert their desired effects. Most AEDs predominantly target voltage-gated cathion channels (α-subunits of voltage-gated Na^+ channels and T-type voltage-gated Ca^{2+} channels) or influence gamma-aminobutyric acid (GABA)-mediated inhibition. Concerning this issue, genetic epileptic syndromes are secondary to mutations produced predominantly on ion channels, which are, in many cases, the same ion channels targeted by most AEDs (Kwan et al. 2001; Meldrum and Rogawski 2007) (Table 4.1).

Some AEDs potently inhibit low-threshold T-type Ca^{2+} channels, which are not expressed presynaptically, but are critically important in controlling excitability of the postsynaptic neuron compartments, both in normal and epileptic conditions. One such interesting pharmacodynamic change is observed as aberrant bursting in CA1 hippocampal neurons in epileptic animals mediated by an increased expression of T-type Ca^{2+} channels (Su et al. 2002) or in thalamic neurons implicated in the generation of spike-wave discharges in absence epilepsy (Huguenard 2002). This type of mechanism could also be applied to other voltage-gated ion channels such as K^+ channels (Remy and Beck 2006).

In humans, these types of modifications that reduce efficacy of a given AED at the "target" level were described in voltage-gated Na^+ channels by downregulation of their accessory β-subunits, altered α-subunit expression, or induction of neonatal Na^+ channel II and III α-isoform mRNAs (Aronica et al. 2001). Similar changes were observed in GABA-A receptors, by decrease of α_1-subunits and increase of α_4-subunits, reducing GABA and benzodiazepines (BZD) affinity for their receptor (Fig. 4.2). These mechanisms resulting in modifications of specific "targets" are associated with seizure activity, producing changes at the transcription level or alternative ion channel subunit mRNA splicing, as well as altered posttranslational

Table 4.1 Antiepileptic drug targets and their features as ABC-transporters (ABC-t) substrates

Antiepileptic drug	Voltage-gated Na^+ channels	HVA Ca^{2+} channels	LVA Ca^{2+} channels	GABA-A receptor	ABC-t substrate
Phenobarbital	–	Yes	–	–	P-gp
Phenytoin	Yes	–	–	–	P-gp/MRP
Carbamazepine	Yes	–	–	–	P-gp/MRP
Valproate	Possible	Possible	Possible	–	P-gp/MRP
Benzodiazepines	Yes	–	–	–	P-gp
Ethosuximide	Yes	–	–	–	–
Vigabatrin	Yes	–	–	–	P-gp
Lamotrigine	Yes	Possible	–	–	P-gp
Gabapentin	–	Possible	–	–	P-gp
Felbamate	Possible	Possible	Possible	Possible	P-gp
Topiramate	Possible	Possible	Possible	Possible	P-gp
Tiagabine	Yes	–	–	–	–
Oxcarbazepine	Yes	–	–	–	–
Levetiracetam	–	–	Possible	–	MRP
Pregabalin	Possible	–	–	–	–

P-gp P-glycoprotein, *MRP* multidrug resistant-associated proteins

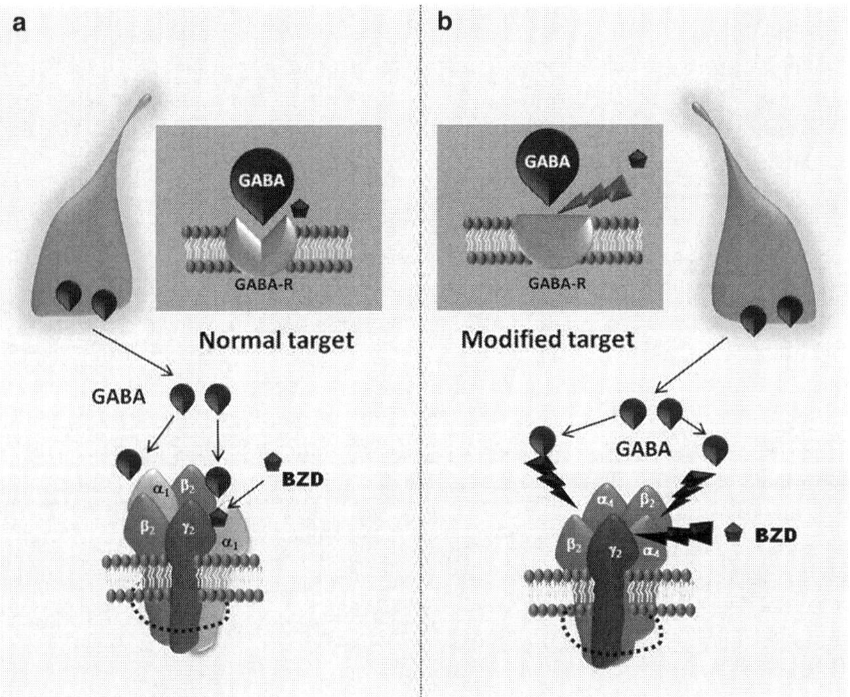

Fig. 4.2 Pharmacodynamic changes in the expression of GABA-R subunits during chronic epilepsies. The normal structure of the GABA-R expressing two α_1-subunits (**a**) can be modified by the expression of two α_4-subunits (**b**), producing a loss of sensibility to GABA and BZD

modification of the protein and/or phosphorylation by protein kinases. One intriguing question is that while carbamazepine, phenytoin (PHT), valproate, and lamotrigine bind to the same target (Na^+ channels) (Kuo 1998), reduced pharmacosensitivity to these drugs following pilocarpine-induced status epilepticus depends on the individual AED (Remy et al. 2003b). An explanation for this dissimilar altered sensitivity in epileptic tissue could be secondary to alterations of subunit composition of Na^+ channels. Indeed, AED-insensitive subunits or subunit combinations are promoted as has been observed in both human and experimental epilepsy (Remy and Beck 2006). Furthermore, downregulation of β1 and β2 accessory subunits of Na^+ channels, or changes secondary to alternative mRNA splicing of pore-forming subunits, have also been observed following induced status epilepticus in experimental models (Nicolas and Cau 1997; Aronica et al. 2001; Ellerkmann et al. 2003). Mutations of the β_1 subunit of Na^+ channels are the cause of generalized epilepsy with febrile seizures plus, an autosomal dominant epilepsy syndrome (Lucas et al. 2005). Interestingly, mutant β_1 subunits of this channel are associated with a dramatic and selective loss of use-dependent blocking effects by PHT (Lucas et al. 2005) and carbamazepine (Remy et al. 2003a, b). Collectively, these pharmacodynamic modifications resulting in loss of sensitivity (or increased refractoriness) have been termed "the target hypothesis of pharmacoresistance" (Remy and Beck 2006). However the "target hypothesis" cannot completely explain refractoriness to polytherapy.

4.3 The Transporters Hypothesis

The *transporters hypothesis* is an emerging concept of pharmacoresistance that is explained by an increased functional expression of multidrug transporter proteins, able to prevent access of AEDs to the brain and decrease concentration at their sites of action (Remy and Beck 2006; Lazarowski et al. 2007b; Löscher 2007; Potschka 2010). Multiple drug resistance (MDR) is a clinical phenotype characterized by insensitivity to a broad spectrum of drugs that presumably act on different mechanisms. Because most AEDs are administered orally, variations in genes related to drug absorption, transport and metabolism might modify the drug's plasmatic levels, body distribution, and access to the CNS. Enterocytes and hepatocytes express the major AEDs-metabolizing enzymes (CYP family), and multidrug transporters such as P-glycoprotein (P-gp), multidrug resistant-associated proteins (MRPs), and breast cancer resistant protein (BCRP). Their over-expression in these and other peripheral organs may play a crucial role by limiting drug absorption as well as regulating metabolism and excretion ratios, resulting in persistently low-AED plasmatic levels (Lazarowski et al. 2004a; Lazarowski and Czornyj 2011).

4.3.1 ABC-Transporters: Functions and Properties

Genes encoding transmembrane proteins that function as drug efflux pumps and belong to the ATP-binding cassette (ABC) transporter superfamily are classified into seven ABC[A-G] subfamilies (Dean et al. 2001). They export not only the drugs but also their metabolites, as well as xenobiotics and endogenous compounds of catabolism. Many transporters that were first characterized in excretory peripheral tissues have also been detected in the brain and are involved in the efflux of a variety of endogenous or exogenous substances (Lee et al. 2001).

Particularly P-gp (the product of MDR-1 gene), MRPs and BCRP, have been associated to the multidrug-resistant phenotype. Most ABC-transporters have two transmembrane domains (TM) and two cytosolic ATP-binding domains. BCRP has only one TM and one ATP-binding domain and is assumed to function as a dimmer (Fig. 4.3) (Dean et al. 2001).

Different agents, hormones, oncogenes, and transcription factors known to be involved in apoptosis, stress, inflammation, and hypoxia (COX-2, p53, NF-IL6, NFkB, AP-1, HIF-1α) (Bauer et al. 2008; Goldsmith et al. 1995; Cornwell and Smith 1993; Combates et al. 1994; Comerford et al. 2002) can upregulate the expression of these transporters in normally non-expressing cells such as neurons (Ramos et al. 2004; Lazarowski et al. 2007a) or cardiomyocytes (Laguens et al. 2007). This group of evidence suggests that P-gp and other MDR-like proteins may also be involved in biological processes related to survival-death mechanisms.

4.3.2 ABC-Transporters in Clinical Refractory Epilepsy

In normal brain, P-gp, MRPs, and BCRP are expressed in the BBB or the blood-cerebrospinal fluid (CSF) barrier (Girardin 2006) playing all together a combined role to reduce brain penetration of many dangerous compounds and drugs. P-gp is expressed on the apical side of the choroids' plexus epithelia, at the luminal membrane of vascular endothelial cells and at the astrocyte-foot-ending-processes of the BBB (Aronica et al. 2012). MRPs and BCRP are expressed in the microvessel endothelial cells of the BBB.

After the first description of P-gp over-expression in the brain of patients with RE (Tishler et al. 1995), several reports have shown high levels of P-gp and MRPs expression in epileptogenic brain areas obtained from patients with different RE syndromes. These studies indicate that P-gp is highly expressed not only in vascular endothelial cells but also in brain parenchymal cells (Lazarowski et al. 1999; Sisodiya et al. 1999; Dombrowski et al. 2001), in which they are not expressed under normal conditions (Lazarowski et al. 2004b).

Several authors have described the role of ABC-transporters in the development of pharmacoresistace in epilepsy (Sisodiya 2007; Lazarowski et al. 2007b; Löscher 2007). A recent review describes cerebral expression patterns of several classes of

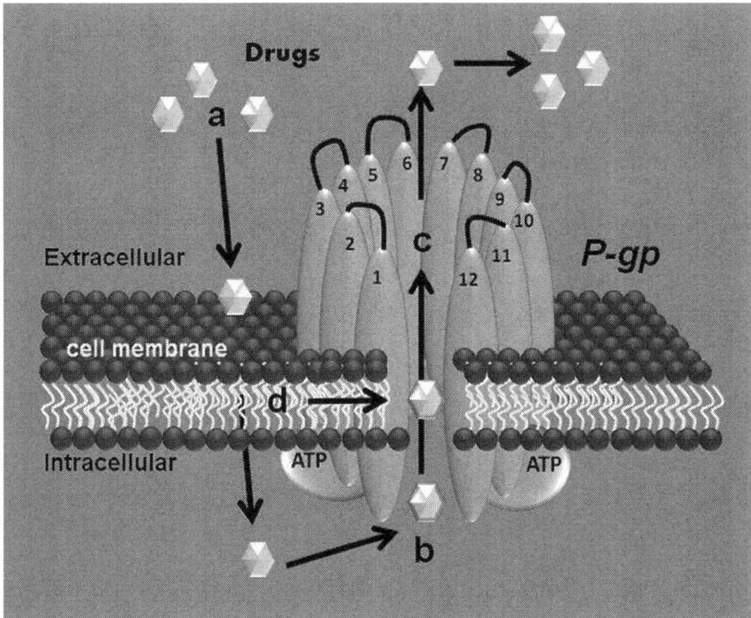

Fig. 4.3 Schematic representation of a typical structure of P-gp and sequential drug movement trough the cell membrane. P-gp is proposed to consist of two equivalent halves, each with six transmembrane segments and a nucleotide binding domain at the cytosolic side on each one. The 12 transmembrane helices together form a central cavity in the lipid bilayer. In the *left* side, it is shown how the extracellular drugs with high liposolubility access the cells (**a**). In the cytosol, drugs bind to the protein (P-gp) at an inward facing high-affinity site (**b**). This binding and hydrolysis of ATP initiate drug extrusion from the intracellular pool that will be expelled via a conformational change that transforms it to a low-affinity outward (extracellular) facing site, producing an active drug efflux (**c**). Alternatively, drugs can also be intercepted and extruded directly from the lipid bilayer (**d**)

ABC-transporters in the epileptogenic brain (Aronica et al. 2012). Over-expression of efflux transporter could be constitutive and exist before the onset of epilepsy, as suggested by the finding of upregulation of drug transporters in abnormal parenchymal cells in epileptogenic tissues from different RE syndromes, such as dysembryoplastic neuro-epithelial tumors, focal cortical dysplasias, hippocampal sclerosis, and cortical tubers (Sisodiya et al. 1999; Lazarowski et al. 2004c). However, they could also be over-expressed as a consequence of epileptic seizures (Seegers et al. 2002; Rizzi et al. 2002; Lazarowski et al. 2004b).

The inducible nature of ABC-transporter genes suggests that over-expression of these proteins can be observed in all excretory organs including BBB, playing a critical role in the modification of both systemic and local pharmacokinetics of AEDs. However, their induced expression in previously non-expressive cells as observed in brain parenchymal cells, particularly in neurons from epileptogenic areas (Aronica et al. 2003; Lazarowski et al. 1999, 2004a) suggests a differential role related to the intrinsic convulsive mechanism, as previously proposed (Lazarowski et al. 2007b).

4.3.3 Experimental Evidences

Several epileptic (or convulsive) experimental models seem to firmly establish that some ABC-transporters, particularly P-gp, are over-expressed secondary to seizure activity. P-gp over-expression that depends on the frequency and intensity of seizures is related to a progressive increase of the pharmacoresistant phenotype [for review see Aronica et al. (2012)]. Furthermore, administration of a P-gp inhibitor such as tariquidar has been shown to revert drug resistance in animal models (van Vliet et al. 2006). Similarly, adjuvant treatment with nimodipine, a calcium channel blocker that also inhibits P-gp activity, is able to restore the normal hippocampal pharmacokinetics of PHT, an effect associated with seizure control (Höcht et al. 2007) avoiding death following repetitive convulsions in PHT-RE models (Lazarowski et al. 2007b). Complex mechanisms associated with excitotoxicity mediated by glutamic acid, including COX2-dependent inflammatory pathways (Bauer et al. 2008) or hypoxia-dependent HIF-1α activation are involved in the induction of P-gp brain over-expression (Ramos et al. 2004; Lazarowski et al. 2007a) and suggest that, even in the absence of seizures, the refractory phenotype could be induced in some epileptic syndromes. In this regard, a group of evidence indicates that P-gp can also decrease the plasma membrane potential of several cell types (Wadkins and Roepe 1997; Roepe 2000) and modify swelling-activated Cl^- currents (Vanoye et al. 1999), situations resulting from brain hypoxia and convulsive stress that may facilitate neuronal excitability.

All these evidences support the notion that induction of neuronal P-gp expression could correlate with a progressive acquisition of refractoriness associated with worsening of clinical features (Lazarowski et al. 2007b). This situation may support a third theory to explain pharmacoresistant epilepsy based on inherent phenotypic severity (Rogawski and Johnson 2008). In a previous study, we found that increased P-gp over-expression in brain of rats submitted to repetitive seizures was associated with membrane depolarization in fresh slices of hippocampus and neocortex, a situation reverted when nimodipine plus PHT were applied (Auzmendi et al. 2008). These results represent unique evidence supporting the notion that progressive P-gp over-expression contributes to membrane depolarization in hippocampus and neocortex, which may play a role in epileptogenesis and refractoriness.

The mechanisms underlying this silent process associated to a progressive functional over-expression of P-gp, particularly in neurons, could represent new therapeutic targets to control pharmacoresistant epilepsy (Hughes 2008; Robey et al. 2008; Potschka 2010).

4.4 Conclusions

Once each of the mechanisms leading to AED resistance are elucidated (target modifications and transporters over-expression), their knowledge may become increasingly important in new drug development and clinical applications. Novel effective treatment strategies to overcome pharmacoresistance would include not only new compounds for new cellular targets but also the development of novel AEDs that would not be substrates for efflux transporters. Regarding the properties of P-gp on membrane potential depolarization, the coadministration of drugs designed to avoid transporter over-expression or specific inhibitors of transporters function could prevent refractoriness and/or epileptogenesis, as suggested above.

References

Aronica E, Yankaya B, Troost D, van Vliet EA, Lopes da Silva FH, Gorter JA. Induction of neonatal sodium channel II and III alpha-isoform mRNAs in neurons and microglia after status epilepticus in the rat hippocampus. Eur J Neurosci. 2001;13:1261–6.

Aronica E, Gorter JA, Jansen GH, van Veelen CW, van Rijen PC, Leenstra S, et al. Expression and cellular distribution of multidrug transporter proteins in two major causes of medically intractable epilepsy: focal cortical dysplasia and glioneuronal tumors. Neuroscience. 2003;118:417–29.

Aronica E, Sisodiya SM, Gorter JA, Bartolomei F, Gastaldi M, Massacrier A, et al. Cerebral expression of drug transporters in epilepsy. Adv Drug Deliv Rev. 2012;64:919–29.

Auzmendi J, Orozco-Suárez S, González-Trujano E, Rocha-Arrieta L, Lazarowski A (2008) P-glycoprotein (P-gp) contribute to depolarization of plasmatic membranes of hippocampal cells in a model of phenytoin-refractory seizures induced by pentyleneterazole (PTZ). V° Latin-American Congress of Epilepsy (ILAE), Montevideo (ROU)

Bauer B, Hartz AM, Pekcec A, Toellner K, Miller DS, Potschka H. Seizure-induced up-regulation of p-glycoprotein at the blood–brain barrier through glutamate and cyclooxygenase-2 signaling. Mol Pharmacol. 2008;73:1444–53.

Benbadis SR. Epileptic seizures and syndromes. Neurol Clin. 2001;19:251–70.

Berg A, Shinnar S, Levy SR, Testa FM, Smith-Rapaport S, Beckerman B. Early development of intractable epilepsy in children: a prospective study. Neurology. 2001;56:1445–52.

Combates N, Rzepka R, Pan Chen Y-N, Cohen D. NF-IL6, a member of the C/EBP family of transcription factors, binds and trans-activates the human MDR1 gene promoter. J Biol Chem. 1994;269:29715–9.

Comerford KM, Wallace TJ, Karhausen J, Louis NA, Montalto MC, Colgan SP. Hypoxia-inducible factor-1-dependent regulation of the multidrug resistance (MDR1) gene. Cancer Res. 2002;62:3387–94.

Cornwell MM, Smith DE. A signal transduction pathway for activation of the mdr1 promoter involves the protooncogene c-raf kinase. J Biol Chem. 1993;268:15347–50.

Dean M, Rzhetsky A, Allikmets R. The human ATP-binding cassette (ABC) transporter superfamily. Genome Res. 2001;11:1156–66.

Dombrowski SM, Desai SY, Marroni M, Cucullo L, Goodrich K, Bingaman W, et al. Overexpression of multiple drug resistance genes in endothelial cells from patients with refractory epilepsy. Epilepsia. 2001;42:1501–6.

Elger C. Pharmacoresistance: modern concept and basic data derivated from human brain tissue. Epilepsia. 2003;44 Suppl 5:9–15.

Ellerkmann RK, Remy S, Chen J, Sochivko D, Elger CE, Urban BW, et al. Molecular and functional changes in voltage-dependent Na^+ channels following pilocarpine-induced status epilepticus in rat dentate granule cells. Neuroscience. 2003;119:323–33.
Girardin F. Membrane transporter proteins: a challenge for CNS drug development. Dialogues Clin Neurosci. 2006;8:311–21.
Goldsmith M, Gudas J, Schneider E, Cowan K. Wild type p53 stimulates expression from the human multidrug resistance promoter in a p53-negative cell line. J Biol Chem. 1995;270: 1894–8.
Höcht C, Lazarowski A, Gonzalez N, Auzmendi J, Opezzo JA, Bramuglia G, et al. Nimodipine restores the altered hippocampal phenytoin pharmacokinetics in a refractory epileptic model. Neurosci Lett. 2007;413:168–72.
Hughes JR. One of the hottest topics in epileptology: ABC proteins. Their inhibition may be the future for patients with intractable seizures. Neurol Res. 2008;30:920–5.
Huguenard JR. Block of T-type calcium channels is an important action of succinimide antiabsence drugs. Epilepsy Curr. 2002;2:49–52.
Kuo CC. A common anticonvulsant binding site for phenytoin, carbamazepine, and lamotrigine in neuronal Na^+ channels. Mol Pharmacol. 1998;54:712–21.
Kwan P, Brodie MJ. Early identification of refractory epilepsy. N Engl J Med. 2000;342:314–9.
Kwan P, Sills GJ, Brodie MJ. The mechanisms of action of commonly used antiepileptic drugs. Pharmacol Ther. 2001;90:21–34.
Laguens R, Lazarowski A, Cuniberti L, Vera Janavel G, Cabeza Meckert P, Yannarelli G, et al. Expression of the MDR-1 gene-encoded P-glycoprotein in cardiomyocytes of conscious sheep undergoing acute myocardial ischemia followed by reperfusion. J Histochem Cytochem. 2007;55:191–7.
Lazarowski A, Czornyj L. Potential role of multidrug resistant proteins in refractory epilepsy and antiepileptic drugs interactions. Drug Metabol Drug Interact. 2011;26(1):21–6.
Lazarowski A, Sevlever G, Taratuto A, Massaro M, Rabinowicz A. Tuberous Sclerosis associated with MDR-1 expression and drug-resistant epilepsy. Pediatr Neurol. 1999;21:731–4.
Lazarowski A, Massaro M, Schteinschnaider A, Intruvini S, Sevlever G, Rabinowicz A. Neuronal MDR-1 gene expression and persistent low levels of anticonvulsants in a child with refractory epilepsy. Ther Drug Monit. 2004a;26:44–6.
Lazarowski A, Ramos AJ, Garcia-Rivello H, Brusco A, Girardi E. Neuronal and glial expression of the multidrug resistance gene product in an experimental epilepsy model. Cell Mol Neurobiol. 2004b;24:77–85.
Lazarowski A, Lubieniecki F, Camarero S, Pomata H, Bartuluchi M, Sevlever G, Taratuto AL. Multidrug resistance proteins in tuberous sclerosis and refractory epilepsy. Pediatr Neurol. 2004c;30:102–6.
Lazarowski A, Caltana L, Merelli A, Rubio MD, Ramos AJ, Brusco A. Neuronal mdr-1 gene expression after experimental focal hypoxia: a new obstacle for neuroprotection? J Neurol Sci. 2007a;258(1–2):84–92.
Lazarowski A, Czornyj L, Lubienieki F, Girardi E, Vazquez S, D'Giano C. ABC transporters during epilepsy and mechanisms underlying multidrug resistance in refractory epilepsy. Epilepsia. 2007b;48:140–9.
Lee G, Dallas S, Hong M, Bendayan R. Drug transporters in the central nervous system: brain barriers and brain parenchyma considerations. Pharmacol Rev. 2001;53:569–96.
Löscher W. Mechanisms of drug resistance in status epilepticus. Epilepsia. 2007;48 Suppl 8:74–7.
Lucas PT, Meadows LS, Nicholls J, Ragsdale DS. An epilepsy mutation in the beta1 subunit of the voltage-gated sodium channel results in reduced channel sensitivity to phenytoin. Epilepsy Res. 2005;64:77–84.
Meldrum BS, Rogawski A. Molecular targets for antiepileptic drug development. Neurotherapeutics. 2007;4(1):18–61.
Nicolas S, Cau P. Changes in the mRNAs encoding subtypes I, II and III sodium channel alpha subunits following kainate-induced seizures in rat brain. J Neurocytol. 1997;26:667–8.

Potschka H. Transporter hypothesis of drug-resistant epilepsy: challenges for pharmacogenetic approaches. Pharmacogenomics. 2010;11(10):1427–38.

Ramos AJ, Lazarowski A, Villar MJ, Brusco A. Transient expression of MDR-1/P-glycoprotein in a model of partial cortical devascularization. Cell Mol Neurobiol. 2004;24:101–7.

Remy S, Beck H. Molecular and cellular mechanisms of pharmacoresistance in epilepsy. Brain. 2006;129:18–35.

Remy S, Gabriel S, Urban BW, Dietrich D, Lehmann TN, Elger CE, et al. A novel mechanism underlying drug-resistance in chronic epilepsy. Ann Neurol. 2003a;53:469–79.

Remy S, Urban BW, Elger CE, Beck H. Anticonvulsant pharmacology of voltage-gated Na^+ channels in hippocampal neurons of control and chronically epileptic rats. Eur J Neurosci. 2003b;17:2648–58.

Rizzi M, Caccia S, Guiso G, Richichi C, Gorter JA, Aronica E, et al. Limbic seizures induce P-glycoprotein in rodent brain: functional implications for pharmacoresistance. J Neurosci. 2002;22:5833–9.

Robey RW, Lazarowski A, Bates SE. P-glycoprotein-a clinical target in drug-refractory epilepsy? Mol Pharmacol. 2008;73:1343–6.

Roepe PD. What is the precise role of human MDR 1 protein in chemotherapeutic drug resistance? Curr Pharm Des. 2000;6:241–60.

Rogawski M, Johnson M. Intrinsic severity as a determinant of antiepileptic drug refractoriness. Epilepsy Curr. 2008;8:127–30.

Seegers U, Potschka H, Loscher W. Expression of the multidrug transporter P-glycoprotein in brain capillary endothelial cells and brain parenchyma of amygdala-kindled rats. Epilepsia. 2002;43:675–84.

Sisodiya SM. Genetics of drug resistance. Epilepsia. 2005;46 Suppl 10:33–8.

Sisodiya SM. Mechanisms of antiepileptic drug resistance. Curr Opin Neurol. 2007;16:197–201.

Sisodiya SM, Heffernan J, Squier MV. Over-expression of P-glycoprotein in malformations of cortical development. Neuroreport. 1999;10:3437–41.

Su H, Sochivko D, Becker A, Chen J, Jiang Y, Yaari Y, et al. Upregulation of a T-type Ca^{2+} channel causes a long-lasting modification of neuronal firing mode after status epilepticus. J Neurosci. 2002;22:3645–55.

Temkin NR. Antiepileptogenesis and seizure prevention trials with antiepileptic drugs: meta-analysis of controlled trials. Epilepsia. 2001;42:515–24.

Tishler DM, Weinberg KI, Hinton DR, Barbaro N, Annett GM, Raffel C. MDR1 gene expression in brain of patients with medically intractable epilepsy. Epilepsia. 1995;36:1–6.

van Vliet EA, van Schaik R, Edelbroek PM, Redeker S, Aronica E, Wadman WJ, et al. Inhibition of the multidrug transporter P-glycoprotein improves seizure control in phenytoin-treated chronic epileptic rats. Epilepsia. 2006;47:672–80.

Vanoye C, Castro A, Pourcher T, Reuss L, Altenberg G. Phosphorylation of P-glycoprotein by PKA and PKC modulates swelling-activated Cl^- currents. Am J Physiol. 1999;276:C370–8.

Wadkins RM, Roepe PD. Biophysical aspect of P-glycoprotein mediated multidrug resistance. Int Rev Cytol. 1997;171:121–65.

Chapter 5
Modifications in the Seizures Susceptibility by Excitotoxic Neuronal Damage and Its Possible Relationship with the Pharmacoresistance

Monica E. Ureña-Guerrero, Alfredo I. Feria-Velasco, Graciela Gudiño-Cabrera, Antoni Camins Espuny, and Carlos Beas-Zárate

Abstract The neuronal damage and seizures are two processes closely related not only as cause and effect in reciprocal way but also through the cellular mechanisms and signaling pathways that they share. Therefore, increments in extracellular levels of the glutamate excitatory neurotransmitter, the over-activation of its receptors and the excessive neuronal excitation, have been described as events associated to both processes. In general, if neurons are not able to recover from its excessive excitation, then they die by excitotoxicity. Our group has showed that the excitotoxicity induced by monosodium glutamate in early developmental stages is able to produce significant modifications in glutamatergic and GABAergic neurotransmission systems. Moreover, preliminary results indicate that those modifications are able to increase the seizure susceptibility in the adulthood, particularly when the convulsive drug 4-aminopyridine and the GABA antagonists are employed to induce the seizures, but not when NMDA agonists are used. Through this chapter the topics mentioned above and the hypothesis about the excitotoxic neonatal damage is able to induce a kind of pharmacoresistance to NMDA analogs will be discussed with in detail.

Keywords Excitotoxicity • Monosodium glutamate • Seizures susceptibility • NMDA receptors • Pharmacoresistance

M.E. Ureña-Guerrero, Ph.D. (✉) • A.I. Feria-Velasco, Ph.D. • G. Gudiño-Cabrera, Ph.D. • C. Beas-Zárate, Ph.D.
Departamento de Biología Celular y Molecular, Centro Universitario de Ciencias Biológicas y Agropecuarias, Universidad de Guadalajara, Km. 15.5 Carretera-Guadalajara-Nogales, Predio Las Agujas, Zapopan, Jalisco 45110, Mexico
e-mail: murena@cucba.udg.mx; monica.urena.guerrero@gmail.com; aferia@cucba.udg.mx; alfredo.feria@redudg.udg.mx; ggudinoc@cucba.udg.mx; carlosbeas@cucba.udg.mx; carlosbeas55@gmail.com

A. Camins Espuny, Ph.D.
Department of Pharmacology and Biomedical Chemistry, University of Barcelona, Avenida Diagonal 643, Barcelona 08028, Spain
e-mail: camins@ub.edu

L. Rocha and E.A. Cavalheiro (eds.), *Pharmacoresistance in Epilepsy: From Genes and Molecules to Promising Therapies*, DOI 10.1007/978-1-4614-6464-8_5,

5.1 Introduction: The Relationship Between Excitotoxicity and Seizures Susceptibility Through Amino Acid Neurotransmitters

Although more than 50 substances have been described as neurotransmitters, 2 of them seem to be particularly important in all neuronal processes: glutamate and gamma-aminobutyric acid (GABA); both are amino acids highly concentrated into the brain, and they are also biochemically related one to each other, but in general, in the adulthood, they have opposite effects over neuronal activity (Deutch and Roth 2008; Kandel and Siegelbaum 2000; Hassel and Dingledine 2006; Olsen and Betz 2006). Glutamate is a dicarboxylic amino acid negatively charged at physiologic pH, synthetized by the enzyme known as phosphate-activated glutaminase (PAG), which hydrolyze the glutamine amine group in a phosphate-dependent manner, and it is considered as the major excitatory neurotransmitter in the nervous vertebrate system (Hassel and Dingledine 2006; Rowley et al. 2012). In contrast, the GABA is a neuter amino acid, synthetized by the glutamic acid decarboxylase enzyme (GAD) through alpha-decarboxylation of glutamate, and it is considered as the major inhibitory neurotransmitter in the mature mammalian nervous system (Olsen and Betz 2006; Rowley et al. 2012). Both glutamate and GABA are considered as classical neurotransmitters because the mechanisms involved in its synthesis, vesicular packing, release, postsynaptic receptor interaction, synaptic inactivation, and neuronal pathways have been clearly identified in the nervous system (Deutch and Roth 2008; Rowley et al. 2012). Interestingly, specific receptors for both amino acids coexist practically along the structures and regions of the nervous system and during all developmental stages (Aronica et al. 2011; Ben-Ari 2001; Manent and Represa 2007). However, in early developmental stages when neurons have not established synaptic definitive contact, GABA induces neuronal excitation and has trophic functions through its interaction with extrasynaptic receptors (Ben-Ari 2001; Ben-Ari et al. 2007; Jensen 2009).

According the essential roles for GABA and glutamate, it is evident that whatever significant alteration in the dynamic balance between these two neurotransmitters could lead to some pathological conditions (Martisova et al. 2012; Rowley et al. 2012). Thus, several experimental and clinical evidences have confirmed the hypothesis that an excess of neuronal excitation mediated by glutamate or a deficiency in the neuronal inhibition mediated by GABA in the adulthood could increase the seizures susceptibility, which in some cases may be related to epilepsy (Mares and Kubová 2008; Rowley et al. 2012; Werner and Coveñas 2011). In general, increments in extracellular cerebral levels of glutamate or reduced concentrations of GABA have been associated with the seizures (Morales-Villagran and Tapia 1996; Tapia et al. 1999; Wilson et al. 1996), which may further be induced by glutamate agonists (Kohl and Dannhardt 2001; Vincent and Mulle 2009) and controlled by its respective antagonists (Kohl and Dannhardt 2001; Morales-Villagran et al. 1996). On the contrary, reductions in GABA release have been related to the seizures (Treiman 2001; Wilson et al. 1996), which are able to be promoted or diminished by GABAergic antagonists

(Löscher 2011; Sperk et al. 2004) and agonists (Biagini et al. 2010; Tolman and Faulkner 2009), respectively. In addition, several alterations in the glutamatergic and GABAergic neurotransmissions also seem to be linked to the seizure activity (Mares and Kubová 2008; Rowley et al. 2012; Treiman 2001; Werner and Coveñas 2011). In this point, it is important to clarify that although GABA and glutamate roles are essentials for the seizures expression, other neurotransmitters and neuromodulators also have relevant implications (Biagini et al. 2010; Manent and Represa 2007; Mares and Kubová 2008; Werner and Coveñas 2011); in particular if the seizures are associated with epilepsy, which is probably one of the more complex neurological syndrome. Furthermore, since neuronal excitation mediated by GABA seems to be a triggering condition for neonatal seizures, recently it has emerged the hypothesis that the immaturity on GABAergic signaling producing neuronal excitation may be a determinant condition for the seizure activity and epilepsies in other developmental stages (Ben-Ari et al. 2007; Briggs and Galanopoulou 2011; Jensen 2009).

On other hand, an excessive neuronal excitation mediated by amino acids leads to neuronal death, through a process known as excitotoxicity (Babot et al. 2005; Dodd 2002; Dong et al. 2009; Zhao et al. 2011). Thus, if during the seizure activity the extracellular levels of glutamate and GABA increase producing neuronal excitation, then the neurons may die by excitotoxicity as a consequence of the seizures (Chen et al. 2010; Fujikawa 2005; Niquet et al. 2012; Vincent and Mulle 2009). Furthermore, the neuronal loss by whatever degenerative process in specific areas of the brain may induce seizures (Chen et al. 2010; Fujikawa 2005; Niquet et al. 2012; Vincent and Mulle 2009). Then, the relationship between seizures and excitotoxicity is very close, reciprocal and essential to regulate both neuronal death and seizures.

5.2 Glutamate-Mediated Excitotoxicity and Neuronal Death in Neurological Illness

The "excitotoxicity" term was coined by J. W. Olney to refer the neuronal death produced by over-activation of sensitive receptors to glutamate (Olney et al. 1971). This kind of death was observed for the first time, during the experimental application of monosodium glutamate (MSG) in high concentrations to treat the retinal atrophy increasing the neuronal excitation (Lucas and Newhouse 1957; Olney 1971; Garattini 1979). Subsequently, the glutamate-mediated excitotoxicity was also related with the over-expression of glutamate receptors (Mishra et al. 2001). Now the term is applied to the neuronal death produced by a neuronal sustained excitation, triggered by an over-activation of the glutamate receptors or by other mechanisms, in which, the GABA receptors over-activation may be implicated, particularly when its immediate effect is the neuronal excitation (Nuñez et al. 2003; Zhao et al. 2011). However, the excitotoxicity triggered by glutamate is the best process known, and it has been broadly associated with the neuronal death observed in several neuropathological conditions (Lipton and Rosenberg 1994; Caudle and Zhang 2009; Dong et al. 2009; Wang and Qin 2010).

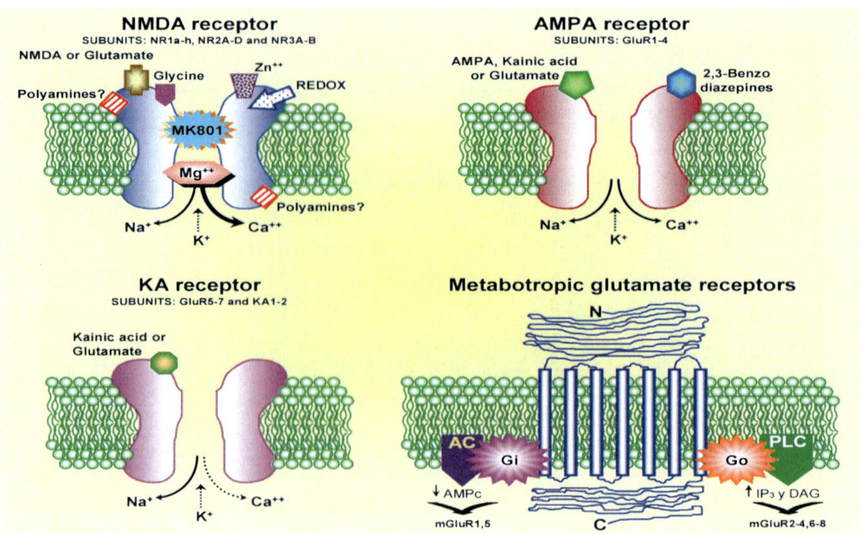

Fig. 5.1 Pharmacological binding sites, conformational subunits, and responses of the glutamate receptors showed schematically. The intensity or continuity of *arrows* is associated with the amplitude of the ionic currents triggered though each ionotropic glutamate receptors when are activated for its particular agonists. In the metabotropic glutamate receptors, different intracellular messengers are activated for each subtype. G_i inhibitory G-protein, *AC* adenylate cyclase, and G_o G-protein that activating to the PLC (phospholipase C)

5.2.1 Glutamate Receptors

The excitatory glutamate effects depend on its specific interaction with cell membrane receptors, functionally classified as ionotropic and metabotropic glutamate receptors, which act as ligand-gated ion channels or as G protein-coupled receptors, respectively (Hassel and Dingledine 2006). In general, the ionotropic glutamate receptors mediate the neuronal fast depolarization allowing the Na^+ and Ca^{2+} influx and the K^+ efflux, through the same ionic pore; and they are classified according their affinity to specific exogenous agonist in sensitive receptors to *N*-methyl-D-aspartate (NMDA-R), alpha-amino-3-hydroxy-5-methyl-4-isoxazolepropionic acid (AMPA-R), and kainic acid (KA-R) (Kohl and Dannhardt 2001; Simeone et al. 2004; Vincent and Mulle 2009; Watkins and Olverman 1987) (Fig. 5.1). Structurally, they are oligomeric macromolecular complexes formed by four polypeptidic subunits, each of which contain an amino-terminal extracellular domain, followed by a transmembrane domain (TM1), a loop partially embedded in the membrane cytosolic face (TM2), other two transmembrane domains (TM3–4) and the carboxy-terminal intracellular domain (Simeone et al. 2004; Vandenberghe and Bredt 2004). The glutamate interacts specifically in the neighborhood between the amino-terminal loop and the extracellular spacer loop of TM3 and TM4 (Wollmuth and Sobolevsky 2004) (Fig. 5.2). For each kind of ionotropic glutamate receptors, there

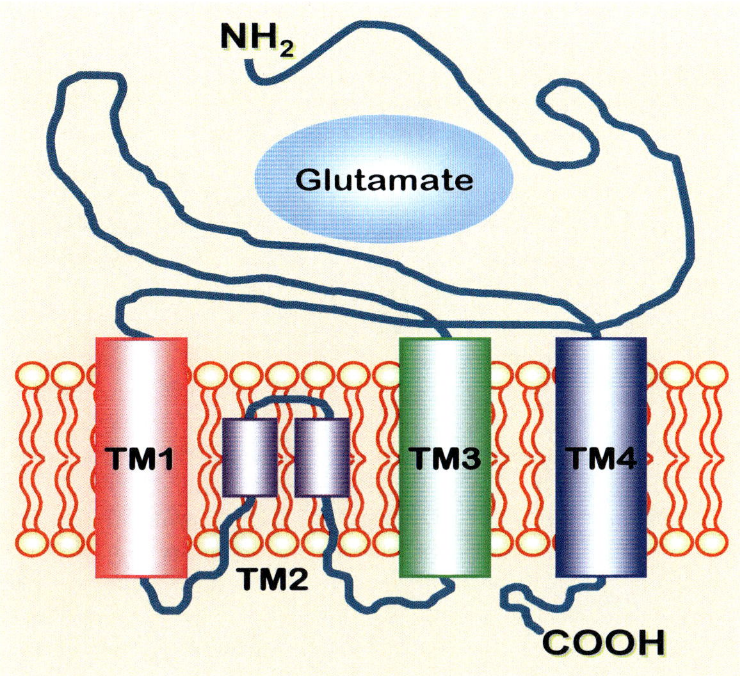

Fig. 5.2 Conformational distribution of transmembrane domains and extracellular and intracellular loops of ionotropic glutamate receptors subunits showed schematically. The extracellular loops build the binding site for glutamate, which may be exchanged by the glutamate agonist analogs in non-NMDA-R and by glycine in the NR1 and NR3 subunits of NMDA-R

are several subunits that differentially associated may originate receptors with diverse pharmacological and electrophysiological properties, but activated for the same endogenous ligand, the glutamate (Holopainen and Laurén 2012; Simeone et al. 2004; Wollmuth and Sobolevsky 2004).

The NMDA-R is characterized by its voltage dependency and high permeability to Ca^{2+}, which according its subunit composition it could be slowly or rapidly inactivated (Popescu and Auerbach 2003; Simeone et al. 2004). It possesses multiple pharmacological sites of regulation, described as binding sites to (1) the glutamate transmitter, its competitive agonists and antagonists; (2) the glycine as coagonist; (3) the phencyclidine and dizocilpine (MK801) as the channel blockers; (4) the Mg^{2+} as the channel blocker removable by depolarization; (5) the Zn^{2+} as positive modulator; (6) the polyamines as positive or negative modulator, depending on the compound and their concentration; and (7) a site sensitive to redox changes (Holopainen and Laurén 2012; Popescu and Auerbach 2003; Simeone et al. 2004; Wollmuth and Sobolevsky 2004). Structurally, this receptor is defined as heterotetramer conformed by combination of NR1 subunit (present in eight variants of editing) with NR2A-D or NR3A-B subunits, where the presence of NR1 determines the existence of a functional ion channel, while NR2A-D and NR3A-B modify the electrophysiological properties of the channel (Holopainen and Laurén 2012; Popescu and Auerbach 2003; Simeone et al. 2004) (Fig. 5.1).

Non-NMDA receptors (AMPA-R and KA-R) do not have voltage dependence and are highly permeable to Na^+, and its response is faster than that of the NMDA-R, but both kinds of receptors coexist in the most of postsynaptic membranes (Holopainen and Laurén 2012). The AMPA-R also recognizes kainic acid but with low affinity in comparison to that of KA-R. It is conformed as homomeric or heteromeric tetramer from the GluR1-4 subunits, which through variations in the editing of Q/R site or during alternative splicing of their messenger RNA could change the selectivity for the ligand and the permeability of the channel, not only in its kinetic properties also allowing the predominant entry of Ca^{2+} (Bettler and Mulle 1995; Simeone et al. 2004; Vandenberghe and Bredt 2004; Vincent and Mulle 2009). Besides, homomeric and heteromeric tetramers of GluR5-7 with KA1-2 proteins build the KA-R, which show a high affinity by kainic acid being predominantly permeable at Na^+ (Bettler and Mulle 1995; Vincent and Mulle 2009) (Fig. 5.1).

On the other hand, metabotropic glutamate receptors (mGlu-R) exist in dimeric associations, where each polypeptide contain seven helical segments that wrap back and forth through the membrane, with the extracellular amino-terminal and the intracellular carboxyl-terminal domains unusually large in comparison with other metabotropic receptors (Holopainen and Laurén 2012; Kunishima et al. 2000; Simeone et al. 2004). Eight different mGlu-R identified in the nervous system have been subdivided into three groups, according to its sequences homologies and its enzymatic coupling. mGlu-R1 and mGlu-R5 of group I, activate a G-protein coupled to phospholipase C activation and IP3 and DAG generation, whereas mGluR2–3 of group II and mGluR4,6–8 of group III inhibit the production of cAMP by inhibitory G-protein activation (Holopainen and Laurén 2012; Kunishima et al. 2000). mGlu-R of the groups I and II have extrasynaptic location, whereas group III are predominantly presynaptic and it is generally accepted that the group I increases the neuronal excitability through inhibition of several K^+ channels, whereas those of groups II and III decrease the release of neurotransmitters such as GABA and Glu (Holopainen and Laurén 2012; Kunishima et al. 2000; Simeone et al. 2004) (Fig. 5.1).

To close this section, it should be pointed out that the synaptic effects mediated by glutamate may be also endogenously exerted by aspartate, another dicarboxylic nonessential amino acid, virtually ubiquitous in the human body, but highly concentrated in the brain, and generated as intermediary metabolite or as neurotransmitter in different metabolic pools (Deutch and Roth 2008; Hassel and Dingledine 2006; Kandel and Siegelbaum 2000).

5.2.2 *Mechanisms Implicated in the Neuronal Death Produced by Glutamate*

Glutamate receptors depolarize the membrane through ionic movements, but when the process is sustained then the osmotic imbalance caused by the massive entry of

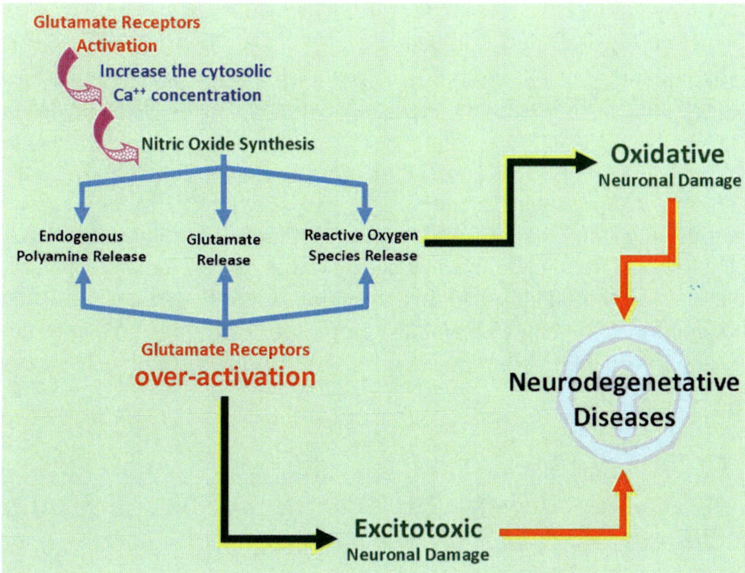

Fig. 5.3 Flow of events that leading to glutamate-receptors over-activation may induce the neuronal damage associated to excitotoxic and oxidative process related to some neurodegenerative disease

Na^+ and Cl^- is followed by an excessive increment in the cytoplasmic Ca^{2+} concentration (Caudle and Zhang 2009; Dong et al. 2009). The Na^+ influx alters the functionality of cotransporters, pumps, and ion channels depending of its electrochemical gradient (Dong et al. 2009; Greene and Greenamyre 1996; Morrison et al. 2012). The influx of Cl^- alters several plasmatic transporters and promotes the glutamate release and then, the over-activation of its receptors potentiates the excitotoxicity (Babot et al. 2005; Zhao et al. 2011). In this conditions, the excessive elevation of the cytoplasmic Ca^{2+} concentration could promote (1) the synthesis of nitric oxide, which could reach to presynaptic glutamatergic terminal to stimulate the additional release of glutamate, through a cGMP-dependent mechanism; (2) the generation of free radicals, as superoxide or peroxynitrites, which promote lipidic peroxidation and destabilization of cell membranes; and (3) the loss of electrochemical mitochondrial potential, altering the oxidative phosphorylation and promoting the free radicals generation until complete invalidation of the mitochondrial metabolism, which could lead to the ending of the energy cellular reserves. Furthermore, the rising in Ca^{2+} cytoplasmic concentration activates various intracellular signaling pathways dependent on protein kinases and phosphatases that could promote proteolysis of the cellular content (Greene and Greenamyre 1996; Arundine and Tymianski 2003; Dong et al. 2009; for more details review Chap. 6) (Fig. 5.3).

The glutamate-mediated excitotoxicity as a continuum process may be too sharp in its initial phase triggering a neuronal death by necrosis, and also it may evolve more slowly producing apoptosis. In this respect, in vitro studies have shown that glutamate may produce the two kinds of death depending on its application scheme (Bonfoco et al. 1995; Portera-Cailliau et al. 1997a, b). Then, a brief exposition at elevated glutamate concentrations could produce the acute neuronal death through degenerative changes immediately associated to an inflammatory tissular process which is characterized by being a Na^+- and Cl^--dependent process. Prolonged exposure to minor glutamate extracellular concentrations could produce delayed neuronal death, which depends on the influx of Ca^{2+} and requires several hours to occur (Bonfoco et al. 1995; Portera-Cailliau et al. 1997a, b). Furthermore, it has been suggested that the glutamate-mediated degenerative process largely depends on the functional mitochondrial state and that when the metabolic cellular rate is reduced, the mitochondria are unable to maintain homeostasis of Ca^{2+} and thus, the neuronal death by apoptosis could occur (Bonfoco et al. 1995; Portera-Cailliau et al. 1997a, b; Niizuma et al. 2010).

5.2.3 Glutamate-Mediated Excitotoxicity and Neurological Illness

Studies carried out in different neural systems, both in vivo and in vitro, about excitotoxic degeneration mediated by glutamate, have demonstrated that in pathological conditions, such as cerebral hypoxia-ischemia (Choi and Rothman 1990), cranial trauma (Bramlett and Dietrich 2004; Wagner et al. 2005), epilepsy (Meldrum 1993a; Friedman et al. 2003; Wilson et al. 1996), and domoic acid poisoning (Meldrum 1993b; Jeffery et al. 2004), the extracellular concentration of glutamate is significantly elevated into the brain, and that the increment is faithfully related with the observed neuronal illnesses. Furthermore, it has been proposed that excitotoxicity participates in the establishment of several neurodegenerative diseases such as Huntington's (Beal et al. 1991; Gardian and Vecsei 2004), Alzheimer's (Ferrarese et al. 2000; Hynd et al. 2004), and Parkinson's diseases (Lipton and Rosenberg 1994; Rego and Oliveira 2003), as well as in schizophrenia (Lipton and Rosenberg 1994), among others degenerative processes. In this regard, experimental trials have shown that glutamate antagonists could protect against neuronal excitotoxic damage, diminishing the neurodegenerative process and also they could control the seizures (Meldrum 1985; Morales-Villagran et al. 1996). In the clinic, this knowledge has been applied with some successes, for example the memantine, one of the therapeutic agents used recently for Alzheimer's disease, acting as NMDA antagonist seems to able to damp the degenerative progression (Moreira et al. 2006; Supnet and Bezprozvanny 2010). Other example is the use of dizocilpine, an ion channel blocker for NMDA-R, that when is applied in combination with nimodipine, in acute excitotoxic neuronal damage generated by a hypoxic-ischemic event seem to decrease the penumbra area, but their neuroprotective effect is variable (Niizuma et al. 2010; Szydlowska and Tymianski 2010).

5.3 Systemic Administration of Monosodium Glutamate as Excitotoxicity Model

Although several glutamate analogs that act as agonists over its receptors have been used to resemble the excitotoxic neuronal damage, the systemic administration of MSG is probably the best election to study the neurodegenerative process induced by glutamate in an integrative way, where all kinds of glutamatergic receptors on all cellular types from the nervous system, are participating in the induction and developing of the process. Further, through this model it is possible to characterize in a temporal way the alterations and adaptive neurophysiological responses induced after the excitotoxic insult. Thus, through the MSG systemically administered it was established that the majority of mammalian species are susceptible to the toxic effects of the glutamate and that the severity of the injury depends on the specie, age, and sex (Garattini 1979). Besides, it is now known that the maximum susceptibility to the glutamate-mediated excitotoxicity is observed in (1) mammalian male neonates in comparison to the adults, females, and other vertebrates (Garattini 1979); (2) in cerebral regions where glutamate receptors density is high such as hippocampus (Meldrum 1993b; Beas-Zarate et al. 2002a; Kim et al. 2009), among others; and (3) in neural and nonneural cells that are expressing glutamate receptors, such as GABA neurons (Reeves et al. 1987; Muller et al. 2001; Ureña-Guerrero et al. 2009) and microglial cells (Brown and Neher 2010), among others.

The immaturity of the blood–brain barrier (Xu and Ling 1994; Ek et al. 2006), the deficient reuptake of glutamate (Thomas et al. 2011), the long amplitude and duration of calcium currents activated by NMDA and voltage (Ben-Ari 2001; Dehorter et al. 2012; Jensen 2009), and the GABA-mediated excitability (Ben-Ari et al. 2007; Dehorter et al. 2012; Nuñez et al. 2003) are some of the conditions associated with the high susceptibility to glutamate-mediated excitotoxicity characteristically observed in newborns. However, MSG systemically administered is also able to induce damage in the adult stage, particularly in the brain areas where the blood–brain barrier is inefficient, such as the arcuate nucleus and other hypothalamic nuclei (Garattini 1979; Hu et al. 1998). Additionally, also it is known that glutamate-mediated excitotoxicity could be associated with seizures (Arauz-Contreras and Feria-Velasco 1984; Lipton and Rosenberg 1994; López-Pérez et al. 2010), obesity (Garattini 1979; Hu et al. 1998; Donaldson et al. 2009), learning deficiencies (Ishikawa et al. 1997; Velázquez-Zamora et al. 2011), and motor impairment (Möykkynen and Korpi 2012), with the males being more susceptible than females, probably due to the neuroprotective effect exerted by steroids (Luoma et al. 2011).

5.3.1 Some Effects Observed After the MSG Systemically Administered to Neonate Rats

In accordance with the above-mentioned points, the MSG systemically administered to newborn male rats induces severe neuronal damage, which could be characterized immediately and later, when the plastic responses have been established to generate more or less permanent changes. Thus, between the immediate changes, Hu et al. (1998) showed that subcutaneously administered MSG at dose of 0.2 mg/g body weight (b.w.) at postnatal day (PD) seven in male mice, produced an elevation of plasma glutamate levels in 17-fold above baseline, which was associated with increments in the expression level of NR1 and GluR2/4 subunits, and minor but significant injury in subependymal neurons near the base of the third ventricle. More recently, it was demonstrated through an enzymatic biosensor stereotaxically implanted in the lateral ventricle that MSG administered subcutaneously at dose of 4 mg/g b.w. at PD1 in male rats, increased glutamate extracellular cerebral levels, reaching mean values between 300 % above of the basal level during the 90 min after injection. Increments in the glutamate extracellular cerebral levels were higher when the same dose of MSG was administrated again at PD3 and PD5, but the increments were not observed at PD7 immediately after the fourth dose of MSG administration. Interestingly, changes in glutamate extracellular cerebral levels were associated to electrographic and behavioral epileptiform activities, as well as increments in the total hippocampal content of glutamate, glutamine, and GABA at 20 h after each MSG administration (López-Pérez et al. 2010). Additionally, using the last described administration scheme, where MSG is subcutaneously administered at doses of 4 mg/g b.w. at PD1, 3, 5, and 7, the neuronal death by apoptosis was observed in CA1 and CA3 hippocampal regions, as well as in the cerebral cortex, 24 h after the last administration (Chaparro-Huerta et al. 2002, 2005; Rivera-Cervantes et al. 2004, 2009). This neuronal loss was also associated with changes in the expression level of NMDA-R and AMPA-R subunits (Rivera-Cervantes et al. 2004, 2009) and with the increment in p38 kinase protein and in TNF-α proinflammatory cytokine (Chaparro-Huerta et al. 2002, 2005; Rivera-Cervantes et al. 2004, 2009).

On the other hand, after the MSG neonatal treatment, the loss of pyramidal neurons (Gonzalez-Burgos et al. 2001; Beas-Zarate et al. 2002a; Velázquez-Zamora et al. 2011) and GABAergic (Ureña-Guerrero et al. 2009) and dopaminergic (López-Pérez et al. 2005) positive cells has been observed in different brain regions of adult rats. This neuronal loss is also associated to the changes in the expression level of the non- and NMDA-R subunits (Beas-Zarate et al. 2001, 2002b, 2007), and of the glutamate transporters (Medina-Ceja et al. 2012); in the binding sites to acetylcholine, and in choline acetyl transferase activity (Ortuño-Sahagún et al. 1997); as well as in dopamine receptors and transporters (López-Pérez et al. 2005); and in the [^{3}H]-GABA release (Beas-Zárate et al. 1998), in glutamic acid decarboxylase activity (Ureña-Guerrero et al. 2003) and in others GABAergic markers (Ureña-Guerrero et al. 2009), all of them observed in different brain regions and ages after treatment until adulthood. Furthermore, the MSG neonatal treatment induces hyperplasia and hypertrophy on astrocytes and microglial cells in the cerebral cortex and hippocampus of adult rats (Martinez-Contreras et al. 2002). Additionally, it is important to do mention, that MSG neonatal treatment produces significant changes in the seizures susceptibility (Ureña-Guerrero and Beas-Zarate 2006), as well as in learning capacity (Gonzalez-Burgos et al. 2001; Velázquez-Zamora et al. 2011), both of which are closely related with the modifications described above.

5.4 Changes in Adulthood Seizure Susceptibility After MSG Neonatal Treatment and Its Possible Relationship with the Pharmacoresistance

When we observed that adult rats neonatally treated with MSG developed an unusual wild running behavior after simple manipulations as cage exchange, and according the significant changes induced on both GABAergic and glutamatergic neurotransmission systems, then we decided to characterize the seizures susceptibility in the adulthood, using several experimental models to induce convulsions, such as (a) 4-aminopyridine as generic convulsive drug acting as blocker of voltage-sensitive potassium channels; (b) iodide-methyl-bicuculline as GABA antagonist; and (c) NMDA as glutamate agonist were evaluated, all of them administered intracerebrally into the lateral ventricle in conscious rats (Ureña-Guerrero and Beas-Zarate 2006). Except to NMDA, all convulsive drugs induced more severe convulsive symptoms in MSG-treated group than in the control group. Moreover, the seizure latency was shorter and the seizures duration was longer in MSG-treated group than in control group (Ureña-Guerrero and Beas-Zarate 2006) (Table 5.1). Intracerebroventricular administration of NMDA (10 nmol) in MSG-treated group produced sudden and intense jumps and tremors, as well as facial and forelimb clonus, but the motor behavioral alterations disappeared during the first 15 min and did not generate any epileptiform discharge in the hippocampus of adult rats, while in the control group behavioral and electrographically the NMDA injection-induced generalized tonic-clonic convulsions, *status epilepticus* and death (Ureña-Guerrero and Beas-Zarate 2006) (Table 5.1). Then, the evidences suggest that after MSG neonatal treatment

Table 5.1 Minimal dose of some convulsive drugs necessary to induce severe convulsive signs in the adulthood after MSG neonatal treatment

	Convulsive drugs (doses)					
	4-Aminopyridine (1, 2, 3, 4, and 5 nmol)		Iodide-methyl bicuculline (0.25, 0.5, 1, 1.5, and 2 nmol)		*N*-Methyl-D-Aspartate (2.5, 5, 7.5, and 10 nmol)	
	Control	MSG-treated	Control	MSG -treated	Control	MSG-treated
Severe convulsive signs						
Wild running	3.0	1.0	1.5	0.5	–	–
Rearing	2.0	1.0	1.0	0.25	5.0	–
Generalized tonic-clonic convulsions	4.0	2.0	2.0	1.0	5.0	–
Status epilepticus establishment	4.0	2.0	–	1.0	7.5	–
Animal death (%)[a]	4.0 (25 %)	2.0 (80 %)	–	1.5 (37.5 %)	10 (50 %)	–

Data indicate the dose in which each severe convulsive sign was observed in each experimental group, such as indicated between the parentheses associated to each convulsive drug

[a]Animal death percentage was estimated from eight animals for each group, convulsive drug and doses

some adaptive changes at the level of NMDA receptors could generate some kind of resistance to NMDA agonists, which remains to clarify. In this sense, it is important to mention that when the MSG neonatal treatment is administered to male rats, the NMDA-R are more numerous than the non-NMDA-R (Simeone et al. 2004; Holopainen and Laurén 2012), particularly in the cerebral cortex and the hippocampus, where any electrographic epileptiform discharges were recorded after intracerebral NMDA administration in adult rats treated with MSG. Furthermore, several experimental evidences have demonstrated that NMDA-R activation could lead to its structural and functional modification resembling some kind of "habituation ligand-receptor" or "preconditioning", where the NMDA-R does not became responsive to NMDA (Boeck et al. 2004; Severino et al. 2011). Then, the MSG neonatal treatment could induce a pronounced preconditioning that is remaining until the adulthood and that probably is conditioning that NMDA intracerebroventricular administration may not induce the epileptiform activity observed in control rats (Ureña-Guerrero and Beas-Zarate 2006). In this sense, the NMDA-R functional modifications have been also suggested in the studies where the learning impairment has been reported after the MSG neonatal treatment (Gonzalez-Burgos et al. 2001; Velázquez-Zamora et al. 2011). Although the pharmacoresistance in epilepsy have been more related to changes in the expression levels of voltage-gated sodium and calcium channels, $GABA_A$ receptor subunits, and efflux transporters (Remy and Beck 2006), it is possible that MSG neonatal treatment may induce some kind of pharmacoresistance, specially for anticonvulsive drugs acting on NMDA-R, such as felbamate (Harty and Rogawski 2000) and lamotrigine (Wang et al. 1996). In this sense, it has been reported that a short preconditioning with NMDA is able to diminish the anticonvulsive efficacy of lamotrigine, without a significant effect on felbamate (Tomczyk et al. 2007).

On other hand, preliminary results obtained for our group suggest that MSG neonatal treatment also induces changes on non-NMDA and GABA receptors, which also be determinant for both augmented seizures susceptibility and NMDA pharmaresistance described above (Lasoń et al. 2011). Then, the modifications induced after MSG neonatal treatment on glutamate and GABA receptors remain to be characterized, particularly its association with the pharmacoresistance.

5.5 Concluding Remarks and Perspectives

Since MSG neonatal treatment resemble the increments in glutamate extracellular levels observed in neonatal illnesses, such as the hypoxic-ischemic and anoxic episodes, as well as cranial trauma, seizures, and other neurodegenerative diseases, then the broad characterization of long time effects induced on glutamatergic and GABAergic neurotransmission systems result important to better understand the mechanisms associated to the seizures susceptibility exacerbation and the pharmacoresistance observed in the humans after the excitotoxic damage. In particular, it is important to considerate the better pharmacological and electrophysiological characterization of glutamate and GABA receptors after the MSG neonatal treatment, since both kinds of receptors have been broadly implicated in the seizures susceptibility and the excitotoxicity as well as in the pharmacoresistance in epilepsy.

References

Arauz-Contreras J, Feria-Velasco A. Monosodium-L-glutamate-induced convulsions–I. Differences in seizure pattern and duration of effect as a function of age in rats. Gen Pharmacol. 1984;15:391–5.

Aronica E, Iyer A, Zurolo E, Gorter JA. Ontogenetic modifications of neuronal excitability during brain maturation: developmental changes of neurotransmitter receptors. Epilepsia. 2011;52 Suppl 8:3–5.

Arundine M, Tymianski M. Molecular mechanisms of calcium-dependent neurodegeneration in excitotoxicity. Cell Calcium. 2003;34:325–37.

Babot Z, Cristofol R, Suñol C. Excitotoxic death induced by releases glutamate in depolarised primary cultures of mouse cerebellar granule cells is dependent on GABAA receptors and ninflumic acid sensitive chloride channels. Eur J Neurosci. 2005;21:103–12.

Beal MF, Ferrante RJ, Swartz KJ, Kowall NW. Chronic quinolenic acid lesions in rats closely resemble Huntington's disease. J Neurosci. 1991;13:4181–92.

Beas-Zárate C, Sánchez-Ruíz MY, Ureña-Guerrero ME, Feria-Velasco A. Effect of neonatal exposure to monosodium L-glutamate on regional GABA release during postnatal development. Neurochem Int. 1998;33:217–32.

Beas-Zarate C, Rivera-Huizar SV, Martinez-Contreras A, Feria-Velasco A, Armendariz-Borunda J. Changes in NMDA-receptor gene expression are associated with neurotoxicity induced neonatally by glutamate in the rat brain. Neurochem Int. 2001;39:1–10.

Beas-Zarate C, Pérez-Vega M, González-Burgos I. Neonatal exposure to monosodium L-glutamate induces loss of neurons and cytoarchitectural alterations in hippocampal CA1 pyramidal neurons of adult rats. Brain Res. 2002a;952:275–81.

Beas-Zarate C, Flores-Soto ME, Armendariz-Borunda J. NMDAR-2C and 2D subunits gene expression is induced in brain by neonatal exposure of monosodium L-glutamate to adult rats. Neurosci Lett. 2002b;321:9–12.

Beas-Zarate C, Ureña-Guerrero ME, Flores-Soto M, Armendariz-Borunda J, Ortuño-Sahagún D. The expression and binding of kainate receptors is modified in different brain regions by glutamate neurotoxicity during postnatal rat development. Int J Dev Neurosci. 2007;25:53–61.

Ben-Ari Y. Developing networks play a similar melody. Trends Neurosci. 2001;24:353–60.

Ben-Ari Y, Gaiarsa JL, Tyzio R, Khazipov R. GABA: a pioneer transmitter that excites immature neurons and generates primitive oscillations. Physiol Rev. 2007;87:1215–84.

Bettler B, Mulle C. Review: neurotransmitter receptors II. AMPA and kainate receptors. Neuropharmacology. 1995;34:123–39.

Biagini G, Panuccio G, Avoli M. Neurosteroids and epilepsy. Curr Opin Neurol. 2010;23:170–6.

Boeck CR, Ganzella M, Lottermann A, Vendite D. NMDA preconditioning protects against seizures and hippocampal neurotoxicity induced by quinolinic acid in mice. Epilepsia. 2004;45:745–50.

Bonfoco E, Krainc D, Ankarcrona M, Nicotera P, Lipton SA. Apoptosis and necrosis: two distinct events induced, respectively, by mild and intense insults with N-methyl-D-aspartate or nitric oxide/superoxide in cortical cell cultures. Proc Natl Acad Sci U S A. 1995;92:7152–66.

Bramlett HM, Dietrich WD. Pathophysiology of cerebral ischemia and brain trauma: similarities and differences. J Cereb Blood Flow Metab. 2004;24:133–50.

Briggs SW, Galanopoulou AS. Altered GABA signaling in early life epilepsies. Neural Plast. 2011;2011:527–605.

Brown GC, Neher JJ. Inflammatory neurodegeneration and mechanisms of microglial killing of neurons. Mol Neurobiol. 2010;41:242–7.
Caudle WM, Zhang J. Glutamate, excitotoxicity, and programmed cell death in Parkinson disease. Exp Neurol. 2009;220(2):230–3.
Chaparro-Huerta V, Rivera-Cervantes M, Torres-Mendoza BM, Beas-Zarate C. Neuronal death and tumor necrosis factor-α response to glutamate induced excitotoxicity in the cerebral cortex of neonatal rats. Neurosci Lett. 2002;333:95–8.
Chaparro-Huerta V, Rivera-Cervantes MC, Flores-Soto ME, Gómez-Pinedo U, Beas-Zárate C. Proinflammatory cytokines and apoptosis following glutamate-induced excitotoxicity mediated by p38 MAPK in the hippocampus of neonatal rats. J Neuroimmunol. 2005;165:53–62.
Chen SD, Chang AY, Chuang YC. The potential role of mitochondrial dysfunction in seizure-associated cell death in the hippocampus and epileptogenesis. J Bioenerg Biomembr. 2010;42(6):461–5.
Choi CW, Rothman SM. The role of glutamate neurotoxicity in hypoxic-ischemic neuronal death. Annu Rev Neurosci. 1990;13:171–82.
Dehorter N, Vinay L, Hammond C, Ben-Ari Y. Timing of developmental sequences in different brain structures: physiological and pathological implications. Eur J Neurosci. 2012;35(12):1846–56.
Deutch AY, Roth RH. Neurotransmitters. In: Squire LR, Bloom F, Spitzer NC, du Lac S, Ghosh A, Berg D, editors. Fundamental neuroscience. 3rd ed. Boston: Elsevier Academic; 2008.
Dodd PR. Excited to death: different ways to lose your neurones. Biogerontology. 2002;3:51–6.
Donaldson LF, Bennett L, Baic S, Melichar JK. Taste and weight: is there a link? Am J Clin Nutr. 2009;90(3):800S–803S.
Dong XX, Wang Y, Qin ZH. Molecular mechanisms of excitotoxicity and their relevance to pathogenesis of neurodegenerative diseases. Acta Pharmacol Sin. 2009;30:379–87.
Ek CJ, Dziegielewska K, Stolp H, Ruthven N. Functional effectiveness of the blood–brain barrier to small water soluble molecules in developing and adult opossum (Monodelphis domestica). J Comp Neurol. 2006;496:13–26.
Ferrarese C, Begni B, Canevari C, Zoia C, Piolti R, Frigo M, et al. Glutamate uptake is decreased in platelets from Alzheimer's disease patients. Ann Neurol. 2000;47:641–3.
Friedman LK, Velísková J, Kaur J, Magrys BW, Liu H. GluR2(B) knockdown accelerates CA3 injury after kainate seizures. J Neuropathol Exp Neurol. 2003;62:733–50.
Fujikawa DG. Prolonged seizures and cellular injury: understanding the connection. Epilepsy Behav. 2005;7 Suppl 3:S3–11.
Garattini S. Evaluation of the neurotoxic effects of glutamic acid. In: Wurtman RJ, Wurtman JJ, editors. Nutrition and the brain, vol. 4. New York: Raven; 1979.
Gardian G, Vecsei L. Huntington's disease: pathomechanism and therapeutic perspectives. J Neural Transm. 2004;111:1485–94.
Gonzalez-Burgos I, Perez-Vega MI, Beas-Zarate C. Neonatal exposure to monosodium glutamate induces cell death and dendritic hypotrophy in rat prefrontocortical pyramidal neurons. Neurosci Lett. 2001;297:69–72.
Greene JG, Greenamyre JT. Bioenergetics and glutamate excitotoxicity. Prog Neurobiol. 1996;48:61–634.
Harty TP, Rogawski MA. Felbamate block of recombinant N-methyl-D-aspartate receptors: selectivity for the NR2B subunit. Epilepsy Res. 2000;39(1):47–55.
Hassel B, Dingledine R. Glutamate. In: Siegel GJ, Albers RW, Brady SP, Price DL, editors. Basic neurochemistry, molecular, cellular, and medical aspects. 7th ed. San Diego: Elsevier Academic; 2006.
Holopainen IE, Laurén HB. Glutamate signaling in the pathophysiology and therapy of prenatal insults. Pharmacol Biochem Behav. 2012;100:825–34.
Hu L, Fernstrom JD, Goldsmith PC. Exogenous glutamate enhances glutamate receptor subunit expression during selective neuronal injury in the ventral arcuate nucleus of postnatal mice. Neuroendocrinology. 1998;68:77–88.

Hynd MR, Scott HL, Dodd PR. Glutamate-mediated excitotoxicity and neurodegeneration in Alzheimer's disease. Neurochem Int. 2004;45:583–95.
Ishikawa K, Kubo T, Shibanoki S, Matsumoto A, Hata H, Asai S. Hippocampal degeneration inducing impairment of learning in rats: model of dementia? Behav Brain Res. 1997;83:39–44.
Jeffery B, Barlow T, Moizer K, Paul S, Boyle C. Amnesic shellfish poison. Food Chem Toxicol. 2004;42:545–57.
Jensen FE. Neonatal seizures: an update on mechanisms and management. Clin Perinatol. 2009;36:881–900.
Kandel ER, Siegelbaum SA. Synaptic integration. In: Kande ER, Schwartz JH, Jesell TM, editors. Principles of neuronal science. 4th ed. New York: Mc Graw-Hill; 2000.
Kim YS, Chang HK, Lee JW, Sung YH, Kim SE, Shin MS, et al. Protective effect of gabapentin on N-methyl-D-aspartate-induced excitotoxicity in rat hippocampal CA1 neurons. J Pharmacol Sci. 2009;109(1):144–7.
Kohl BK, Dannhardt G. The NMDA receptor complex: a promising target for novel antiepileptic strategies. Curr Med Chem. 2001;8:1275–89.
Kunishima N, Shimada Y, Tsuji Y, Sato T, Yamamoto M, Kumasaka T, et al. Structural basis of glutamate recognition by a dimeric metabotropic glutamate receptor. Nature. 2000;407: 971–7.
Lasoń W, Dudra-Jastrzębska M, Rejdak K, Czuczwar SJ. Basic mechanisms of antiepileptic drugs and their pharmacokinetic/pharmacodynamic interactions: an update. Pharmacol Rep. 2011;63:271–92.
Lipton SA, Rosenberg PA. Excitatory amino acids a final common pathway for neurologic disorders. N Engl J Med. 1994;330:613–22.
López-Pérez SJ, Vergara P, Ventura-Valenzuela JP, Ureña-Guerrero ME, Segovia J, Beas-Zárate C. Modification of dopaminergic markers expression in the striatum by neonatal exposure to glutamate during development. Int J Dev Neurosci. 2005;23:335–42.
López-Pérez SJ, Ureña-Guerrero ME, Morales-Villagrán A. Monosodium glutamate neonatal treatment as a seizure and excitotoxic model. Brain Res. 2010;1317:246–456.
Löscher W. Critical review of current animal models of seizures and epilepsy used in the discovery and development of new antiepileptic drugs. Seizure. 2011;20:359–68.
Lucas DR, Newhouse JP. The toxic effect of sodium L-glutamate on the inner layers of the retina. Arch Ophthalmol. 1957;58:193–204.
Luoma JI, Kelley BG, Mermelstein PG. Progesterone inhibition of voltage-gated calcium channels is a potential neuroprotective mechanism against excitotoxicity. Steroids. 2011;76:845–55.
Manent JB, Represa A. Neurotransmitters and brain maturation: early paracrine actions of GABA and glutamate modulate neuronal migration. Neuroscientist. 2007,13.268–79.
Mares P, Kubová H. What is the role of neurotransmitter systems in cortical seizures? Physiol Res. 2008;57 Suppl 3:S111–20.
Martinez-Contreras A, Huerta M, Lopez-Perez S, Garcia-Estrada J, Luquin S, Beas-Zarate C. Astrocytic and microglia cells reactivity induced by neonatal administration of glutamate in cerebral cortex of adult rats. J Neurosci Res. 2002;67:200–10.
Martisova E, Solas M, Horrillo I, Ortega JE, Meana JJ, Tordera RM, et al. Long lasting effects of early-life stress on glutamatergic/GABAergic circuitry in the rat hippocampus. Neuropharmacology. 2012;62:1944–53.
Medina-Ceja L, Sandoval-García F, Morales-Villagrán A, López-Pérez SJ. Rapid compensatory changes in the expression of EAAT-3 and GAT-1 transporters during seizures in cells of the CA1 and dentate gyrus. J Biomed Sci. 2012;19:78.
Meldrum B. Possible therapeutic applications of antagonists of excitatory amino acid neurotransmitters. Clin Sci. 1985;68:118–22.
Meldrum B. Excitotoxicity and selective neuronal loss in epilepsy. Brain Pathol. 1993a;3:405–12.
Meldrum B. Amino acids as dietary excitotoxins: a contribution to understanding neurodegenerative disorders. Brain Res Rev. 1993b;18:293–314.

Mishra OP, Fritz KI, Delivoria-Papadopoulos M. NMDA receptor and neonatal hypoxic brain injury. Ment Retard Dev Disabil Res Rev. 2001;7:249–53.

Morales-Villagran A, Tapia R. Preferential stimulation of glutamate release by 4-aminopyridine in rat striatum in vivo. Neurochem Int. 1996;28:35–40.

Morales-Villagran A, Ureña-Guerrero ME, Tapia R. Protection by NMDA receptor antagonist seizures induced by intracerebral administration of 4-aminopyridine. Eur J Pharmacol. 1996;305:87–93.

Moreira PI, Zhu X, Nunomura A, Smith MA, Perry G. Therapeutic options in Alzheimer's disease. Expert Rev Neurother. 2006;6(6):897–910.

Morrison G, Fraser DD, Cepinskas G. Mechanisms and consequences of acquired brain injury during development. Pathophysiology. 2012; doi:10.1016/j.pathophys.2012.02.006.

Möykkynen T, Korpi ER. Acute effects of ethanol on glutamate receptors. Basic Clin Pharmacol Toxicol. 2012;111:4–13.

Muller GJ, Moller A, Johansen FF. Stereological cell counts of GABAergic neurons in rat dentate hilus following transient cerebral ischemia. Exp Brain Res. 2001;141:380–8.

Niizuma K, Yoshioka H, Chen H, Kim GS, Jung JE, Katsu M, et al. Mitochondrial and apoptotic neuronal death signaling pathways in cerebral ischemia. Biochim Biophys Acta. 2010;1802:92–9.

Niquet J, Lopez-Meraz ML, Wasterlain CG. Programmed necrosis after status epilepticus. In: Noebels JL, Avoli M, Rogawski MA, Olsen RW, Delgado-Escueta AV, editors. Jasper's basic mechanisms of the epilepsies [Internet]. 4th ed. Bethesda, MD: National Center for Biotechnology Information, USA; 2012.

Nuñez JL, Alt JJ, McCarthy MM. A new model for prenatal brain damage. I. GABAA receptor activation induces cell death in developing rat hippocampus. Exp Neurol. 2003;181:258–69.

Olney JW. Glutamate induces neuronal necrosis in the infant mouse hypothalamus. J Neuropathol Exp Neurol. 1971;30:75–90.

Olney JW, Ho OL, Rhee V. Cytotoxic effects of acidic and sulphur containing amino acids on the infant mouse central nervous system. Exp Brain Res. 1971;14(1):61–76.

Olsen RW, Betz H. GABA and glycine. In: Siegel GJ, Albers RW, Brady SP, Price DL, editors. Basic neurochemistry, molecular, cellular, and medical aspects. 7th ed. San Diego: Elsevier Academic; 2006.

Ortuño-Sahagún D, Beas-Zárate C, Adame-Gonzalez G, Feria-Velasco A. Effect of L-glutamate on cholinergic neurotransmission in various brain regions and during the development of rats, when administered perinatally. Neurochem Int. 1997;31:683–92.

Popescu G, Auerbach A. Modal gating of NMDA receptors and the shape of their synaptic response. Nat Neurosci. 2003;6:476–783.

Portera-Cailliau C, Price DL, Martin LJ. Excitotoxic neuronal death in the immature brain is an apoptosis-necrosis morphological continuum. J Comp Neurol. 1997a;378:70–87.

Portera-Cailliau C, Price DL, Martin LJ. Non-NMDA and NMDA receptor-mediated excitotoxic neuronal death in adult brain are morphologically distinct: further evidence for an apoptosis-necrosis continuum. J Comp Neurol. 1997b;378:88–104.

Reeves TM, Lyeth BG, Phillips LL, Hamm RJ, Povlishock JT. The effects of traumatic brain injury on inhibition in the hippocampus and dentate gyrus. Brain Res. 1987;757:119–32.

Rego AC, Oliveira CR. Mitochondrial dysfunction and reactive oxygen species in excitotoxicity and apoptosis: implications for the pathogenesis of neurodegenerative diseases. Neurochem Res. 2003;28:1563–74.

Remy S, Beck H. Molecular and cellular mechanisms of pharmacoresistance in epilepsy. Brain. 2006;129:18–35.

Rivera-Cervantes MC, Torres JS, Feria-Velasco A, Armendariz-Borunda J, Beas-Zárate C. NMDA and AMPA receptor expression and cortical neuronal death are associated with p38 in glutamate-induced excitotoxicity in vivo. J Neurosci Res. 2004;76:678–87.

Rivera-Cervantes MC, Flores-Soto ME, Chaparro-Huerta V, Reyes-Gómez J, Feria-Velasco A, Schliebs R, et al. Changes in hippocampal NMDA-R subunit composition induced by exposure of neonatal rats to L-glutamate. Int J Dev Neurosci. 2009;27:197–204.

Rowley NM, Madsen KK, Schousboe A, White HS. Glutamate and GABA synthesis, release, transport and metabolism as targets for seizure control. Neurochem Int. 2012;61:546–58.

Severino PC, Muller Gdo A, Vandresen-Filho S, Tasca CI. Cell signaling in NMDA preconditioning and neuroprotection in convulsions induced by quinolinic acid. Life Sci. 2011;89:570–6.

Simeone TA, Sanchez RM, Rho JM. Molecular biology and ontogeny of glutamate receptors in mammalian central nervous system. J Child Neurol. 2004;19:343–60.

Sperk G, Furtinger S, Schwarzer C, Pirker S. GABA and its receptors in epilepsy. Adv Exp Med Biol. 2004;548:92–103.

Supnet C, Bezprozvanny I. The dysregulation of intracellular calcium in Alzheimer disease. Cell Calcium. 2010;47:183–9.

Szydlowska K, Tymianski M. Calcium, ischemia and excitotoxicity. Cell Calcium. 2010;47: 122–9.

Tapia R, Medina-Ceja L, Peña F. On relationship between extracellular glutamate, hyperexcitation and neurodegeneration, in vivo. Neurochem Int. 1999;34:23–31.

Thomas CG, Tian H, Diamond JS. The relative roles of diffusion and uptake in clearing synaptically released glutamate change during early postnatal development. J Neurosci. 2011;31: 4743–54.

Tolman JA, Faulkner MA. Vigabatrin: a comprehensive review of drug properties including clinical updates following recent FDA approval. Expert Opin Pharmacother. 2009;10:3077–89.

Tomczyk T, Haberek G, Zuchora B, Jarosławska-Zych A, Kowalczyk MS, Wielosz M, et al. Enhanced glutamatergic transmission reduces the anticonvulsant potential of lamotrigine but not of felbamate against tonic-clonic seizures. Pharmacol Rep. 2007;59:462–6.

Treiman DM. GABAergic mechanisms in epilepsy. Epilepsia. 2001;42 Suppl 3:8–12.

Ureña-Guerrero ME, Beas-Zarate C. Modificaciones en la susceptibilidad convulsive por degeneración excitotóxica. In: De Celis R, editor. Investigación en Neurociencias (Homenaje al Dr. Alfredo Feria-Velasco). Guadalajara: Bios-Medica Editores; 2006.

Ureña-Guerrero ME, López-Pérez SJ, Beas-Zárate C. Neonatal monosodium glutamate treatment modifies glutamic acid decarboxylase activity during rat brain postnatal development. Neurochem Int. 2003;42:269–76.

Ureña-Guerrero ME, Orozco-Suárez S, López-Pérez SJ, Flores-Soto ME, Beas-Zárate C. Excitotoxic neonatal damage induced by monosodium glutamate reduces several GABAergic markers in the cerebral cortex and hippocampus in adulthood. Int J Dev Neurosci. 2009;27:845–55.

Vandenberghe W, Bredt DS. Early events in glutamate receptor trafficking. Curr Opin Cell Biol. 2004;16:134–9.

Velázquez-Zamora DA, González-Ramírez MM, Beas-Zárate C, González-Burgos I. Egocentric working memory impairment and dendritic spine plastic changes in prefrontal neurons after NMDA receptor blockade in rats. Brain Res. 2011;1402:101–8.

Vincent P, Mulle C. Kainate receptors in epilepsy and excitotoxicity. Neuroscience. 2009;158(1):309–23.

Wagner AK, Fabio A, Puccio AM, Hirschberg R, Li W, Zafonte RD, et al. Gender associations with cerebrospinal fluid glutamate and lactate/pyruvate levels after severe traumatic brain injury. Crit Care Med. 2005;33:407–13.

Wang Y, Qin ZH. Molecular and cellular mechanisms of excitotoxic neuronal death. Apoptosis. 2010;15:1382–402.

Wang SJ, Huang CC, Hsu KS, Tsai JJ, Gean PW. Presynaptic inhibition of excitatory neurotransmission by lamotrigine in the rat amygdalar neurons. Synapse. 1996;24:248–55.

Watkins JC, Olverman H. Agonists and antagonists for excitatory amino acid receptors. Trends Neurosci. 1987;10:265–72.

Werner FM, Coveñas R. Classical neurotransmitters and neuropeptides involved in generalized epilepsy: a focus on antiepileptic drugs. Curr Med Chem. 2011;18(32):4933–48.

Wilson CL, Maidment NT, Shomer MH, Behnke EJ, Ackerson L, Fried I, et al. Comparison of seizure related amino acid release in human epileptic hippocampus versus chronic kainate rat model of hippocampal epilepsy. Epilepsy Res. 1996;26:245–54.

Wollmuth LP, Sobolevsky AI. Structure and gating of the glutamate receptor ion channel. Trends Neurosci. 2004;27:321–8.

Xu J, Ling EA. Studies of the ultrastructure and permeability of the blood–brain barrier in the developing corpus callosum in postnatal rat brain using electron dense tracers. J Anat. 1994;184:227–37.

Zhao YL, Xiang Q, Shi QY, Li SY, Tan L, Wang JT, et al. GABAergic excitotoxicity injury of the immature hippocampal pyramidal neurons' exposure to isoflurane. Anesth Analg. 2011;113:1152–60.

Chapter 6
Intracellular Pathways Associated with Neuronal Survival and Death in Epilepsy

Martha Rivera-Cervantes, Alfredo I. Feria-Velasco, Felix Junyent, Antoni Camins Espuny, and Carlos Beas-Zárate

Abstract Epilepsy has been characterized a disease whose social and occupational behavioural has had devastating economical consequences and is associated with great cumulative brain damage and neurological deficits. From different forms of epilepsy, the most frequent type is temporal lobe epilepsy (TLE), being the most common form of drug refractory epilepsy. Although there are a great amount of studies about the mechanisms involved in neuronal damage and death during critical phases of epileptogenesis, it is crucial to construct strategies for neuroprotection that may prevent the development of epilepsy. In this chapter, some molecular mechanisms involved in the neuronal death, which are induced by excitotoxicity phenomena following the signalling pathways activation and studied in animal models under seizure conditions or expressed in the epilepsy are discussed, mainly those as the mitogen-activated protein kinases, Jak/Stat, and Pi3k/Akt pathways those genes responsible to participate in the apoptosis and cell cycle regulation are also analysed.

M. Rivera-Cervantes (✉)
Departamento de Biologia Celular y Molecular, Centro Universitario de Ciencias Biologicas y Agropecuarias, Universidad de Guadalajara, Km. 14.5 Carretera A Nogales, Predio Las Agujas Nextipac, Zapopan, Jalisco 45110, México
e-mail: mrivera939@gmail.com

A.I. Feria-Velasco • C. Beas-Zárate
Departamento de Biologia Celular y Molecular, Centro Universitario de Ciencias Biologicas y Agropecuarias, Universidad de Guadalajara, Km. 15.5 Carretera-Guadalajara-Nogales, Predio Las Agujas, Zapopan, Jalisco 45110, México
e-mail: alfredoferia1340@hotmail.com; carlosbeas55@gmail.com

F. Junyent
Unitat de Bioquimica, Facultat de Medicina i Ciencies de la Salut, Universitat Rovira i Virgili, C./ St. Llorenc 21 Reus (Tarragona), Barcelona 46201, Spain
e-mail: felixjunyent@ub.edu

A. Camins Espuny
Department of Pharmacology and Biomedical Chemistry, University of Barcelona, Avenida Diagonal 643, Barcelona 08028, Spain
e-mail: camiins@ub.edu

L. Rocha and E.A. Cavalheiro (eds.), *Pharmacoresistance in Epilepsy: From Genes and Molecules to Promising Therapies*, DOI 10.1007/978-1-4614-6464-8_6,

In summary, the structural and molecular changes at cellular level are believed to play a key role in the generation of convulsive seizures and its possible identification should facilitate the develop of potential therapeutic targets heading towards of specific genes, proteins, and signalling pathways altered during the different stages of epileptogenesis process.

Keywords TLE • Epileptogenesis • Apoptosis • Excitotoxicity • Cell death • Cell damage • Intrinsic pathway • Extrinsic pathway

6.1 Introduction

Epilepsy has devastating behavioural, social, and occupational consequences and is associated with cumulative brain damage and neurological deficits. In addition, it is characterized by the occurrence of repeated and sudden transitory episodes of motor, sensory, autonomic, and physical origin known as seizures, which at the cellular level are characterized by synchronized discharges of large groups of neurons that interfere their functions. Temporal lobe epilepsy (TLE) is the most common form of partial epilepsy and affects 40% of the patients. Seizures arising from the mesial temporal lobe structures (i.e., amygdala and hippocampus) can be progressive and often becomes refractory to drug treatment. It is characterized by the presence of complex partial seizures and generalized tendency to produce multiple epileptic foci. One of the most common histologic abnormalities observed in approximately 66% of patients with TLE is hippocampal sclerosis or mesial temporal sclerosis, characterized by a remarkable loss of neurons in the hippocampus leading to excessive glial proliferation, particularly in the hilar region of the dentate gyrus and the CA1 and CA3 regions (Thom et al. 2005). The majority of the patients with TLE suffer from symptomatic focal epilepsies, which are frequently a consequence of brain trauma, complicated febrile convulsions, prolonged seizures (*status epilepticus*—SE), ischemic lesions and brain tumours, encephalitis or childhood febrile seizures (Cendes 2002; Engel 2001; French et al. 2004). It has been established that each of these initial events leads to the activation of molecular signalling cascades, which in turn induce selective cell death that is directly related to the epileptogenic process, although even now it is not well known if cell death is the cause or effect of the establishment of the phenomenon of epilepsy. Hippocampal sclerosis (HS), also known as Ammon's horn sclerosis, is characterized by the loss of pyramidal cells and gliosis in CA1 (Ammon's horn) and end folium, dispersion of the granule cell layer of the dentate gyrus (DG), neurogenesis of granule cells, axonal sprouting, and synaptic reorganization of the mossy fibres (Wieser 2004; Thom et al. 2005). Cell loss is typically asymmetric between the hippocampus; the most affected regions are the CA1 and CA3 subfields and hilar region of the DG, while the CA2 subfield and granule cells of the DG usually show much less cell loss (Mathern et al. 1997). In spite of damage to other limbic regions, the cerebellum and cerebral cortex are also commonly affected.

TLE represents the final stage of a long and complex process of cellular and molecular events that are determined by the initial stimulus that triggers the process. There is usually a latent period of several years between this injury and the emergence of the chronic TLE characterized by spontaneous recurrent seizures originating from the temporal lobe, as well as learning and memory impairments (Bartolomei et al. 2005; Detour et al. 2005; Devinski 2004).

The TLE can be reproduced in laboratory animals (typically rodents) by the systemic or intracerebral administration of powerful convulsant agents such as glutamatergic (kainic acid) or cholinergic (pilocarpine) agonists (Pitkänen et al. 2005; Covolan et al. 2000). Over the last few decades, there has been considerable progress in the pharmacotherapy of epilepsy, including the introduction of several new antiepileptic drugs (AEDs) (McCabe 2000). The mechanisms of action of most clinically used drugs in human epilepsies are based upon the synchronized neuronal activity and imbalance between inhibitory and excitatory neurotransmission, events commonly linked to the pathogenesis of epilepsy (Dalby and Mody 2001). However, approximately 30–40% of all patients with TLE are estimated to be drug resistant, therefore identification of specific biological processes and biochemical pathways that trigger cell death during critical phases of epileptogenesis is crucial to design strategies for neuroprotection that may prevent epileptogenesis process.

6.2 Epileptogenesis and Animal Models

The term epileptogenesis refers to the transformation through the normal process of the plastic neuronal network into a chronically hyperexcitable state. The epileptogenic processes emerge after precipitating insults (i.e., local infections, *SE*, ischemia, or trauma) in concert with genetic susceptibility factors, which they are possible to trigger such persistent pathophysiological changes (Coulter and DeLorenzo 1999). However, the study of human epileptic hippocampus does not allow revealing the sequence of events leading to neuronal loss and the regulation of plastic events. For this reason, different animal models have been designed using electrical or drug stimulation, among which include systemic administration of kainic acid, an analogue of glutamate, or cholinergic agonist-pilocarpine (Pitkänen et al. 2005). Both experimental models and postmortem human studies support the idea that cell death is a common pathological feature of insult to the brain, which triggers a chronic epileptic condition (Sutula 2004). Briefly, such injuries invariably set in signal various cell and molecular processes including gliosis, inflammation and vascular changes, neurogenesis and rewiring, axonal reorganization, dispersion of granule cells, and changes in expression of ion channels and signalling molecules including neuronal death. Collectively, this process is identified as epileptogenesis (Blumcke et al. 1999; Mathern et al. 1993; Sloviter 1999).

In the animal models of TLE, the damage within the hippocampus precedes the appearance of spontaneous seizures. Moreover *SE* induced by systemic injection of pilocarpine or kainic acid or by repeated electrical stimulation-caused structural brain damage in rats (Sloviter 2008). Cell loss has been observed in these models in the hilus and CA3 regions, as well as amygdala and entorhinal cortex (Turski et al. 1989; Bartolomei et al. 2005). Moreover, prominent mossy fibre sprouting occurred. The primary cause of neuronal death following seizures is probably over-activation of ion channels gated by glutamate, the principal excitatory neurotransmitter in the brain (Meldrum 1991; Fujikawa 2006). In these conditions, biological processes, including activation of signalling pathways related to stress response, ion transport, signal transduction, and synaptic transmission are triggered (Aronica and Gorter 2007).

6.3 Mechanisms of Cell Death

6.3.1 *Excitotoxicity*

The *excitotoxicity* is a pathological process into the cells. The pioneering work of Meldrum (1993) provided evidence that seizure-induced cell death and other events that induce neurodegeneration result from over-activation of ionotropic glutamate receptors which leads to increased intracellular levels of Ca^{2+} and Na^{+} and causes swelling and cell lysis. There is also energy failure, production of free radicals, activation of enzymatic complex, and cell death (Smolders et al. 2009). The death of cells has been classified generally into two distinct types: apoptosis and necrosis. Both forms of cell death can be induced by excitotoxicity. It has been shown that the excitotoxic damage induced by seizures activates programmed cell death pathways through changes in the expression of specific genes (Engel and Henshall 2009).

6.3.2 *Apoptotic Pathways*

Apoptotic signals are given through a highly ordered molecular cascade that is energy dependent. Several different stimuli can initiate the apoptotic death of neurons. Complex intracellular and intercellular cell-death-regulatory pathways are increasingly recognized as important contributors to seizure-induced neuronal death; however, apoptotic pathways converge on a restricted number of common effector (Sastry and Rao 2000; Engel and Henshall 2009). Two principal pathways have been described as apoptotic death. These two signalling pathways and the final caspase executor activation pathway are also regulated by several proteins such as glycogen synthase kinase (GSK3), ataxia-telangiectasia-mutated protein (ATM)/p53, Bcl-2, cyclin-dependent kinases (CDKs), and mitogen-activated protein kinases (MAPKs), which act on both pathways (Wang et al. 2007; Kroemer et al. 2007).

There are two main cell-signalling pathways that have been identified in the control of apoptosis: the intrinsic pathway, or core pathway, and the extrinsic pathway.

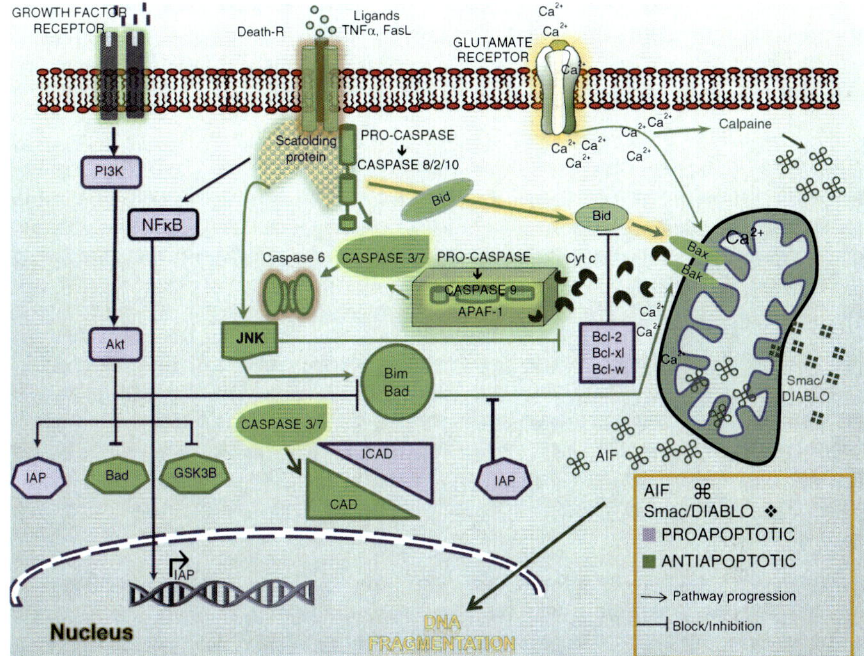

Fig. 6.1 Major apoptosis pathways activated by seizures. Both the excitotoxicity which may directly trigger mitochondrial dysfunction or activate enzymatic pathways (e.g., mitogen activated protein kinases-MAPK) and the pathway activated by death receptors (DR) converge in the activation of modulators (e.g., inhibitor of caspase-activated DNase-ICAD) and executors proteins of death process (e.g., caspases). Other pathways may compensate these processes (e.g., pathway mediated by Growth-factor receptor or cytokines) promoting activity or expression (e.g., inhibitors of apoptosis proteins-IAP) of anti-apoptotic proteins or decreasing their activity (e.g., Bad and glycogen synthase kinase-3β (GSK-3β))

The extrinsic pathway mediates cell death in response to extracellular stimuli and is initiated by cell-surface receptors called death receptors (DR) of the tumour necrosis factor (TNF) superfamily (Wajant 2002). Ligands for these receptors include TNFα, Fas ligand, and TNF receptor apoptosis-inducing ligand (TRAIL). Activation follows binding of the ligand to its receptor and oligomerization of the receptor. In the case of Fas, the cell death signal is propagated inside the cell by recruitment of Fas-Associated protein with Death Domain (FADD) and an initiator caspase (e.g., 8 or 10 caspases) to the intracellular side of the plasma membrane, resulting in formation of a death-inducing signalling complex (DISC). In contrast, activation of TNFR1 leads to direct association with TNF receptor-associated death domain (TRADD); the recruited to this complex can then modulate the nuclear factor-κB pathway (Fig. 6.1) (Wajant 2002; Strasser et al. 2000).

Extrinsic pathway activation after seizures is documented in various seizure models where the presence or activity for 2 and 8 caspases has been reported (Henshall et al. 2001a, b). While death receptors are constitutively expressed in the brain, their participation has been linked to the activity of caspase 8 observed after seizures through scaffolding proteins and receptors for TNFα and FasL, both present in the adult rat hippocampus before and after seizures (Shinoda et al. 2003; Henshall et al. 2001a, b).

On the other hand, *an intrinsic pathway* that is associated to apoptosis is regulated by mitochondria, which integrates a lethal or pro-survival signal that eventually determines the cell density. It is initiated after cell stressors that perturb intracellular organelle function (Danial and Korsmeyer 2004; Xu et al. 2005) and include raised intracellular Ca^{2+} and reactive oxygen species (ROS) (Orrenius et al. 2003). Mitochondrial apoptosis in neurons can be triggered by a variety of structurally related agents (Sastry and Rao 2000). A key event in this pathway is the release of apoptogenic molecules from mitochondria, which is caused by a change in permeability of the outer mitochondrial membrane and the release of molecules from mitochondria, and in particular *cytochrome c* (*cyt c*), binds the apoptotic protease, activating factor 1 (Apaf1) and recruiting caspase 9. This forms the so-called apoptosome, which processes downstream effector caspases such as caspase 3, culminating in cleavage of various structural and other proteins (Fig. 6.1) (Bratton and Salvesen 2010).

The permeability of the mitochondrial outer membrane (MOMP) is regulated by the activity of several proteins that belong to the Bcl2 family. The Bcl-2 gene family comprises more than 20 different members that either positively or negatively regulate apoptosis primarily by affecting the mitochondria (Cory and Adams 2002; Liou et al. 2003; Kroemer et al 2007). The proteins of this family with anti-apoptotic function include Bcl-2, Bcl-X_L, and Mcl-1, which preserve the integrity of the outer mitochondrial membrane. The major pro-apoptotic proteins here include Bad, Bid, Bik, Bim, Noxa, p53-upregulated mediator of apoptosis (PUMA), Bax, and Bak. Interestingly, Bid protein constitutes one link between the extrinsic and intrinsic pathways through the cleavage of caspase-8, which further amplifies the apoptotic death signal. Bid interacts with Bax–Bak, which forms pores that allow the release of *cyt c* (Cory and Adams 2002). The anti-apoptotic Bcl-2 and Bcl-X_L proteins can prevent Bax translocation towards the mitochondria, but additionally Bcl-X_L may bind to Apaf-1 and in doing so suppresses caspase-9 activation (Fig. 6.1) (Kroemer et al. 2007; Stavrovskaya and Kristal 2005).

As previously mentioned, ROS production is another common stressor factor that is triggered by excitotoxicity. One target of ROS is DNA, which is extremely sensitive to oxidative stress. One of the sensors of DNA damage is the ATM, which belongs to the family of phosphatidylinositol-3 kinases (PI3K) (Roos and Kaina 2006; Chipuk and Green 2009). Once activated, ATM stimulates p53 (a nuclear transcription factor). Thus, DNA damage and the subsequent p53 activation; both contribute to other apoptotic signals that the mitochondria receive through the intrinsic pathway. In fact, if the neuronal DNA damage cannot be repaired, overactivation of p53 triggers the neuronal apoptotic process. In a second step, p53 mainly induces the expression of the pro-apoptotic Bcl-2 family members PUMA (Roos and Kaina 2006; Chipuk and Green 2009). Noxa is another p53-activated mediator that can contribute to apoptosis. Interestingly, PUMA activates the intrinsic apoptotic pathway by binding to Bax, which acts directly on the mitochondria (Chipuk and Green 2009). In addition, PUMA can bind with and consequently inhibit anti-apoptotic Bcl-2 family members, including Bcl-2, Bcl-X_L, Bcl-w, and Mcl-1 (Fig. 6.1) (Roos and Kaina 2006). A tight balance exists between the activities of pro- and anti-apoptotic Bcl-2 family members in resting conditions. The cell's fate will progress to apoptosis only when this equilibrium is altered toward enhanced activity of pro-apoptotic proteins.

While both extrinsic and intrinsic pathways have different beginnings, they eventually converge in the massive activation of catabolic enzymes (including a class proteases known as caspases, no caspases proteases, lipases, and endonucleases); at present there are 14 known mammalian caspases (named from cysteinyl-aspartate-specific proteases) that are enzymes that cleave other proteins next to an aspartate residue. The apoptosis regulatory caspases are divided into initiators of apoptosis that include caspases 8, 9, and 10, and the apoptotic executioners are caspases 3, 6, and 7 (Schindler et al. 2006; Bozzi et al. 2011). Each caspase is initially synthesized as a zymogen and requires processing at specific cleavage sites to generate the active enzymes. The caspases that are the first to be activated trigger downstream other caspases giving rise to a proteolytic cascade that culminates in the execution of apoptosis. Different subsets of caspases are activated depending on the pro-apoptotic stimulus (Salvesen and Riedl 2007). For example, caspases 3, 6, and 8 are part of the Fas/TNFα-mediated death pathway, while caspases 3 and 9 together with apoptosis protease-activated factor 1 (Apaf1) and *cyt c* participate in mitochondria-associated cell death (see Fig. 6.1) (Bratton and Salvesen 2010).

Activation of intrinsic, mitochondria-dependent cell death pathways after seizures would be predicted based on the assumed significance of glutamate excitotoxicity and mitochondrial dysfunction due to both calcium (Ca^{2+}) and ROS loading (Orrenius et al. 2003). Several authors have observed that neuroprotection is also less pronounced when mitochondrial-activated caspase-9 is blocked after seizures, and other data suggests the extrinsic cell death pathway-associated caspase 8 is activated following seizures in vitro (Henshall et al. 2001b, c; Meller et al. 2006).

6.3.3 Apoptosis and Cell Cycle Regulation

The biochemical mechanisms of the different phases of the cell cycle are highly regulated by intracellular signalling elements such as protein kinases (e.g., MAPKs) as well as their target substrates in particular cell cycle regulators. A family of cyclins act as regulatory subunits for CDKs, and thus regulate passage through the four phases of the cell cycle. The activities of the various cyclin/CDK complexes regulate the progression through G1/S/G2/M phases of the cell cycle (Nigg 1995). MAPKs are involved in regulating the protein expression of cell cycle regulators; in particular those that regulate passage of cells of phase G_0 to G_1 (Yeste-Velasco et al. 2009).

In particular, the differentiated neurons are post-mitotic cells and completely lacking in replicative capability. These cells enter a phase of mitotic quiescence commonly referred to as the Go phase, and as such were believed to be unable to re-enter the cell cycle. Postmortem studies have revealed pathological evidence of aberrant cell cycle re-entry occurring in neurons of patients with Alzheimer's disease (Yang et al. 2001, 2003), epilepsy (Nagy and Esiri 1998), and Parkinson's disease (Jordan-Sciutto et al. 2003). Moreover, it has been observed experimentally that cell cycle regulators such as CDKs are produced and abnormally activated in different models of induction of cell damage (e.g., ischemia, epilepsy, excitotoxicity, and trauma) (Timsit and Menn 2007; Sutula 2004). The activation of these events leads to cell death. Various markers of this event have been detected before neuronal death occurs suggesting its participation as an initiator of the execution of the cell death program (Katchanov et al. 2001; Timsit and Menn 2007). The atypical expression of mitogenic genes may promote entry and progression of neurons into the cell cycle through an increase in the expression level of cyclin D and phosphorylation of the retinoblastome protein (Rb), regulating the E2F activity which induces modifications to the transcription of pro-apoptotic molecules as caspases 3, 8, and 9, as well as Apaf-1 or members of the Bcl-2 family (Greene et al. 2004).

Although few studies have evaluated the role of cell cycle regulators in epilepsy, there is enough evidence to link changes in the expression and activity of these molecules in epileptogenesis. A study following kainate-induced seizures showed that the cyclin D1 mRNA was induced in the vulnerable CA3 region, and to a lesser extent, in non-vulnerable regions, while that the expression of CDK4 and cyclin D1 was upregulated in neurons of the rat piriform cortex and amygdala 1–3 days after KA administration in vivo. CDK4 and cyclin D1 proteins were induced in the cytoplasm and nuclei of neurons, with a concomitant increase of CDK4- and cyclin D1-positive microglia in the affected areas; these results suggest that CDK4 and cyclin D1 are essential for KA-induced neuronal apoptosis *in vivo* (Timsit and Menn 2007; Ino and Chiba 2001).

6.4 Signal Pathways in Survival or Cell Damage

Epilepsy activates several signalling cascades that are essential to regulate the survival or cell damage, which are evoked by multiple stimuli, including excitotoxicity, oxidative stress, and inflammation processes (Henshall and Murphy 2008; Okamoto et al. 2010). Particularly the inflammatory processes, including activation microglia and astrocytes and production of proinflammatory cytokines and related molecules, have been described in human epilepsy patients as well as in experimental models of epilepsy (Vezzani et al. 2008). A number of proinflammatory mediators, thus initiating a cascade of processes in brain tissue, alter neuronal excitability and affect the physiological functions of glia by paracrine or autocrine actions, thus interfering with the neuronal communications and may compromise neuronal survival (Riazi et al. 2010; Vezzani et al. 2008). Chronic brain inflammation may also contribute to susceptibility to seizures and comorbidity in chronic epilepsy patients. Prototypical inflammatory cytokines such as interleukine-1β (IL-1β), TNF-alpha, and interleukine-6 (IL-6) are over-expressed in experimental models of seizures in brain areas of seizure generation and propagation, and are prominent in glia, and to a lesser extent by neurons. Cytokines receptors are also upregulated, and the related intracellular signalling is activated in both cell populations highlighting autocrine and paracrine actions of cytokines in the brain (Riazi et al. 2010; Vezzani et al 2008). The recent demonstration of functional interactions between cytokines and classical neurotransmitters such as glutamate and gamma amino butyric acid (GABA), as well as intracellular signalling mechanisms, suggest the possibility that these interactions underlie the cytokine-mediated changes in neuronal excitability, thus promoting seizure phenomena and the associated neuropathology (Balosso et al. 2008, 2009; Stellwagen et al. 2005; Pickering et al. 2005).

6.4.1 Protein Kinases Activated by Mitogen

Extracellular stimuli evoked by neurotransmitters, neurotrophins, and growth factors in the brain regulate critical cellular events, including synaptic transmission, neuronal plasticity, morphological differentiation, and survival. A pathway known to influence seizure-induced neuronal damage and epileptogenesis includes the MAPK cascades (Liou et al. 2003; Shinoda et al. 2003). The MAPK pathways are used by eukaryotic cells for the transduction of extracellular signals to the nucleus and other intracellular targets (Chang and Karin 2001).

There are two known major pathways of MAPK including the extracellular signal-regulated kinases (ERK) and stress-activated protein kinases (SAPK). The latter is divided into the kinases c-Jun NH_2-terminal (JNK/SAPK) and p38 kinase pathway (p38/SAPK) (Pearson et al. 2001; Okuno et al. 2004). The MAPKs are also involved in apoptosis and may, therefore, play a role in neurodegeneration (Borsello and Forloni 2007; Guan et al. 2006; Kyosseva 2004). These kinases are activated by phosphorylation on threonine and tyrosine residues. Subsequently, phosphorylated and other intracellular enzymes or transcription factors regulate the expression of genes involved in cellular response (Kyosseva 2004). The substrates that are identified are phosphorylated; for MAPKs in the nucleus they include some hormone receptors, as well as transcription factors such as the activator protein-1 (AP-1), the family of Jun factors (c-Jun, Jun-B, and Jun-D), Elk-1, p53, transcription factor-2 (ATF-2), JDP2, c-Myc, the NAFT family, the STAT family, and the PAX family (Chen et al. 2001; Kyosseva 2004).

Commonly the activation of signalling pathways JNK/SAPK and p38/SAPK has been associated with the promotion of cell damage (Borsello and Forloni 2007; Guan et al. 2006; Kyosseva 2004). Nevertheless, extracellular signal-regulated kinase1/2 (ERK1/2) has been implicated in several cellular functions including regulation of cell proliferation, differentiation, survival, and apoptosis in response to a wide variety of external stimuli (Cheung and Slack 2004; Miller and Gauthier 2007; Yoon and Seger 2006).

ERK pathway exhibits dynamic changes following several types of seizure activity and may function in the regulation of neuronal excitability (Dudek and Fields 2001; Houser et al. 2008). This signalling pathway is strongly activated in neurons following severe, chemically induced seizures. In an initial *SE* episode-increased ERK activation may be neuroprotective and limit the damage of some neurons, such as dentate granule cells (Choi et al. 2008). Conversely, a lack of ERK activation in other neurons may contribute to their vulnerability to excitotoxic damage (Choi et al. 2007). At later stages, ERK phosphorylation may decrease as a compensatory mechanism to control increased network excitability (Dudek and Fields 2001).

Certain evidence has shown that neuronal activity-dependent modulation of the ERK signalling pathway plays an important role in synaptic plasticity (Yoon and Seger 2006).

Moreover, *in vivo* studies have implicated that the SAPKs play an important role in mediating glutamate receptor (GluR) responses, possibly involving the normal physiology of glutamate and associated pathophysiology. For example, the activation of the *N*-methyl-D-aspartate (NMDA) receptor stimulates JNK and p38 MAPK in cultured CGCs (Kawasaki et al. 1997); and in hippocampal neurons α-amino-3-hydroxy-5-methyl-4-isoxazolepropionic acid (AMPA) and kainite (KA) receptors stimulate ERKs, JNK, and p38 kinase (Mukherjee et al. 1999).

The JNK pathway has a central position in cellular damage particularly in apoptosis and participates in the death cell program through regulation of the function of pro-apoptotic activators members of bcl-2 family (BH3-only) or phosphorylates Bim- and Bcl2-associated agonist of cell death (Bad) at distinct serine residues (Donovan et al. 2002; Putcha et al. 2003). Moreover, JNK enhances *bim*-gene expression through activation of the transcription factor c-Jun. Therefore, the deletion or inhibition of JNKs components substantially limits the cellular potential to undergo death in neuronal and non-neuronal cells, principally the caspases dependent. The most convincing evidence to suggest that JNK is implicated in excitotoxic neuronal death has come from studies using JNK3 knockout mice, where KA-mediated seizures in vivo failed to cause apoptosis in hippocampal neurons, coincident with the reduction of *c-Jun* phosphorylation (Yang et al. 1997). The principal substrate for JNK is c-Jun; however, it is not known which isoform is responsible for its phosphorylation. High expression of both the gene and protein of c-Jun precedes or coincides with periods of cell death, such as that occurring during embryonic development (Sun et al. 2005), after trauma (Raivich et al. 2004), cerebral ischemia (Wessel et al. 1991), and seizures (Morgan and Curran 1991).

This dual role of MAPKs may make it possible to design alternative and/or synergistic approaches to the management of degenerative diseases, either by using specific inhibitors of the MAPKs involved in apoptosis or by increasing the activation of the MAPKs involved in neuronal survival and differentiation.

6.4.2 JAK/STAT and PI3K/AKT Pathways

The Janus kinases (JAKs) are a family of non-receptor protein tyrosine kinases. They are activated in a variety of different ways. In the canonical pathway, two JAK molecules bind to two receptors that dimerized in response to ligand binding and the juxtaposed JAKs trans and/or autophosphorylate resulting in their activation (Yamaoka et al. 2004). This mode of activation applies, for example, to cytokine receptors, growth hormone-like receptors, and the leptin receptor. Alternatively, JAKs may be activated following stimulation of G protein-coupled receptors and/or via intracellular Ca^{2+} changes. Once activated, JAKs phosphorylate and activate downstream targets. For instance, the recruitment of JAK2 mediates the activation of several signalling pathways, including STAT5, ERK/MAPK, and PI3K/Akt (Silva et al. 1999; Kretz et al. 2005). The best-established downstream effector of JAK is the signal transducer and activator of transcription (STAT) family. Seven STAT isoforms, named STAT1 to STAT4, STAT5A, STAT5B, and STAT6, have been identified (Battle and Frank 2002). Once phosphorylated by JAK, STATs dimerize and are translocated to the nucleus where they regulate the expression of numerous genes (Aaronson and Horvath 2002). The JAK/STAT pathway is involved in many physiological processes including those governing cell survival, proliferation, differentiation, development, and inflammation. There is increasing evidence that this pathway also has neuronal specific functions in the central nervous system (Yadav et al. 2005). The cellular and molecular mechanism by which the JAK/STAT pathway is involved in neuronal function is unknown. However, it has been shown that STAT can regulate the expression or function of several neurotransmitter receptors, including GABA (Lund et al. 2008), muscarinic acetylcholine (Chiba et al. 2009), and NMDA and AMPA receptors. Particularly, STAT5 is a predominantly pro-survival signal (Debierre-Grockiego 2004).

A role for Akt in mediating neuronal survival was first demonstrated by Datta and colleagues (Datta et al. 1997) in a primary postnatal cerebellar granule cell culture model, in which apoptosis is induced by either low potassium or growth factor withdrawal (D'Mello et al. 1993). Moreover, Akt is a serine/threonine kinase with diverse roles related to the regulation of cell growth, proliferation, migration, glucose metabolism, transcription, protein synthesis, and angiogenesis (Bazil et al. 2002). Activation of Akt occurs following the binding of a protein growth factor to its receptor on the cell surface. Ligand binding induces autophosphorylation of tyrosine residues in the cytoplasmic portion of the receptor, resulting in the recruitment and activation of phosphatidylinositol 3-kinase (PI3K).

One best-characterized signalling survival mediated by Akt is activated by NMDA receptors (Datta et al. 1997); the inhibition of this kinase activity contributes to NMDA receptor-mediated apoptosis. Moreover the protein kinase serine/threonine (Akt), also known as protein kinase B (PKB) has two sites of phosphorylation that determine the regulation of Akt activity: threonine 308 (Thr308), located in the kinase domain, and serine 473 (Ser473), which is in the regulatory domain (Coffer and Woodgett 1991; Song et al. 2005).

The activation of Akt by trophic factors depends on PI3-K (Burgering and Coffer 1995). When the trophic factor specifically binds to its receptor, PI3-K is recruited by activating Akt modulating, and an anti-apoptotic effect may be through:

1. Direct regulation of the apoptotic pathway
2. Transcriptional control of molecules that promote cell survival, and
3. Regulation of cellular metabolism (Song et al. 2005)

With respect to direct regulation, Akt can phosphorylate different members of the pro-apoptotic Bcl-2 family such as Bad (Datta et al. 1997) and Bim. Once phosphorylated bind to proteins called chaperones 14-3-3 in the cytoplasm; they are thereby inactive in a pro-apoptotic function. Other direct effects involve the inactivation of caspase-9 by phosphorylation or the negative regulation of JNK/SAPK. Regarding the transcriptional control, Akt can phosphorylate different transcription factors indirectly by modulating its activity. Phosphorylation of the family of FoxO transcription factors, whose function includes the induction of apoptosis through the redistribution of these factors from the nucleus to the cytoplasm, prevents its activity (Huang and Tindal 2007).

6.5 Mechanisms of Neuronal Death in Both Experimental Models and Patients with Intractable TLE

6.5.1 Experimental Models of TLE and Cell Signalling

Molecular analyses of epilepsy-induced hippocampal plasticity have largely focused on individual candidate genes, with particular emphasis on genes with known functions for specific pathogenetic aspects (Aronica and Gorter 2007; Mefford et al. 2010). Various studies have reported changes in gene expression in the *SE* induced by kainic acid (Hunsberger et al. 2005) and pilocarpine (Becker et al. 2003), as well as by electric stimulation (Gorter et al. 2006; Engel and Henshall 2009). Moreover, the analyses of these studies have shown an overlap in gene expression profiling in epileptogenesis revealing that the biological process emerges as the most frequently encountered in this context and is related to glial activation, immune response (e.g., inflammation), signal transduction, synaptic transmission (e.g., dopaminergic, glutamatergic, and GABAergic), and the induction of immediate early genes (IEGs) (De Lanerolle and Lee 2005; Aronica and Gorter 2007; Okamoto et al. 2010).

In the work of Okamoto et al. (2010), all possible changes in the rat transcriptome were monitored at distinct time points corresponding from the latent to chronic phase of the pilocarpine model of epilepsy, one the most extensively studied models of TLE. Genes identified as being differentially expressed were classified based on their respective biological functions to envisage processes and pathways likely implicated in epileptogenesis. The hyper-expression of 128 genes was described in this model, indicating stable modulation of the p38/MAPK, JAK/STAT, and PI3K signalling pathways (Okamoto et al. 2010), some of which displaying a parallel expression pattern in humans with epilepsy.

The involvement of caspases in *SE*-induced neurodegeneration has also been studied after systemic injection of kainic acid or lithium-pilocarpine, both of which produce vast and severe neuronal damage (Fujikawa et al. 1999, 2000). Henshall et al (2001b) and Li et al (2006) reported that caspases-8 and -9 are activated in the hippocampus after focal *SE* was induced by kainic acid. The expression of activated caspase-3 in hippocampal neurons and astrocytes have been also detected after pilocarpine-induced *SE* (Narkilahti et al. 2003; Weise et al. 2005). The different location of caspase after *SE* suggests different functions in the brain.

Additionally, López–Meraz et al. (2010) using the lithium–pilocarpine model of *SE* in 2-week-old rat pups showed that dying neurons in the DG and CA1-subiculum area do not share the same mechanism of death. In CA1-subiculum, caspase-8 upregulation preceded caspase-3 activation in morphologically necrotic neurons, while in the DG dying neurons were caspases-9 and -3 immunoreactive and morphologically apoptotic. *SE*-induced neuronal necrosis can be an active mechanism involving the activation of a caspase cascade (Niquet et al. 2007; Lopez-Meraz et al. 2010).

Weak evidence for apoptotic mitochondrial pathways has been described after lithium–pilocarpine-induced *SE* in degenerating neuronal populations (Fujikawa et al. 2002). Some works have shown that *SE* triggered by intra-amygdala kainic acid in mice causes rapid p53 accumulation and subsequent hippocampal damage. Expression of PUMA, a pro-apoptotic protein under p53 control, was increased within a few hours of *SE*. Induction of PUMA was blocked by pharmacologic inhibition of p53, and hippocampal damage was also reduced. Compared to PUMA-expressing mice, PUMA-deficient mice had significantly smaller hippocampal lesions after *SE*. Moreover, PUMA-deficient mice were found to develop fewer epileptic seizures than wild-type animals after *SE* (Engel et al. 2010). Nevertheless, functional-proteomics studies are needed to determine which molecules are active during the process of epileptogenesis or after *SE* (Engel and Henshall 2009).

On the other hand, the neuronal stem cells in the hippocampus appear to be sensitive to a prolonged seizure resulting in an increase in stem or progenitor cell numbers (Walker et al. 2008). In agreement, a quantitative real-time PCR analysis of cell cycle genes confirmed hyper-expression of Cdk1, a gene regulating the G1 to S and G2 to M transition of the cell cycle, and Nestin, a marker of neural stem cells and neural progenitor cells. However, expression of the cell cycle inhibitor *p18*(*INK4c*) was paradoxically enhanced after *SE* induced by pilocarpine and coincided with the peak of Cdk1 and Nestin expression at day 3 post-*SE* (Okamoto et al. 2010). These findings suggest that the proliferative stage may be inhibited by such activation *p18* in pilocarpine model.

Cells born after seizure have altered synaptic inputs and neurotransmitter expression (Jessberger et al. 2007; Parent et al. 2006; Jakubs et al. 2006). These alterations have also been shown in neurogenesis in pilocarpine-induced *SE* (Radley and Jacobs 2003). Experimental TLE is associated with an increase in neurogenesis following amygdala kindling (Parent et al. 1998, 2006; Scott et al. 1998); since many of the newborn neurons eventually integrate into hippocampal circuitry and they may either contribute to the hippocampal network plasticity associated with epilepsy or, possibly, limit seizure activity (Jakubs et al. 2008; Overstreet-Wadiche et al. 2006).

Moreover, phosphorylated ERK (pERK) is increased in many hippocampal neurons following recurrent spontaneous seizures in pilocarpine-treated mice (Houser et al. 2008). Its activity appears to be involved in regulation of seizure-induced neurogenesis during the first few days after *SE*, since ERK activation returns to control levels within 1 week (Choi et al. 2008).

Experimental evidence suggests that seizures evoked by microinjection of kainic acid into the amygdala of the rat activate multiple cell death pathways involving Bcl-2 and caspase family proteins in brain regions destined to die, whereas survival promoting responses predominate in cortical populations that survive (Henshall 2001a). Pro-apoptotic BAD and the counteractive effects of Akt-pathway may underlie in part, the cell death outcome after seizures, providing a more complete understanding of the mechanisms by which seizures damage brain and highlighting novel targets for treatment of brain injury associated with seizure disorders (Henshall 2001a, b). Moreover, the end effector of the signalling pathway regulated by STAT5 proteins includes Bcl-xL and XIAP. Both have shown anti-apoptotic effects in diverse damage animal models (Okamoto et al. 2010).

In summary, although there are several models for the study of epileptogenesis, *SE*, and convulsive seizures, it is important to continue with additional studies for search potential molecular elements that can participate in the process of neuroprotection and/or as therapeutic targets for the treatment of epilepsy.

6.5.2 Studies of Signalling in Patients with Pharmacoresistant TLE

Studies have shown that both pro- and anti-apoptotic proteins, as well as death receptors are found in surgically removed brain samples from patients with pharmacoresistant TLE (Nagy and Esiri 1998; Henshall et al. 2000a, b; Dorr et al 2002).

Analysis of hippocampus from patients with intractable TLE from several groups has confirmed altered expression of Bcl-2 and caspase family genes. In particular, it has been observed that the Bcl-2 and bax immunoreactivity increases predominantly in cells with the morphologic appearance of neurons, whereas bcl-x_L immunoreactivity augments in cells with the appearance of glia (for review Engel and Henshall 2009). In another studies, the expression of anti-apoptotic proteins Bcl-2, Bcl-x, and Bcl-w has been reported to be higher in brain tissue obtained from patients with intractable seizures; however, some pro-apoptotic changes are also seen in this gene family. It may suggest the possible predominance of apoptotic protective pathway-Bcl2 in human epileptic brain (Henshall et al. 2000a, b; Shinoda et al. 2004). DNA fragmentation was also detected in some but not all brain sections from patients undergoing temporal lobectomy for intractable seizures (Henshall et al. 2000a, b).

Nagy and Esiri (1998) described cell cycle disturbances and a possible apoptotic mechanism of hippocampal neuronal cell death in hippocampus obtained from patients with pharmacoresistant epilepsy, suggesting that neurons have re-entered the cell division cycle and reached the G_2 phase. Another interaction was described between the cell cycle machinery and the intrinsic processes in apoptotic neurons, with evidence that Cdk1 activates pro-apoptotic bad protein. Moreover, that interaction has also been associated with different pathological conditions such as stress, depression, and epilepsy (Becker and Bonni 2004).

Other studies trying to prove a causal relationship between changes in neurogenesis and the disease state (i.e., depression and epilepsy) have been controversial (Jung et al. 2006; Malberg et al. 2000; Scharfman et al. 2000).

6.6 Conclusions and Perspectives

In TLE, structural changes in the hippocampus are believed to play a key role in the generation of epileptic seizures. However, given the complexity of hippocampal circuitry and cell damage in case of hippocampal sclerosis, structural repair of epileptic hippocampal networks will require complex strategies in which proper integration and rewiring of the implanted neurons will be of crucial importance. The activation of cell-signalling pathways in response to acute seizures has dramatic consequences such as neuronal loss and irreversible loss of function. In the past 10 years, researchers have found molecular "signatures" of gene-directed cell death signalling strategy linked to apoptosis in brain samples from a subpopulation of patients with pharmacoresistant epilepsy who experience frequent seizures. Using animal models, researchers have shown that evoked seizures or epilepsy often activates the same signalling pathways, and drugs or genetic modulation of these cascades can reduce brain injury.

The analysis of molecular responses to seizure is not simple because biological processes are not uniform and experimental protocols differ. The identification of potential therapeutic targets should be facilitated by the knowledge of genes, proteins, and altered signalling pathways during the different stages of epilepsy development.

It is important to consider that most of the functional studies reviewed here support targeting apoptosis signalling pathways to prevent seizure-induced neuronal death. However, not all groups detect an apoptotic signature (Henshal and Murphy 2008). Also, protection of some cell populations may be more critical than others. Translating short-term to long-term neuroprotection will also be challenging. Apoptosis-regulatory genes with neuromodulatory properties may be particularly promising but, of course, raises concerns of its effects on brain function that targeting apoptosis pathways was originally expected to avoid.

A deep understanding of signalling pathways involved in both acute and long-term responses to seizures continues to be crucial to unravel the origins of epileptic behaviours. Therefore, additional studies would be necessary to identify those genes related to neuroprotection and/or those involved in neuronal activities related to epileptogenesis and could potentially represent target genes in design new preventive drugs for epilepsy.

Acknowledgements This work was partially supported by grants: CYTED (http://www.cyted.org/) through Group study of neuroscience Iberoamerican Network and CONACyT 00177594 to CBZ.

References

Aaronson DS, Horvath CM. A road map for those who don't know JAK-STAT. Science. 2002;296:1653–5.

Aronica E, Gorter JA. Gene expression profile in temporal lobe epilepsy. Neuroscientist. 2007;151:272–92.

Balosso S, Maroso M, Sanchez-Alavez M, Ravizza T, Frasca A, Bartfai T, et al. A novel non-transcriptional pathway mediates the proconvulsive effects of interleukin-1beta. Brain. 2008;131:3256–65.

Balosso S, Ravizza T, Pierucci M, Calcagno E, Invernizzi R, Di Giovanni G, et al. Molecular and functional interactions between tumor necrosis factor-alpha receptors and the glutamatergic system in the mouse hippocampus: implications for seizure susceptibility. Neuroscience. 2009;161:293–300.

Bartolomei F, Khalil M, Wendling F, Sontheimer A, Regis J, Ranjeva JP. Entorhinal cortex involvement in human mesial temporal lobe epilepsy: an electrophysiologic and volumetric study. Epilepsia. 2005;46:677–87.

Battle TE, Frank DA. The role of STATs in apoptosis. Curr Mol Med. 2002;2:381–92.

Bazil DP, Park J, Hemmings BA. PKB binding proteins: getting in on the Akt. Cell. 2002;111:293–303.

Becker EB, Bonni A. Cell cycle regulation of neuronal apoptosis in development and disease. Prog Neurobiol. 2004;72:1–25.

Becker AJ, Chen J, Zien A, Sochivko D, Normann S, Schramm J, et al. Correlated stage- and subfield-associated hippocampal gene expression patterns in experimental and human temporal lobe epilepsy. Eur J Neurosci. 2003;18:2792–802.

Blumcke I, Beck H, Lie AA, Wiestler OD. Molecular neuropathology of human mesial temporal lobe epilepsy. Epilepsy Res. 1999;36:205–23.

Borsello T, Forloni G. JNK signalling: a possible target to prevent neurodegeneration. Curr Pharm Des. 2007;13:1875–86.

Bozzi Y, Dunleavy M, Henshall DC. Cell signaling underlying epileptic behavior. Front Behav Neurosci. 2011;5:1–11.

Bratton SB, Salvesen GS. Regulation of the Apaf-1-caspase-9 apoptosome. J Cell Sci. 2010;123:3209–14.

Burgering PJC, Coffer PJ. Protein kinase B (c-Akt) in phosphatidylinositol-3-OH kinase signal transduction. Nature. 1995;376:599–602.

Cendes F. Febrile seizures and mesial temporal sclerosis. Curr Opin Neurol. 2002;17:161–4.

Chang L, Karin M. Mammalian MAP kinase signalling cascades. Nature. 2001;410:37–40.

Chen Z, Gibson TB, Robinson F, Silvestro L, Pearson G, Xu B, et al. MAP kinases. Chem Rev. 2001;101:2449–76.

Cheung EC, Slack RS. Emerging role for ERK as a key regulator of neuronal apoptosis. Sci STKE. 2004;2004(251):pe45.

Chiba T, Yamada M, Aiso S. Targeting the JAK2/STAT3 axis in Alzheimer's disease. Expert Opin Ther Targets. 2009;13:1155–67.

Chipuk JE, Green DR. PUMA cooperates with direct activator proteins to promote mitochondrial outer membrane permeabilization and apoptosis. Cell Cycle. 2009;8:2692–6.

Choi YS, Lin SL, Lee B, Kurup P, Cho HY, Naegele JR, et al. Status epilepticus induced somatostatinergic hilar interneuron degeneration is regulated by striatal enriched protein tyrosine phosphatase. J Neurosci. 2007;27:2999–3009.

Choi YS, Cho HY, Hoyt KR, Naegele JR, Obrietan K. IGF-1 receptor-mediated ERK/MAPK signaling couples status epilepticus to progenitor cell proliferation in the subgranular layer of the dentate gyrus. Glia. 2008;56:791–800.

Coffer PJ, Woodgett JR. Molecular cloning and characterisation of a novel putative protein-serine kinase related to the cAMP-dependent and protein kinase C families. Eur J Biochem. 1991;13:1401–9.

Cory S, Adams JM. The bcl2 family: regulators of the cellular life-or-death switch. Nat Rev Cancer. 2002;2:647–56.

Coulter DA, DeLorenzo RJ. Basic mechanisms of status epilepticus. Adv Neurol. 1999;79: 725–33.

Covolan L, Ribeiro LT, Longo BM, Mello LE. Cell damage and neurogenesis in the dentate granule cell layer of adult rats after pilocarpine- or kainate-induced status epilepticus. Hippocampus. 2000;10:169–80.

D'Mello SR, Galli C, Ciotti T, Calissano P. Induction of apoptosis in cerebellar granule neurons by low potassium: inhibition of death by insulin-like growth factor I and cAMP. Proc Natl Acad Sci USA. 1993;3(171):1–9.

Dalby NO, Mody I. The process of epileptogenesis: a pathophysiological approach. Curr Opin Neurol. 2001;14:187–92.

Danial NN, Korsmeyer SJ. Cell death: critical control points. Cell. 2004;116:205–19.

Datta SR, Dudek H, Tao X, Masters S, Fu H, Gotoh Y, et al. Akt phosphorylation of BAD couples survival signals to the cell-intrinsic death machinery. Cell. 1997;91:231–41.

De Lanerolle NC, Lee TS. New facets of the neuropathology and molecular profile of human temporal lobe epilepsy. Epilepsy Behav. 2005;7:190–203.

Debierre-Grockiego F. Anti-apoptotic role of STAT5 in haematopoietic cells and in the pathogenesis of malignancies. Apoptosis. 2004;9:717–28.

Detour J, Schroeder H, Desor D, Nehlig A. A 5-month period of epilepsy impairs spatial memory, decreases anxiety, but spares object recognition in the lithium-pilocarpine model in adult rats. Epilepsia. 2005;46:499–508.

Devinski O. Diagnosis and treatment of temporal lobe epilepsy. Rev Neurol Dis. 2004;1:2–9. http://ukpmc.ac.uk/abstract/MED/16397445.

Donovan N, Becker EB, Konishi Y, Bonni A. JNK phosphorylation and activation of BAD couples the stress-activated signaling pathway to the cell death machinery. J Biol Chem. 2002;277:40944–9.

Dorr J, Bechmann I, Waiczies S, Aktas O, Walckzac H, Krammer PH, et al. Lack of tumor necrosis factor-related apoptosis-inducing ligand but presence of its receptors in human brain. J Neurosci. 2002;22:RC209.

Dudek SM, Fields RD. Mitogen-activated protein kinase/extracellular signal-regulated kinase activation in somatodendritic compartments: roles of action potentials, frequency, and mode of calcium entry. J Neurosci. 2001;21:RC122.

Engel J. Mesial temporal lobe epilepsy: what have we learned? Neuroscientist. 2001;7:340–52.

Engel T, Henshall DC. Apoptosis, Bcl-2 family proteins and caspases: the ABCs of seizure-damage and epileptogenesis? Int J Physiol Pathophysiol Pharmacol. 2009;8:267–71.

Engel T, Murphy BM, Hatazaki S, Jimenez-Mateos EM, Concannon CG, Woods I, et al. Reduced hippocampal damage and epileptic seizures after status epilepticus in mice lacking proapoptotic Puma. FASEB J. 2010;24:853–61.

French JA, Kanner AM, Bautista J, About- Khalil B, Browne T, Harden CL, et al. Efficacy and tolerability of the new antiepileptic drugs I: Treatment of new onset epilepsy. Neurology. 2004; 62(8):1252–60.

Fujikawa DG. Neuroprotective strategies in status epilepticus. In: Wasterlain CG, Treiman DM, editors. Status epilepticus: mechanisms and management. Cambridge: MIT Press; 2006. p. 463–80.

Fujikawa DG, Shinmei SS, Cai B. Lithium-pilocarpine-induced status epilepticus produces necrotic neurons with internucleosomal DNA fragmentation in adults rats. Eur J Neurosci. 1999;11:1605–14.

Fujikawa DG, Shinmei SS, Cai B. Kainic acid-induced seizures produce necrotic, not apoptotic neurons with internucleosomal DNA cleavage: implications for programmed cell death mechanisms. Neuroscience. 2000;98:41–53.

Fujikawa DG, Ke X, Trinidad RB, Shinmei SS, Wu A. Caspase-3 is not activated in seizure-induced neuronal necrosis with internucleosomal DNA cleavage. J Neurochem. 2002;83: 229–40.

Gorter JA, van Vliet EA, Aronica E, Breit T, Rauwerda H, Lopes da Silva FH, et al. Potential new antiepileptogenic targets indicated by microarray analysis in a rat model for temporal lobe epilepsy. J Neurosci. 2006;26:11083–110.

Greene LA, Biswas SC, Liu DX. Cell cycle molecules and vertebrate neuron death: E2F at the hub. Cell Death Differ. 2004;11:49–60.

Guan QH, Pei DS, Zong YY, Xu TL, Zhang GY. Neuroprotection against ischemic brain injury by a small peptide inhibitor of c-Jun N-terminal kinase (JNK) via nuclear and non-nuclear pathways. Neuroscience. 2006;139:609–27.

Henshall DC, Murphy BM. Modulators of neuronal cell death in epilepsy. Curr Opin Pharmacol. 2008;8:75–81.

Henshall DC, Araki T, Schindler CK, Lan J-Q, Tiekoter KL, Taki W, et al. Activation of Bcl-2-associated death protein and counter-response of Akt within cell populations during seizure-induced neuronal death. Neurology. 2000a;55:250–7.

Henshall DC, Clark RS, Adelson PD, Chen M, Simon RP, Watkins SC. Alterations in bcl2 and caspases gene family protein expression in human temporal lobe epilepsy. Neurology. 2000b;55:250–7.

Henshall DC, Bonislawski DP, Skradski SL, Meller R, Lan J-Q, Simon RP. Cleavage of Bid may amplify caspase-8-induced neuronal death following focally evoked limbic seizures. Neurobiol Dis. 2001a;8:568–80.

Henshall DC, Bonislawski DP, Skradski SL, Araki T, Lan J-Q, Schindler CK, et al. Formation of the Apaf-1/cytochrome c complex precedes activation of caspase-9 during seizure induced neuronal death. Cell Death Differ. 2001b;8:1169–81.

Henshall DC, Skradski SL, Bonislawski DP, Lan JQ. Simon RP (2001c) Caspase-2 activation is redundant during seizure-induced neuronal death. J Neurochem. 2001c;77:886–95.

Houser CR, Huang CS, Peng Z. Dynamic seizure-related changes in extracellular signal-regulated kinase activation in a mouse model of temporal lobe epilepsy. Neuroscience. 2008;156:222–37.

Huang H, Tindal DJ. Dynamic FoxO transcription factors. J Cell Sci. 2007;120:2479–87.

Hunsberger JG, Bennett AH, Selvanayagam E, Duman RS, Newton SS. Gene profiling the response to kainic acid induced seizures. Brain Res Mol Brain Res. 2005;141:95–112.

Ino H, Chiba T. Cyclin-dependent kinase 4 and Cyclin D1 are required for excitotoxin-induced neuronal cell death *in vivo*. J Neurosci. 2001;21:6086–94. http://www.jneurosci.org/content/21/16/6086.short.

Jakubs K, Nanobashvili A, Bonde S, Ekdahl CT, Kokaia Z, Kokaia M, et al. Environment matters: synaptic properties of neurons born in the epileptic adult brain develop to reduce excitability. Neuron. 2006;52:1047–59.

Jakubs K, Bonde S, Iosif RE, Ekdahl CT, Kokaia Z, Kokaia M, et al. Inflammation regulates functional integration of neurons born in adult brain. J Neurosci. 2008;28:12477–88.

Jessberger S, Zhao C, Toni N, Clemenson Jr GD, Li Y, Gage FH. Seizure-associated, aberrant neurogenesis in adult rats characterized with retrovirus-mediated cell labeling. J Neurosci. 2007;27:9400–7.

Jordan-Sciutto KL, Dorsey R, Chalovich EM, Hammond RR, Achim CL. Expression patterns of retinoblastoma protein in Parkinson disease. J Neuropathol Exp Neurol. 2003;62:68–74.

Jung KH, Chu K, Lee ST, Kim J, Sinn DI, Kim JM, et al. Cyclooxygenase-2 inhibitor, celecoxib, inhibits the altered hippocampal neurogenesis with attenuation of spontaneous recurrent seizures following pilocarpine-induced status epilepticus. Neurobiol Dis. 2006;23:237–46.

Katchanov J, Harms C, Gertz K, Hauck L, Waeber C, Hirt L, et al. Mild cerebral ischemia induces loss of cyclin-dependent kinase inhibitors and activation of cell cycle machinery before delayed neuronal cell death. J Neurosci. 2001;21:5045–53.

Kawasaki H, Morooka T, Shimohama S, Kimura J, Hirano T, Gotoh Y, Nishida E. Activation and involvement of p38 mitogen-activated protein kinase in glutamate-induced apoptosis in rat cerebelar granulle cells. J Biol Chem. 1997;272:18518–521.

Kretz A, Happold CJ, Marticke JK, Isenmann S. Erythropoietin promotes regeneration of adult CNS neurons via Jak2/Stat3 and PI3K/AKT pathway activation. Mol Cell Neurosci. 2005;29:569–79.

Kroemer G, Galluzzi L, Brenner C. Mitochondrial membrane permeabilization in cell death. Physiol Rev. 2007;87:99–163.

Kyosseva SV. Mitogen-activated protein kinase signaling. Int Rev Neurobiol. 2004;59:201–20.

Li T, Lu C, Xia Z, Xiao B, Luo Y. Inhibition of caspase-8 attenuates neuronal death induced by limbic seizures in a cytochrome c-dependent and Smac/DIABLOindependent way. Brain Res. 2006;1098:204–11.

Liou AKF, Clark RS, Henshall DC, Yin XM, Chen J. To die or not to die for neurons in ischemia, traumatic brain injury and epilepsy: a review on the stress-activated signaling pathways and apoptotic pathways. Prog Neurobiol. 2003;69:103–42.

Lopez-Meraz ML, Niquet J, Wasterlain CG. Distinct caspase pathways mediate necrosis and apoptosis in subpopulations of hippocampal neurons after status epilepticus. Epilepsia. 2010;51:56–60.

Lund IV, Hu Y, Raol YH, Benham RS, Faris R, Russek SJ, et al. BDNF selectively regulates $GABA_A$ receptor transcription by activation of the JAK/STAT pathway. Sci Signal. 2008;1:ra9.

Malberg JE, Eisch AJ, Nestler EJ, Duman RS. Chronic antidepressant treatment increases neurogenesis in adult rat hippocampus. J Neurosci. 2000;20:9104–10.

Mathern GW, Cifuentes F, Leite JP, Pretorius JK, Babb TL. Hippocampal EEG excitability and chronic spontaneous seizures are associated with aberrant synaptic reorganization in the rat intrahippocampal kainate model. Electroencephalogr Clin Neurophysiol. 1993;87:326–39.

Mathern GW, Babb TL, Armstrong DL. Hippocampal sclerosis. In: Engel JJ, Pedley TA, editors. Epilepsy: a comprehensive textbook. Philadelphia: Lippincott-Raven Publishers; 1997. p. 133–55.

McCabe PH. New anti-epileptic drugs for the 21st century. Expert Opin Pharmacother. 2000;1: 633–74.

Mefford HC, Muhle H, Ostertag P, von Spiczak S, Buysse K, Baker C, et al. Genome-wide copy number variation in epilepsy: novel susceptibility loci in idiopathic generalized and focal epilepsies. PLoS Genet. 2010;6:e1000962.

Meldrum B. Excitotoxicity and epileptic brain damage. Epilepsy Res. 1991;10:55–61.

Meldrum B. Excitotoxicity and selective neuronal loss in epilepsy. Brain Pathol. 1993;3:405–12.

Meller R, Clayton C, Torrey DJ, Schindler CK, Lan JQ, Cameron JA, et al. Activation of the caspase 8 pathway mediates seizure-induced cell death in cultured hippocampal neurons. Epilepsy Res. 2006;70:3–14.

Miller FD, Gauthier AS. Timing is everything: making neurons versus glia in the developing cortex. Neuron. 2007;54:357–69.

Morgan JI, Curran T. Proto-oncogene transcription factors and epilepsy. Trends Pharmacol Sci. 1991,12:459–62.

Mukherjee PK, Decoster M, Campbell FZ, Davis RJ, Bazan NG. Glutamate receptor signaling interplay modulates stress-sensitive mitogen-activated protein kinases and neuronal cell death. J Biol Chem. 1999;274:6493–8.

Nagy Z, Esiri MM. Neuronal cyclin expression in the hippocampus in temporal lobe epilepsy. Exp Neurol. 1998;150:240–7.

Narkilahti S, Pirttila TJ, Lukasiuk K, Tuunanen J, Pitkanen A. Expression and activation of caspase 3 following status epilepticus in the rat. Eur J Neurosci. 2003;18:1486–96.

Nigg A. Cyclin-dependent protein kinases: key regulation of the eukaryotic cell cycle. Bioessays. 1995;17:471–80.

Niquet J, Auvin S, Archie M, Seo DW, Allen S, Sankar R, et al. Status epilepticus triggers caspase-3 activation and necrosis in the immature rat brain. Epilepsia. 2007;48:1203–6.

Okamoto OK, Janjoppi L, Bonone FM, Pansani AP, Da Silva AV, Scorza FA, et al. Whole transcriptome analysis of the hippocampus: toward a molecular portrait of epileptogenesis. BMC Genomics. 2010;11:230.

Okuno S, Saito A, Hayashi T, Chan PH. The c-Jun N-terminal protein kinase signaling pathway mediates Bax activation and subsequent neuronal apoptosis through interaction with Bim after transient focal cerebral ischemia. J Neurosci. 2004;24(36):7879–87.

Orrenius S, Zhivotovsky B, Nicotera P. Regulation of cell death: the calcium–apoptosis link. Nat Rev Mol Cell Biol. 2003;4:552–65.
Overstreet-Wadiche LS, Bromberg DA, Bensen AL, Westbrook GL. Seizures accelerate functional integration of adult-generated granule cells. J Neurosci. 2006;26:4095–103.
Parent JM, Janumpalli S, McNamara JO, Lowenstein DH. Increased dentate granule cell neurogenesis following amygdala kindling in the adult rat. Neurosci Lett. 1998;247:9–12.
Parent JM, Elliott RC, Pleasure SJ, Barbaro NM, Lowenstein DH. Aberrant seizure-induced neurogenesis in experimental temporal lobe epilepsy. Ann Neurol. 2006;59:81–91.
Pearson G, Robinson F, Beers Gibson T, Xu BE, Karandikar M, Berman K, Cobb MH. Mitogen-activated protein (MAP) kinase pathways: regulation and physiological functions. Endocr Rev. 2001;22(2):153–83.
Pickering M, Cumiskey D, O'Connor JJ. Actions of TNFalpha on glutamatergic synaptic transmission in the central nervous system. Exp Physiol. 2005;90:663–70.
Pitkänen A, Schwartzkroin P, Moshé S. Models of seizures and epilepsy. 1st ed. Burlington, MA: Academic; 2005.
Putcha GV, Le S, Frank S, Besirli CG, Clark K, Chu B, et al. JNK-mediated BIM phosphorylation potentiates BAX-dependent apoptosis. Neuron. 2003;38:899–914.
Radley JJ, Jacobs BL. Pilocarpine-induced status epilepticus increases cell proliferation in the dentate gyrus of adult rats via a 5-HT_{1A} receptor-dependent mechanism. Brain Res. 2003;966:1–12.
Raivich G, Bohatschek M, Da Costa C, Iwata O, Galiano M, Hristova M, et al. The AP-1 transcription factor c-Jun is required for efficient axonal regeneration. Neuron. 2004;43:7–67.
Riazi K, Galic MA, Pittman QJ. Contributions of peripheral inflammation to seizure susceptibility: cytokines and brain excitability. Epilepsy Res. 2010;89:34–42.
Roos WP, Kaina B. DNA damage-induced cell death by apoptosis. Trends Mol Med. 2006;12:440–50.
Salvesen GS, Riedl SJ. Programmed cell death in cancer progression and therapy. Adv Exp Med Biol. 2007;615:13–23.
Sastry PS, Rao KS. Apoptosis and the nervous system. J Neurochem. 2000;74(1):1–20.
Scharfman HE, Goodman JH, Sollas AL. Granule-like neurons at the hilar/CA3 border after status epilepticus and their synchrony with area CA3 pyramidal cells: functional implications of seizure induced neurogenesis. J Neurosci. 2000;20:6144–58.
Schindler CK, Pearson EG, Bonner HP, So NK, Simon RP, Prehn JH, et al. Caspase-3 cleavage and nuclear localization of caspase-activated DNase in human temporal lobe epilepsy. J Cereb Blood Flow Metab. 2006;26:583–9.
Scott BW, Wang S, Burnham WM, De BU, Wojtowicz JM. Kindling-induced neurogenesis in the dentate gyrus of the rat. Neurosci Lett. 1998;248:73–6.
Shinoda S, Skradski SL, Araki T, Schindler CK, Meller R, Lan J-Q. Formation of a tumour necrosis factor receptor 1 molecular scaffolding complex and activation of apoptosis signal-regulating kinase 1 during seizure-induced neuronal death. Eur J Neurosci. 2003;17:2065–76.
Shinoda S, Schindler CK, Meller R, So NK, Araki T, Yamamoto A, et al. Bim regulation may determine hippocampal vulnerability after injurious seizures and in temporal lobe epilepsy. J Clin Invest. 2004;113:1059–68.
Silva M, Benito A, Sanz C. Erythropoietin can induce the expression of bcl-x(L) through Stat5 in erythropoietin-dependent progenitor cell lines. J Biol Chem. 1999;274:22165–9.
Sloviter RS. Status epilepticus-induced neuronal injury and network reorganization. Epilepsia. 1999;40:s34–9.
Sloviter RS. Hippocampal epileptogenesis in animal models of mesial temporal lobe epilepsy with hippocampal sclerosis: the importance of the "latent period" and other concepts. Epilepsia. 2008;49:85–92.
Smolders I, Khan GM, Manil J, Ebinger G, Michotte Y. NMDA receptor-mediated pilocarpine-induced seizures: characterization in freely moving rats by microdialysis. Br J Pharmacol. 2009;121:1171–9.
Song G, Ouyang G, Bao S. The activation of Akt/PKB signaling pathway and cell survival. J Cell Mol Med. 2005;9:59–71.

Stavrovskaya IG, Kristal BS. The powerhouse takes control of the cell: is the mitochondrial permeability transition a viable therapeutic target against neuronal dysfunction and death? Free Radic Biol Med. 2005;38:687–97.

Stellwagen D, Beattie EC, Seo JY, Malenka RC. Differential regulation of AMPA receptor and GABA receptor trafficking by tumor necrosis factor-alpha. J Neurosci. 2005;25(12):3219–28.

Strasser A, O'Connor L, Dixit VM. Apoptosis signaling. Annu Rev Biochem. 2000;69:217–45.

Sun W, Gould TW, Newbern J, Milligan C, Choi SY, Kim H, et al. Phosphorylation of c-Jun in avian and mammalian motoneurons in vivo during programmed cell death: an early reversible event in the apoptotic cascade. J Neurosci. 2005;25:5595–603.

Sutula TP. Mechanisms of epilepsy progression: current theories and perspectives from neuroplasticity in adulthood and development. Epilepsy Res. 2004;60:161–71.

Thom M, Martinian L, Williams G, Stoeber K, Sisodiya SM. Cell proliferation and granule cell dispersion in human hippocampal sclerosis. J Neuropathol Exp Neurol. 2005;64:194–201.

Timsit S, Menn B. Cerebral ischemia, cell cycle elements and Cdk5. Biotechnol J. 2007;2: 958–66.

Turski L, Ikonomidou CH, Turski WA, Bortolotto ZA, Cavalheiro EA. Cholinergic mechanisms and epileptogenesis. The seizures induced by pilocarpine: a novel experimental model of intractable epilepsy. Synapse. 1989;3:154–71.

Vezzani A, Balosso S, Ravizza T. The role of cytokines in the pathophysiology of epilepsy. Brain Behav Immun. 2008;22:797–803.

Wajant H. The Fas signaling pathway: more than a paradigm. Science. 2002;296(5573):1635–6.

Walker TL, White A, Black DM, Wallace RH, Sah P, Bartlett PF. Latent stem and progenitor cells in the hippocampus are activated by neural excitation. J Neurosci. 2008;28:5240–7.

Wang W, Yang Y, Ying C, Li W, Ruan H, Zhu X, et al. Inhibition of glycogen synthase kinase-3beta protects dopaminergic neurons from MPTP toxicity. Neuropharmacology. 2007;52:1678–84.

Weise J, Engelhorn T, Dorfler A, Aker S, Bahr M, Hufnagel A. Expression time course and spatial distribution of activated caspase-3 after experimental status epilepticus: contribution of delayed neuronal cell death to seizure-induced neuronal injury. Neurobiol Dis. 2005;18:582–90.

Wessel TC, Joh TH, Volpe BT. In situ hybridization analysis of c-fos and c-jun expression in the rat brain following transient forebrain ischemia. Brain Res. 1991;567:231–40.

Wieser HG. ILAE Commission report. Mesial temporal lobe epilepsy with hippocampal sclerosis. Epilepsia. 2004;45:695–714.

Xu C, Bailly-Maitre B, Reed JC. Endoplasmic reticulum stress: cell life and death decisions. J Clin Invest. 2005;115(10):2656–64.

Yadav A, Kalita A, Dhillon S, Banerjee K. JAK/STAT3 pathway is involved in survival of neurons in response to insulin-like growth factor and negatively regulated by suppressor of cytokine signaling-3. J Biol Chem. 2005;280:31830–40.

Yamaoka K, Saharinen P, Pesu M, Holt V, Silvennoinen O, O'Shea JJ. The Janus kinases (Jaks). Genome Biol. 2004;5:253.

Yang DD, Kuan CY, Withmarsh AJ, Rincon M, Zheng TS, Davis RJ, et al. Absence of excitotoxicity-induced apoptosis in the hippocampus of mice lacking the jnk3 gene. Nature. 1997;389: 865–70.

Yang Y, Geldmacher DS, Herrup K. DNA replication precedes neuronal cell death in Alzheimer's disease. J Neurosci. 2001;21:2661–8.

Yang Y, Mufson EJ, Herrup K. Neuronal cell death is preceded by cell cycle events at all stages of Alzheimer's disease. J Neurosci. 2003;23:2557–63.

Yeste-Velasco M, Folch J, Pallàs M, Camins A. The p38(MAPK) signaling pathway regulates neuronal apoptosis through the phosphorylation of the retinoblastoma protein. Neurochem Int. 2009;54:99–105.

Yoon S, Seger R. The extracellular signal-regulated kinase: multiple substrates regulate diverse celular functions. Growth Factors. 2006;24:21–44.

Chapter 7
The Role of JNK Pathway in the Process of Excitotoxicity Induced by Epilepsy and Neurodegeneration

Carme Auladell, Felix Junyent, Aurelio Vazquez de la Torre, Maria Luisa de Lemos, Mercè Pallàs, Ester Verdaguer Cardona, and Antoni Camins Espuny

Abstract The c-Jun N-terminal kinases (JNKs) are members of the MAPK family and can be activated in neurons by different neurotoxins such as kainic acid (an experimental model of epilepsy), beta amyloid, and nitropropionic acid. Although JNKs have different physiological functions they have been linked mainly to the apoptotic process in neurons and other cell types. Therefore, the JNK signaling pathway constitutes an important target to prevent the apoptotic cell death in epilepsy and neurodegeneration. In the present chapter, the role of JNKs, specifically the JNK3 isoform, as a potential target for epilepsy and neurodegenerative diseases will be discussed. In addition, the pharmacological compounds that inhibit the JNKs signaling pathway constitutes a potential therapeutic intervention to prevent neuronal death.

Keywords C-Jun N-terminal kinase • JNK3 • Epilepsy • Alzheimer's disease • Neurodegeneration • Apoptosis

---

C. Auladell • E. Verdaguer Cardona
Departament de Biologia Cellular, Universitat de Barcelona, Avenida Diagonal 645, Barcelona 08028, Spain

F. Junyent
Unitat de Bioquimica, Facultat de Medicina i Ciencies de la Salut, Universitat Rovira i Virgili, C./St. Llorenc 21 Reus (Tarragona), Barcelona 46201, Spain

A. Vazquez de la Torre • M.L. de Lemos • M. Pallàs • A. Camins Espuny (✉)
Institute of Biomedicine, Department of Pharmacology and Biomedical Chemistry, University of Barcelona, Avenida Diagonal 643, Barcelona 08028, Spain
e-mail: camins@ub.edu

L. Rocha and E.A. Cavalheiro (eds.), *Pharmacoresistance in Epilepsy: From Genes and Molecules to Promising Therapies*, DOI 10.1007/978-1-4614-6464-8_7,

7.1 Introduction

One of the biggest health problems that we have today is the development of effective drugs for the treatment of neurodegenerative diseases and epilepsy. The cause is clear, in the case of the neurodegenerative diseases the population over 65 is growing, at least in developed countries and favors the emergence of neurological diseases (Smith et al. 1999). In the treatment of epilepsy, the pharmacoresistance is probably one of the main problems in the treatment of this neurological disease. Thus, in next coming years, the aims will be develop effective drugs for the prevention of neuronal death process that occurs in neurological diseases.

Although it is well known the participation of more than one pathway in the process of neuronal loss, for example the cell cycle activation, GSK3β, cdk5, oxidative stress among them, c-Jun N-terminal kinase (c-JNKs) constitutes one of the main pathway related with cell death (McCubrey et al. 2006; Levy et al. 2009). Thus c-JNKs are an interesting target for the development of drugs for the treatment of neurodegenerative disorders (Borsello and Forloni 2007; Braithwaite et al. 2010).

It is well know that c-JNKs is a member of the family of serine and threonine mitogen-activated protein kinases (MAPKs) which participates in numerous physiological processes such as tissue differentiation, cancer, diabetes, cell survival and apoptosis, and other pathogenic processes (Bevilaqua et al. 2003; Borsello and Bonny 2004; Eshraghi et al. 2007; Borsello et al. 2003). Thus, MAPKs allows the cell to respond to exogenous and endogenous stimuli integrating signals into complex cytoplasmic and nuclear processes. Currently, it has been characterized four mammalian MAPK cascades: (a) extracellular signal-regulated kinase 1 and 2 (ERK1/2), (b) c-Jun N-terminal kinases (c-JNKs), (c) p38 consisting of four isoforms (α, β, γ, and δ), and (d) ERK5 (Bozyczko-Coyne et al. 2002; Brecht et al. 2005; Borsello and Forloni 2007).

Three genes encoding for c-JNKs have been characterized in humans (*Jnk1*, *Jnk2*, and *Jnk3*). Some differences exist among the three isoforms codified by these genes, since whereas JNK1 and JNK2 are widely distribute in all organism tissues, JNK3 mainly shows a neuronal localization and thus constitutes a target for neuronal death prevention (Brecht et al. 2005; de Lemos et al. 2010). MAPK pathways are activated either as a result of a series of interactions between the kinase components or through the formation of a signaling complex that contains multiple kinases, driven by a scaffold protein (Behrens et al. 1999; Morrison and Davis 2003; Björkblom et al. 2008; Borsello et al. 2003). C-JNKs are activated by phosphorylation of Thr and Tyr residues in the activation loop by mitogen-activated protein kinase kinase 4 (MKK4) and kinase kinase 7 (MKK7) (Weston and Davis, 2007). Interactions between proteins and scaffold proteins are crucial for MAPK function and regulation in the cell. For instance, kinase suppressor of Ras-1 (KSR) and MEK partner 1 (MP1) act as scaffold proteins for the ERK signaling pathway, whereas JNK-interacting proteins (JIPs) serve as scaffold proteins for the c-JNK pathway. Likewise, β-arrestin 2 acts as a scaffold protein for both the ERK and the JNK signaling pathways. Following activation, c-JNKs can phosphorylate and modulate the activities of hundreds of substrates (Borsello and Forloni 2007). Among the substrates identified that are phosphorylated in the nucleus include some hormone receptors, as well as transcription factors such as the activator protein-1 (AP-1), the family of Jun factors (c-Jun, JunB, Jund), Elk-1, p53, the anti-activation transcription factor-2 (ATF-2), JDP2, c-Myc, the NAFT family, the STAT family, and the PAX family (Bogoyevitch and Kobe). For many of these factors, phosphorylation increases its activity and induces transcriptional gene expression. Currently, the most studied substrate for c-JNKs is c-Jun; however, it is not known which isoform is responsible for its phosphorylation. Interestingly, the high expression of both *c-Jun* gene and the great protein levels precedes or coincides with periods of cell death, such as that occurring during embryonic development (Herdegen et al. 1997; Coffey et al. 2000), after trauma (Bozyczko-Coyne et al. 2002; Suckfuell et al. 2007), cerebral ischemia (Tian et al. 2005; Hu et al. 2008), and seizures (Gass et al. 1993; de Lemos et al. 2010). This link of c-JNKs to neuronal death have attracted enormous interest of this pathway in several neurodegenerative disorders such as Alzheimer diseases (AD) and Parkinson diseases (PD) (Resnick and Fennell 2004). In this chapter, we reviewed the progress in understanding the role of c-JNKs in the pathophysiology of neurodegenerative diseases and the potential role of JNK inhibitors to treat neurodegenerative disorders.

7.2 Role of c-Jun N-Terminal Kinase Activation in Apoptosis

Some mechanisms have been proposed to explain how the c-JNKs pathway governs the whole process of neuronal death by apoptosis. For example, c-JNKs directly phosphorylate and regulate the pro- and anti-apoptotic activity of members of the B-cell lymphoma 2 (Bcl-2) families (Sun et al. 2005; Vogel et al. 2009; Donovan et al. 2002; Björkblom et al. 2008). The Bcl-2 family proteins can be divided into three major subgroups: (1) Anti-apoptotic proteins, such as Bcl 2, Bcl-XL, and Mcl-1, which typically share four conserved motifs termed Bcl-2 homology (BH) domains and can form heterodimers with Bax, inhibiting mitochondrial cytochrome c release and protecting against cell death; (2) The pro-apoptotic proteins, such as Bax, Bak, and Bok, which typically have three BH domains but promote cytochrome *c* release and apoptosis; (3) The BH3-only proteins, including Dp5/HRK (death protein 5/harakiri), Bim (Bcl2-interacting mediator of cell death), Bid, Bad, Puma, and Noxa, which share the BH3 domain. Thus BH3-only proteins are critical initiators of apoptosis and during this process are stringently regulated at the transcriptional and posttranslational levels depending on the cell type and apoptotic stimulus (Morishima et al. 2001; Puthalakath and Strasser 2002) (Fig. 7.1).

Dp5 is one of the BH3-only proteins of particular interest to studies of apoptosis in the nervous system. Dp5 was the first found to be induced by NGF deprivation in sympathetic neurons. The induction of Dp5 is also observed in cerebellar granule neurons (CGNs) deprived of potassium, cortical neurons exposed to toxic concentrations of β-amyloid protein, retinal ganglion cells of axotomized rat retinas, and

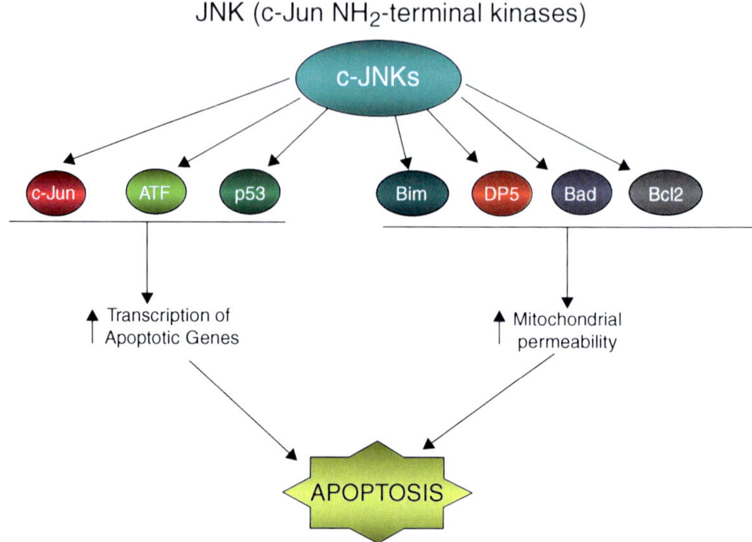

Fig. 7.1 Proposed mechanisms by which JNKs could regulate the apoptotic process. JNKs can induce the expression of nuclear genes that promote neuronal apoptosis. Furthermore, pro-apoptotic proteins can be phosphorylate by JNKs and are translocate to the mitochondrial and induce neuronal apoptosis

postnatal mouse motoneurons (Ma et al. 2007). Over expression of Dp5 in sympathetic neurons or CGNs induces apoptosis in a Bax-dependent manner, and this effect can be attenuated by co-expression of anti-apoptotic Bcl-2. Deletion of Dp5 delays sympathetic neuron apoptosis triggered by NGF withdrawal and rescues motoneurons from axotomy-induced apoptosis (Coultas et al. 2007). These studies suggest that Dp5 plays a critical role in neuronal apoptosis.

Studies from several laboratories have demonstrated that JNK is involved in *dp5* upregulation during neuronal injury or apoptosis. Although JNK has been shown to be involved in *dp5* upregulation, the mechanism of how JNK regulates *dp5* expression is not clarified.

c-JNKs phosphorylate and decrease the anti-apoptotic activity of both Bcl-2 and Bcl-XL. In addition, these kinases phosphorylate the pro-apoptotic protein BAD at Ser-128, thereby potentiating its pro-apoptotic effect (Donovan et al. 2002; Bogoyevitch and Kobe 2006). Similarly, c-JNKs phosphorylate the pro-apoptotic proteins Bim and Bcl-2-modifying factor (Bmf), causing their release and translocation to the mitochondria, where they promote the release of mitochondrial proteins such as cytochrome c, apoptosis-inducing factor (AIF), and other mitochondrial pro-apoptotic death mediators. Therefore, the release of cytochrome c and other pro-apoptotic proteins from the mitochondria is regulated by the Bcl-2 protein family. Finally, all these processes favor the process of cell death by activation of a caspase-dependent or independent pathway.

7.3 Experimental Data with JNK Inhibitors

Since the activation of the c-JNKs pathway may be a common step in neurodegeneration the pharmacological inhibition of c-JNKs is a potential strategy to protect against neuronal loss. In this sense, we highlight three chemical inhibitors: CEP-1347, an inhibitor of the MLK family of the c-JNKs pathway, and SP600125 and AS601245, both selective inhibitors of c-JNKs activity (Chen et al. 2010; Chambers et al. 2011).

The main limitation of the CEP-1347 inhibitor is its poor selectivity because it acts upstream of JNK activators, namely the MLKs (Saporito et al. 2002). This compound has shown neuroprotective effects both in vitro and in vivo against β-amyloid toxicity, trophic withdrawal in PC12 cells, MPP+ exposure and apoptosis in cerebellar granule cells following serum and potassium deprivation (Maroney et al. 1999). Moreover, in addition to inhibiting the pro-apoptotic JNK pathway, this drug activates neurotrophic pathways, including the neurotrophin BDNF in a mouse model of Huntington disease (HD). Specifically, CEP-1347 increases BDNF mRNA levels in the brain compared to vehicle, which correlates with a reduction of disease progression in R6/2 mice, an experimental model of HD (Apostol et al. 2008).

However, although the PRECEPT clinical trial showed that CEP-1347 was safe and well-tolerated in a randomized placebo-controlled study in PD subjects, it was concluded that this drug was not effective to treat PD. Nevertheless, further studies are needed to assess why this drug was not effective (The Parkinson Study Group PRECEPT Investigators 2007).

SP600125 is a reversible ATP-competitive inhibitor that can inhibit JNK, including JNK-1, -2, and -3 isoforms, with high selectivity. The neuroprotective effect of SP600125 has been seen in ischemic processes (Guan et al. 2005). Other studies have further demonstrated that SP600125 can inhibit the phosphorylation of c-Jun and prevent the expression of IL-2, IFN-γ, TNF-α, and COX-2, while inactivating Bcl-2 and blocking IL-1-induced accumulation of p-c-Jun and inducing c-Jun transcription (Guan et al. 2005; Choi et al. 2010; Chen et al. 2010; Chambers et al. 2011).

SP600125 blocked the induction of BH3-only protein Bim after seizures in mice, suggesting that the JNK pathway may be critical in epilepsy/neurodegeneration. Interestingly, Chen and colleagues (2010) reported that SP600125 was effective in the treatment of experimental temporal lobe epilepsy (TLE) in rats (Murphy et al. 2010). Moreover, SP600125 exerts neuroprotective effects against MPTP-induced neurotoxicity in mice, inhibiting JNK signaling and also reducing COX-2 expression (Wang et al. 2004). Likewise, SP600125 displays neuroprotective functions in β-amyloid-injected rats, as it has potent memory-enhancing effects and blocks learning deficits induced by β-amyloid (Ramin et al. 2011). In addition to the neuroprotective properties of SP600125, this compound also improves neuroplasticity. Effectively, this JNK inhibitor increases synaptic transmission in the hippocampus after treatment with β-amyloid in the CA1 area, suggesting a role of JNK in regulating short-term memory formation. More studies are required to evaluate the effects of SP600125 in β-amyloid production in AD models; however, its low water solubility limits its usefulness in human treatment.

AS601245 is also a reversible ATP-competitive inhibitor that inhibits the three JNK isoforms, with a higher affinity for JNK3. This compound exhibits neuroprotective effects in models of ischemia (Carboni et al. 2004). It also decreases microglial activation and exerts beneficial effects on memory deficits.

As mentioned above, JNK activity can be regulated by JNK-interacting proteins, such as JIP-1, a protein that integrates the positive and negative regulators of JNK, facilitating the activity of the JNK signaling pathway. In mice, JIP-1 contains a JNK-binding domain (JBD) that mediates the sequestration of JNK in the cytoplasm, thus inhibiting the expression of genes that are activated via the JNK signaling pathway and acts as a functional inhibitor of JNK. Therefore, in addition to chemical inhibitors, JIP-derived peptides have been developed to inhibit JNK activity b*ased* on the properties of the protein JIP-1. The peptide is XG-102, also called D-JNK-permeable peptide 1 (D-JNKI), exerts neuroprotective effects against different models of excitotoxicity in vitro and plays a neuroprotective role in experimental models of ischemia, preventing cell death by apoptosis (Pan et al. 2010; Liu et al. 2010). Thus, rather than inhibiting the enzymatic activity of JNKs as classical chemical inhibitors do, XG-102 selectively blocks the access of JNK to different substrates, preventing protein–protein interactions without interfering with its activation. Moreover, XG-102 has been observed to show beneficial effects on both hair cell death and the permanent loss of hearing induced by sound trauma (Wang et al. 2007). A phase I/II clinical study with XG-102 are currently underway to evaluate the efficacy of this compound in patients with acute acoustic trauma; the study will be completed in 2012. Therefore, in the coming years, more clinical data will shed light on the neuroprotective potential of these compounds.

7.4 Role of the JNK3 Pathway in Epilepsy

Knockouts for the mammalian Jnk genes *Jnk1*, *Jnk2*, and *Jnk3* are viable and have enabled the study of the physiological and pathological roles of the JNK pathway (de Lemos et al. 2010). The first evidence of the role of *Jnk3* in neurotoxicity was provided by Yang and colleagues (1997), who demonstrated that in comparison to wild-type mice, *Jnk3* (–/–) mice were less sensitive to seizures induced by kainic acid and to neuronal death in the hippocampal CA1 and CA3 areas. Furthermore, *Jnk3* (–/–) mice remain viable during development and show normal brain structure. These studies were the first which demonstrated that *Jnk3* deletion is a suitable target to prevent both neuronal cell death and seizures elicited (Yang et al. 1997). Subsequent studies demonstrated that *Jnk3* (–/–) mice had increased p110-beta protein levels and PI3K activity because of an upregulation of the *pik3cb*. This gene selectively increases neuroprotective cell pathways; however, it is unknown how the PI3K/Akt signaling pathway is activated in the absence of JNK3 (Junyent et al. 2011). On the other hand, *Jnk1* (–/–) null mice did not shown any changes in AKT activity in the hippocampus and probably could explain why loss of *Jnk1* or *Jnk2* did not show any effects against KA treatment (Brecht et al. 2005).

All these experimental data suggest that JNK3 is required to induce neuronal stress and apoptosis in adult hippocampus. The disruption of *Jnk1* or *Jnk2* does not affect the nervous system, but double knockout Jnk1 (−/−) Jnk2 (−/−) mice die during embryonic development with major alterations in the neural phenotype (Kuan et al. 1999). This is because the neural tube fails to close due to a deficiency in apoptosis. However, the opposite effect has been observed in the developing cortex brain, where there is an increase in apoptosis (Kuan et al. 1999). This indicates that *Jnk1* and *Jnk2* are necessary for the development of cell death in the neural tube and, in turn, for promoting cell survival during cerebral cortex development. Thus, although c-JNKs and c-Jun proteins are pro-apoptotic in different cell types, they may have other functions, as already mentioned. Furthermore, induction of axonal regeneration in axotomised peripheral neurons in an adult organism appears to be associated with increased expression of c-Jun, suggesting that this transcription factor regulates the expression of genes related to regeneration (Herdegen et al. 1997).

As we have commented above, the first evidence of the involvement of c-JNKs in experimental epilepsy models was derived from the reduction of seizures activity and prevention of apoptosis in JNK3-deficient mice treated with kainic acid (Yang et al. 1997). In addition, mice with an inactive form of the c-jun gene (Jun AA: alanine instead of serine at positions 63 and 73) showed resistance to excitotoxic neuronal death. These data opened the study of a specific target to protect against epilepsy seizures and also neurodegenerative disorders. Thus, blocking the access of c-JNKs to their substrate c-Jun may offer a suitable target in neuroprotection (Behrens et al. 2001).

Interestingly Murphy and colleagues demonstrate that Bim has a causal role in the status epilepticus-induced cell death process because neurodegeneration was reduced in bim(−/−) mice (Murphy et al. 2010). Bim is a downstream BH3-only protein target regulated by JNKs. These data indicate that loss of a specific BH3-only can reduce seizure damage in vivo.

7.5 Role of JNK3 in Alzheimer's Disease

Alzheimer's disease (AD) is currently the leading global cause of dementia in the elderly. At the initial stages, AD is characterized by a mild loss of memory and then progresses to a severe loss of cognitive performance in the advanced stages (Xu et al. 2009; Zhu et al. 2001; Mondragón-Rodríguez et al. 2010). AD is characterized by a series of histological markers that include neurofibrillary tangles, senile plaques, and a large loss of neurons (Castellani et al. 2009). Apart from these markers, the loss of neurons is associated with apoptosis, which is probably mediated by several inducers such as reactive oxygen species, β-amyloid, mitochondrial alteration, and an inflammatory process that induces microglial activation in the AD brain (Su et al. 2008). In this process of neuronal demise in AD, different signaling pathways are activated and among them, the c-JNKs pathway plays a prominent role. This is based on several lines of evidence: (a) c-JNKs can phosphorylate tau and

(b) β-amyloid activates the c-JNKs pathway that then promotes neuronal loss and this activation mediates β-amyloid toxicity (Ramin et al. 2011; Morishima et al. 2001; Colombo et al. 2009; Mazzitelli et al. 2011). Furthermore, it has been previously reported that expression of c-Jun increases in the AD brain and neurons from c-Jun-null mice are resistant to β-amyloid toxicity (Mazzitelli et al. 2011).

Morishima and colleagues were the first to demonstrate that neuronal hippocampal and cortical cultures of JNK3 knockout mice were partially protected from neuronal apoptosis mediated by β-amyloid (Morishima et al. 2001). However, c-Jun phosphorylation was not completely inhibited, indicating that JNK1 or JNK2 may be involved in this phosphorylation (Morishima et al. 2001). On the other hand, a very important point in AD is the formation of β-amyloid fragments that are derived from amyloid precursor protein (APP) after cleavage by beta/gamma secretase. The C-terminal intracellular region (AICD) of APP plays an important functional role in regulating APP metabolism (Slomnicki et al. 2008). AICD contains eight potential phosphorylation sites, but one of them, specifically T668, is phosphorylated by several kinases including GSK3β, JNK3, Cdc2, and Cdk5. Likewise, these kinases are associated with neurotoxicity and have been implicated in neurodegenerative diseases. Interestingly, JNK3 is specifically involved in the physiological regulation of AICD during neuronal differentiation, suggesting a role of JNK3 in synaptogenesis (Kimberly et al. 2005).

Moreover, Colombo and colleagues used the JNK inhibitor peptide (D-JNKI1) to demonstrate that JNK plays a prominent role in APP production and that the extracellular β-amyloid fragments are also reduced (Colombo et al. 2009). It has been observed that β-secretase (BACE1) is regulated by BACE1 gene transcription through the JNK/c-Jun signaling pathway (Sclip et al. 2011). This is important because it has been hypothesized that β-amyloid fragments are mainly responsible for the neurodegeneration in AD.

Studies performed in neuronal cell cultures have shown that JNK3 is involved in the apoptotic process mediated by β-amyloid. This process involves MLK3–MKK7–JNK3 activation, as well as downstream events including p-JNK nuclear localization, c-Jun phosphorylation and Bad translocation to the mitochondria, with the mitochondria then releasing pro-apoptotic proteins (Sclip et al. 2011).

7.6 Role of JNK3 in Experimental Models of Parkinson's Disease

Parkinson's disease (PD) is the second most common neurodegenerative disease. The mechanisms involved in its pathogenesis include oxidative stress production, mitochondrial dysfunction, and protein aggregation, which promote the loss of dopaminergic neurons in the substantia nigra pars compacta (Levy et al. 2009). Currently, the main problem of PD and all neurodegenerative diseases is that therapy is focused on symptomatic relief. It is necessary to develop neuroprotective therapies that will slow disease progression. The investigation of cell death mechanisms common to several models of experimental PD may identify new drug targets for treatment.

It has been reported that in mice exposed to MPTP, a PD neurotoxin that inhibits mitochondrial complex I, dopaminergic neurons degenerate in the substantia nigra (Peng and Andersen 2003; Saporito et al. 2000; Hunot et al. 2004; Pan et al. 2009; Choi et al. 2010). Inhibiting c-JNKs or their upstream signals may reduce dopamine-mediated neuronal death induced by MPTP, suggesting a possible therapeutic application for c-JNK inhibitors in PD (Pan et al. 2010). Additionally, dopaminergic neuronal death induced by MPTP, rotenone, paraquat, and 6-hydroxydopamine all require JNK3 activation (Hunot et al. 2004; Pan et al. 2007; Pan et al. 2009; Pan et al. 2010). Therefore, JNK3 is a critical and common mediator of dopaminergic neuronal death in PD experimental models.

Hunot and colleagues demonstrated that mice treated with MPTP showed increased COX-2 expression that was mediated by JNK (Hunot, et al. 2004). Interestingly, COX-2 expression is upregulated in PD brains and is generally induced by stress stimuli. Moreover, COX-2 localizes in neurons and its expression is upregulated in numerous pathological conditions, including Alzheimer's disease. Therefore, COX-2 induction might represent an important step in the cascade of molecular events leading to neuronal loss in PD.

Disappointingly, a clinical trial using CEP1347 to treat PD was terminated because it failed to produce significant improvements. The main problem of this compound is its poor selectivity against JNK3, the main target involved in apoptosis. As we previously discussed, JNK1 and 2 are ubiquitously expressed in adult tissues and have important physiological functions; hence, the side effects associated with inhibiting these enzymes limit the tolerable doses of JNK inhibitors. Accordingly, general inhibition of all JNK isoforms, such as that achieved by CEP1347, may be of limited benefit to treat neurodegenerative diseases. On the other hand, JNK3 is neural-specific and does not exhibit high basal activity in the brain. Therefore, selective or specific inhibition of the JNK3 isoform may be more specific to slow down PD progression.

7.7 JNK and Huntington's Disease

Huntington's disease (HD) is a progressive neurodegenerative disorder caused by an autosomal dominant mutation in either of the two copies of the huntingtin gene. Specifically, this disorder is caused by an abnormal expansion of a CAG codon in exon-1 of the gene (Liu 1998; Garcia et al. 2002).

Systemic administration of mitochondrial toxin 3-nitropropionic acid (3-NPA) to experimental animals, such as nonhuman primates and rodents, produces symptoms similar to those of human HD. The toxin irreversibly inhibits the succinate dehydrogenase (SDH) enzyme, the main constituent of the mitochondrial respiratory chain complex (MCC) II (Garcia et al. 2002). Treatment of rats and in vitro primary striatal cultures with 3-NPA activates the JNK pathway and contributes to neuronal death (Perrin et al. 2009). This neuronal loss depends on c-Jun because expression of dominant negative c-Jun protects striatal neurons from cell death mediated by this complex II inhibitor. Likewise, JNK activation appears to be a major factor in the apoptotic death of HN33 cells induced by polyglutamine-expanded huntingtin (Liu 1998). Mutated huntingtin with 48 or 89 polyglutamine repeats enhances JNK activation and may trigger apoptosis, while normal huntingtin with 16 repeats fails to activate the JNK pathway.

However, a recent study demonstrated that the intraperitoneal administration of 3-NPA to Jnk3(−/−) mice was not neuroprotective in contrast to the neurotoxin KA (Junyent et al. 2012). This suggests that although the JNK pathway may be activated in this model, JNK3 is probably not mainly responsible for neuronal death and other pathways may be involved in neuronal loss.

7.8 Role of JNK3 and Ischemia

Pirianov and colleagues were the first to describe the neuroprotective role of the specific isoform of JNK3 in a model of hypoxic–ischemic injury (Pirianov et al. 2007). They demonstrated that the deletion of JNK3 had a neuroprotective role by reducing ATF-2 phosphorylation, which was associated with the size of the infarct. Therefore, it was proposed that the JNK3/c-Jun/ATF-2 pathway was likely to be the main route in neural cell death induced by hypoxic–ischemic injury. Moreover, the authors demonstrated that JNK3 activation phosphorylated c-Jun, which has been shown to trigger the transcription of a large number of death genes including the pro-apoptotic Bcl-2 family member, Bim, and the death receptors TNFR (p55) and CD95/Fas (Qi et al. 2010). Furthermore, JNK3 signaling is implicated in the mitochondrial release of cytochrome c, leading to caspase-3 activation either via a Bim-dependent mechanism or through direct targeting of the mitochondria (Morishima et al. 2001; Murphy et al. 2010). Jnk3 knockout in perinatal brain injury has been linked to a decrease in caspase-3 activity, as well as a reduction in the levels of the pro-apoptotic proteins PUMA and Bim (Tian et al. 2005; Pirianov et al. 2007; Qi et al. 2010).

The postsynaptic density protein 95 (PSD-95) is a scaffold protein characterized by the presence of several protein-binding domains, including three N-terminal PDZ domains, a signal Src homology region 3 domain, and a C-terminal guanylate kinase-like domain (Han et al. 2008; Hu et al. 2008). Moreover, the PDZ domains bind to the C-terminus of the NMDA receptor NR2 and KA receptor GluR6 subunit, which is crucial for the grouping of NMDA receptors and KA receptors in the post-synaptic membrane. It has been reported that brain ischemia alters the GluR6-PSD-95-MLK3 complex in the hippocampus, which affects JNK3 phosphorylation and activation. Likewise, inhibition of the JNK3 signaling pathway is involved in the neuroprotective role of GABA against ischemic injury.

7.9 Future Perspectives of Inhibiting the c-JNKs Pathway in the Treatment of Neurological Disorders

The development of neuroprotective drugs is undoubtedly an area of increasing relevance due to the high incidence and prevalence of neurological disorders and the lack of effective treatments. However, since the exact mechanism of neuronal cell death in neurological disorders is not known, this limits the success in searching for effective drugs. Given that the process of neuronal death is complex, to at least find a drug that effectively blocks a pathway involved in cell death or delays the progress of AD, PD, or HD is considered a success. Apart from c-JNKs activation in neurodegenerative diseases, other biochemical parameters such as oxidative stress, mitochondrial alteration, cell cycle reentry, cytoskeletal alteration, GSK-3 activation, and inhibition of pro-survival pathways (such as the AKT pathway) might also contribute to the neurodegenerative process. Therefore, targeting the c-JNKs pathway with effective inhibitors at least provides a powerful way to experimentally achieve neuroprotection, as well as preserving cognitive function, inhibiting apoptosis, and having a trophic function. Unfortunately, clinical studies with CEP-1347 in PD have failed, but the loss of drug efficacy could have been due to multiple causes, such as whether the clinical trial (selected patients) for the specific compound was well designed or not. Other possible causes could have been a failure of the dose, administering the drug when the neurons were already dead, or the drug rescuing nonfunctioning neurons that could not perform their physiological roles. Therefore, it is necessary to conduct more clinical studies with inhibitors of the c-JNK pathway. It would probably be interesting to consider clinical trials with two drugs, such as an antioxidant, a GSK3β inhibitor, or other c-JNKs antagonists, since more than one pathway may be involved in neuronal death and this might be more effective in treating neurodegenerative diseases.

However, the inhibition of the c-JNK pathway has limitations due to the biological functions involved. For example, it has been reported that c-JNK inhibitors can rescue axotomised neurons, but prevent its regeneration. A possible alternative would be to develop direct targets against specific molecules of the c-JNK pathway; however, this requires more information about the individual actions of the different c-JNK isoforms. In this sense, the work of Zhao and colleagues demonstrated that inhibiting the mitochondrial complex MKK: JNK3 attenuated apoptosis without affecting cellular functions (Zhao et al. 2012). Likewise, the study of Björkblom and colleagues suggests that the nuclear localization of c-JNKs is the main factor responsible for cell death, while the cytoplasmic localization is responsible for its physiological functions (Björkblom 2005). This is an important factor to consider when designing drugs to treat neurological disorders.

Acknowledgements This study was funded by grant 2009/SGR00853 from the *Generalitat de Catalunya* (autonomous government of Catalonia), grants BFU2010-19119/BFI, SAF2011-23631, and SAF2009-13093 from the Spanish *Ministerio de Ciencia e Innovación*, grant PI080400 and PS09/01789 from the Instituto de Salud Carlos III, and grant 610RT0405 from Programa Iberoamericano de Ciencia y Tecnologia para el Desarrollo (CYTED).

References

Apostol BL, Simmons DA, Zuccato C, Illes K, Pallos J, Casale M, Conforti P, et al. CEP-1347 reduces mutant huntingtin-associated neurotoxicity and restores BDNF levels in R6/2 mice. Mol Cell Neurosci. 2008;39:8–20.

Behrens A, Sabapathy K, Graef I, Cleary M, Crabtree GR, Wagner EF.Jun N-terminal kinase 2 modulates thymocyte apoptosis and T cell activation through c-Jun and nuclear factor of activated T cell (NF-AT). Proc Natl Acad Sci USA. 2001;98:1769–74.

Behrens A, Sibilia M, Wagner EF. Amino-terminal phosphorylation of c-Jun regulates stress-induced apoptosis and cellular proliferation. Nat Genet. 1999;21:326–9.

Bevilaqua LR, Kerr DS, Medina JH, Izquierdo I, Cammarota M. et al. Inhibition of hippocampal Jun N-terminal kinase enhances short-term memory but blocks long-term memory formation and retrieval of an inhibitory avoidance task. Eur J Neurosci. 2003;17:897–902.

Björkblom B, Vainio JC, Hongisto V, Herdegen T, Courtney MJ, Coffey ET. et al. All JNKs can kill, but nuclear localization is critical for neuronal death. J Biol Chem. 2008;283:19704–13.

Björkblom B, Ostman N, Hongisto V, Komarovski V, Filén JJ, Nyman TA, Kallunki T, Courtney MJ, Coffey ET. Constitutively active cytoplasmic c-Jun N-terminal kinase 1 is a dominant regulator of dendritic architecture: role of microtubule-associated protein 2 as an effector. J Neurosci. 2005;25:6350–61.

Bogoyevitch MA, Kobe B. Uses for JNK: the many and varied substrates of the c-Jun N-terminal kinases. Microbiol Mol Biol Rev. 2006;70:1061–95.

Borsello T, Bonny C. Use of cell-permeable peptides to prevent neuronal degeneration. Trends Mol Med. 2004;10:239–44.

Borsello T, Forloni G. JNK signalling: a possible target to prevent neurodegeneration. Curr Pharm Des. 2007;13:1875–86.

Borsello T, Clarke PG, Hirt L, Vercelli A, Repici M, Schorderet DF, et al. A peptide inhibitor of c-Jun N-terminal kinase protects against excitotoxicity and cerebral ischemia. Nat Med. 2003;9:1180–6.

Bozyczko-Coyne D, Saporito MS, Hudkins RL. Targeting the JNK pathway for therapeutic benefit in CNS disease. Curr Drug Targets CNS Neurol Disord. 2002;1:31–49.

Braithwaite SP, Schmid RS, He DN, Sung ML, Cho S, Resnick L, et al. Inhibition of c-Jun kinase provides neuroprotection in a model of Alzheimer's disease. Neurobiol Dis. 2010;39:311–7.

Brecht S, Kirchhof R, Chromik A, Willesen M, Nicolaus T, Raivich G, et al. Specific pathophysiological functions of JNK isoforms in the brain. Eur J Neurosci. 2005;21:363–77.

Carboni S, Hiver A, Szyndralewiez C, et al. AS601245 (1,3-benzothiazol-2-yl (2-[[2-(3-pyridinyl) ethyl] amino]-4 pyrimidinyl) acetonitrile): a c-Jun NH2-terminal protein kinase inhibitor with neuroprotective properties. J Pharmacol Exp Ther. 2004;310:25–32.

Castellani RJ, Lee HG, Siedlak SL, et al. Reexamining Alzheimer's disease: evidence for a protective role for amyloid-beta protein precursor and amyloid-beta. J Alzheimers Dis. 2009;18:447–52.

Chambers JW, Pachori A, Howard S, et al. Small molecule c-jun-N-terminal kinase (JNK) inhibitors protect dopaminergic neurons in a model of parkinson's disease. ACS Chem Neurosci. 2011;2:198–206.

Chen X, Wu J, Hua D, Shu K, et al. The c-Jun N-terminal kinase inhibitor SP600125 is neuroprotective in amygdala kindled rats. Brain Res. 2010;1357:104–14.

Choi WS, Abel G, Klintworth H, Flavell RA, Xia Z, et al. JNK3 mediates paraquat- and rotenone-induced dopaminergic neuron death. J Neuropathol Exp Neurol. 2010;69:511–20.

Coffey ET, Hongisto V, Dickens M, Davis RJ, Courtney MJ. Dual roles for c-Jun N-terminal kinase in developmental and stress responses in cerebellar granule neurons. J Neurosci. 2000;20:7602–13.

Colombo A, Bastone A, Ploia C, et al. JNK regulates APP cleavage and degradation in a model of Alzheimer's disease. Neurobiol Dis. 2009;33:518–25.

Coultas L, Terzano S, Thomas T, et al. Hrk/DP5 contributes to the apoptosis of select neuronal populations but is dispensable for haematopoietic cell apoptosis. J Cell Sci. 2007;15:2044–52.

de Lemos L, Junyent F, Verdaguer E, et al. Differences in activation of ERK1/2 and p38 kinase in Jnk3 null mice following KA treatment. J Neurochem. 2010;114:1315–22.

Donovan N, Becker EB, Konishi Y, Bonni A. JNK phosphorylation and activation of BAD couples the stress-activated signaling pathway to the cell death machinery. J Biol Chem. 2002;277:40944–9.

Eshraghi AA, Wang J, Adil E, et al. Blocking c-Jun-N-terminal kinase signaling can prevent hearing loss induced by both electrode insertion trauma and neomycin ototoxicity. Hear Res. 2007;226:168–77.

Garcia M, Vanhoutte P, Pages C, et al. The mitochondrial toxin 3-nitropropionic acid induces striatal neurodegeneration via a c-Jun N-terminal kinase/c-Jun module. J Neurosci. 2002;22:2174–84.

Gass P, Kiessling M, Bading H. Regionally selective stimulation of mitogen activated protein (MAP) kinase tyrosine phosphorylation after generalized seizures in the rat brain. Neurosci Lett. 1993;162:39–42.

Guan, QH., Pei, DS., Zhang, QG., Hao, ZB., Xu, TL., Zhang, GY. The neuroprotective action of SP600125, a new inhibitor of JNK, on transient brain ischemia/reperfusion-induced neuronal death in rat hippocampal CA1 via nuclear and non-nuclear pathways. Brain Res. 2005;1035: 51–9.

Han D, Zhang QG, Yong-Liu, Li C, Zong YY, Yu CZ, et al. Co-activation of GABA receptors inhibits the JNK3 apoptotic pathway via the disassembly of the GluR6-PSD95-MLK3 signalling module in cerebral ischemic-reperfusion. FEBS Lett. 2008;582:1298–306.

Herdegen T, Skene P, Bahr M. The c-Jun transcription factor–bipotential mediator of neuronal death, survival and regeneration. Trends Neurosci. 1997;20:227–31.

Hu WW, Du Y, Li C, Song YJ, Zhang GY. Neuroprotection of hypothermia against neuronal death in rat hippocampus through inhibiting the increased assembly of GluR6-PSD95-MLK3 signaling module induced by cerebral ischemia/reperfusion. Hippocampus. 2008;18:386–97.

Hunot S, Vila M, Teismann P, Davis RJ, Hirsch EC, Przedborski S, et al. JNK-mediated induction of cyclooxygenase 2 is required for neurodegeneration in a mouse model of Parkinson's disease. Proc Natl Acad Sci USA. 2004;101:665–70.

Junyent F, de Lemos L, Verdaguer E, Folch J, Ferrer I, Ortuño-Sahagún D, et al. Gene expression profile in JNK3 null mice: a novel specific activation of the PI3K/AKT pathway. J Neurochem. 2011;117:244–52.

Junyent F, de Lemos L, Verdaguer E, Pallàs M, Folch J, Beas-Zárate C, et al. Lack of Jun-N-terminal kinase 3 (JNK3) does not protect against neurodegeneration induced by 3-nitropropionic acid. Neuropathol Appl Neurobiol. 2012;38:311–21.

Kimberly WT, Zheng JB, Town T, Flavell RA, Selkoe DJ. Physiological regulation of the beta-amyloid precursor protein signaling domain by c-Jun N-terminal kinase JNK3 during neuronal differentiation. J Neurosci. 2005;25:5533–43.

Kuan CY, Yang DD, Samanta Roy DR, Davis RJ, Rakic P, Flavell RA. The Jnk1 and Jnk2 protein kinases are required for regional specific apoptosis during early brain development. Neuron. 1999;22:667–76.

Levy OA, Malagelada C, Greene LA. Cell death pathways in Parkinson's disease: proximal triggers, distal effectors, and final steps. Apoptosis. 2009;14:478–500.

Liu YF. Expression of polyglutamine-expanded Huntingtin activates the SEK1-JNK pathway and induces apoptosis in a hippocampal neuronal cell line. J Biol Chem. 1998;273:28873–7.

Liu JR, Zhao Y, Patzer A. The c-Jun N-terminal kinase (JNK) inhibitor XG-102 enhances the neuroprotection of hyperbaric oxygen after cerebral ischaemia in adult rats. Neuropathol Appl Neurobiol. 2010;36:211–24.

Ma C, Ying C, Yuan Z, Song B, Li D, Liu Y, et al. dp5/HRK is a c-Jun target gene and required for apoptosis induced by potassium deprivation in cerebellar granule neurons. J Biol Chem. 2007; 282: 30901–9.

Maroney AC, Finn JP, Bozyczko-Coyne D, O'Kane TM, Neff NT, Tolkovsky AM, et al. CEP-1347 (KT7515), an inhibitor of JNK activation, rescues sympathetic neurons and neuronally differentiated PC12 cells from death evoked by three distinct insults. J Neurochem. 1999;73:1901–12.

Mazzitelli S, Xu P, Ferrer I, Davis RJ, Tournier C. The loss of c-Jun N-terminal protein kinase activity prevents the amyloidogenic cleavage of amyloid precursor protein and the formation of amyloid plaques in vivo. J Neurosci. 2011;31:16969–76.

McCubrey JA, Lahair MM, Franklin RA. Reactive oxygen species-induced activation of the MAP kinase signaling pathways. Antioxid Redox Signal. 2006;8:1775–89.

Mondragón-Rodríguez S, Basurto-Islas G, Lee HG, Perry G, Zhu X, Castellani RJ, et al. Causes versus effects: the increasing complexities of Alzheimer's disease pathogenesis. Expert Rev Neurother. 2010;10:683–91.

Morishima Y, Gotoh Y, Zieg J. Beta-amyloid induces neuronal apoptosis via a mechanism that involves the c-Jun N-terminal kinase pathway and the induction of Fas ligand. J Neurosci. 2001;21:7551–60.

Morrison DK, Davis RJ. Regulation of MAP kinase signaling modules by scaffold proteins in mammals. Annu Rev Cell Dev Biol. 2003;19:91–118.

Murphy BM, Engel T, Paucard A, Hatazaki S, Mouri G, Tanaka K, et al. Contrasting patterns of Bim induction and neuroprotection in Bim-deficient mice between hippocampus and neocortex after status epilepticus. Cell Death Differ. 2010;17:459–68.

Pan J, Wang G, Yang HQ, Hong Z, Xiao Q, Ren RJ, et al. K252a prevents nigral dopaminergic cell death induced by 6-hydroxydopamine through inhibition of both mixed-lineage kinase 3/c-Jun NH2-terminal kinase 3 (JNK3) and apoptosis-inducing kinase 1/JNK3 signaling pathways. Mol Pharmacol. 2007;72:1607–18.

Pan J, Xiao Q, Sheng CY, Hong Z, Yang HQ, Wang G, et al. Blockade of the translocation and activation of c-Jun N-terminal kinase 3 (JNK3) attenuates dopaminergic neuronal damage in mouse model of Parkinson's disease. Neurochem Int. 2009;54:418–25.

Pan J, Qian J, Zhang Y, Ma J, Wang G, Xiao Q, et al. Small peptide inhibitor of JNKs protects against MPTP-induced nigral dopaminergic injury via inhibiting the JNK-signaling pathway. Lab Invest. 2010;90:156–67.

Peng J, Andersen JK. The role of c-Jun N-terminal kinase (JNK) in Parkinson's disease. IUBMB Life. 2003;55:267–71.

Perrin V, Dufour N, Raoul C. Implication of the JNK pathway in a rat model of Huntington's disease. Exp Neurol. 2009;215:191–200.

Pirianov G, Brywe KG, Mallard C, Edwards AD, Flavell RA, Hagberg H, et al. Deletion of the c-Jun N-terminal kinase 3 gene protects neonatal mice against cerebral hypoxic-ischaemic injury. J Cereb Blood Flow Metab. 2007;27:1022–32.

Puthalakath H, Strasser A. Keeping killers on a tight leash: transcriptional and post-translational control of the pro-apoptotic activity of BH3-only proteins. Cell Death Differ. 2002;9:505–12.

Qi SH, Liu Y, Hao LY, Guan QH, Gu YH, Zhang J, et al. Neuroprotection of ethanol against ischemia/reperfusion-induced brain injury through decreasing c-Jun N-terminal kinase 3 (JNK3) activation by enhancing GABA release. Neuroscience. 2010;167:1125–37.

Ramin M, Azizi P, Motamedi F, Haghparast A, Khodagholi F. Inhibition of JNK phosphorylation reverses memory deficit induced by β-amyloid (1-42) associated with decrease of apoptotic factors. Behav Brain Res. 2011;217:424–31.

Resnick L, Fennell M. Targeting JNK3 for the treatment of neurodegenerative disorders. Drug Discov Today. 2004;9:932–9.

Saporito MS, Thomas BA, Scott RW. MPTP activates c-Jun NH(2)-terminal kinase (JNK) and its upstream regulatory kinase MKK4 in nigrostriatal neurons in vivo. J Neurochem. 2000;75:1200–8.

Saporito MS, Hudkins RL, Maroney AC. Discovery of CEP-1347/KT-7515, an inhibitor of the JNK/SAPK pathway for the treatment of neurodegenerative diseases. Prog Med Chem. 2002;40:23–62.

Sclip A, Antoniou X, Colombo A, Camici GG, Pozzi L, Cardinetti D, et al. c-Jun N-terminal kinase regulates soluble Aβ oligomers and cognitive impairment in AD mouse model. J Biol Chem. 2011;286(51):43871–80.

Slomnicki J, Lesniak LP, Slomnicki W, Lesniak D. A putative role of the Amyloid Precursor Protein Intracellular Domain (AICD) in transcription. Acta Neurobiol Exp (Wars). 2008;68:219–28.

Smith J, Jones Jr M, Houghton L, et al. Future of health insurance. N Engl J Med. 1999;965: 325–9.

Su B, Wang X, Nunomura A, Moreira PI, Lee HG, Perry G, et al. Oxidative stress signaling in Alzheimer's disease. Curr Alzheimer Res. 2008;5:525–32.

Suckfuell M, Canis M, Strieth S, Scherer H, Haisch A. Intratympanic treatment of acute acoustic trauma with a cell-permeable JNK ligand: a prospective randomized phase I/II study. Acta Otolaryngol. 2007;127:938–42.

Sun W, Gould TW, Newbern J, Milligan C, Choi SY, Kim H, et al. Phosphorylation of c-Jun in avian and mammalian motoneurons in vivo during programmed cell death: an early reversible event in the apoptotic cascade. J Neurosci. 2005;25:5595–603.

The Parkinson Study Group PRECEPT Investigators. Mixed lineage kinase inhibitor CEP-1347 fails to delay disability in early Parkinson disease. Neurology. 2007;69:1480–90.

Tian H, Zhang QG, Zhu GX, Pei DS, Guan QH, Zhang GY. Activation of c-Jun NH2-terminal kinase 3 is mediated by the GluR6.PSD-95.MLK3 signaling module following cerebral ischemia in rat hippocampus. Brain Res. 2005;1061:57–66.

Vogel J, Anand VS, Ludwig B, Nawoschik S, Dunlop J, Braithwaite SP. The JNK pathway amplifies and drives subcellular changes in tau phosphorylation. Neuropharmacology. 2009;57: 539–50.

Wang W, Shi L, Xie Y, Ma C, Li W, Su X, et al. SP600125, a new JNK inhibitor, protects dopaminergic neurons in the MPTP model of Parkinson's disease. Neurosci Res. 2004;48:195–202.

Wang J, Ruel J, Ladrech S, Bonny C, van de Water TR, Puel JL. Inhibition of the c-Jun N-terminal kinase-mediated mitochondrial cell death pathway restores auditory function in sound-exposed animals. Mol Pharmacol. 2007;71:654–66.

Weston CR, Davis RJ. The JNK signal transduction pathway. Curr Opin Cell Biol. 2007;19: 142–9.

Xu Y, Hou XY, Liu Y, Zong YY. Different protection of K252a and N-acetyl-L-cysteine against amyloid-beta peptide-induced cortical neuron apoptosis involving inhibition of MLK3-MKK7-JNK3 signal cascades. J Neurosci Res. 2009;87:918–27.

Yang DD, Kuan CY, Whitmarsh AJ, Rincón M, Zheng TS, Davis RJ, et al. Absence of excitotoxicity-induced apoptosis in the hippocampus of mice lacking the Jnk3 gene. Nature. 1997;389:865–70.

Zhao Y, Spigolon G, Bonny C, Culman J, Vercelli A, Herdegen T. The JNK inhibitor D-JNKI-1 blocks apoptotic JNK signaling in brain mitochondria. Mol Cell Neurosci. 2012;49:300–10.

Zhu X, Raina AK, Rottkamp CA, Aliev G, Perry G, Boux H, et al. Activation and redistribution of c-jun N-terminal kinase/stress activated protein kinase in degenerating neurons in Alzheimer's disease. J Neurochem. 2001;76:435–41.

Chapter 8
Proteomics-Based Strategy to Identify Biomarkers and Pharmacological Targets in Temporal Lobe Epilepsy

Maria José da Silva Fernandes, Rebeca Padrão Amorim, Jose Eduardo Marques Carneiro, Michelle Gasparetti Leão Araújo, and Daniele Suzete Persike

Abstract Temporal lobe epilepsy (TLE), the most common type of epilepsy in humans, is frequently associated with hippocampal sclerosis, cognitive deficit, and pharmacoresistant seizures. A major difficulty in designing new treatments to block seizures or epileptogenesis is the sequence of events involved in the development of the epileptic circuitry after an initial insult in the brain. The neuroproteomics emerges as a powerful tool for researchers interested in pursuing biomarkers for neurodegenerative diseases, including TLE. In this chapter, we present data obtained from studies employing proteomics technology to determine differential expression of proteins in brain tissue or cerebrospinal fluid of patients with TLE and in experimental models of epilepsy. Based on the findings it is possible to identify similarities of protein changes related to TLE in humans and models. Data obtained with proteomics are very useful to understand the pathophysiology of TLE and in the future may assist in finding target proteins for new therapies.

Keywords Temporal lobe epilepsy • Proteomics • Neuroproteomics • Pharmacoresistant seizures • Hippocampus • Pilocarpine • Status epilepticus

---

M.J. da Silva Fernandes (✉) • R.P. Amorim • J.E.M. Carneiro • M.G.L. Araújo • D.S. Persike
Department of Neurology and Neurosurgery,
Universidade Federal de São Paulo-UNIFESP,
Rua Pedro de Toledo, 669 - 2° andar, CEP 04039-032,
São Paulo, SP, Brazil
e-mail: fernandes.nexp@epm.br

L. Rocha and E.A. Cavalheiro (eds.), *Pharmacoresistance in Epilepsy: From Genes and Molecules to Promising Therapies*, DOI 10.1007/978-1-4614-6464-8_8,

8.1 Introduction

Proteomics is a science or method developed to study the proteome. Proteome is a term used to refer the amount of protein expressed in a cell or tissue of an organism. While the genome reflects the sum of genes, the proteome does not exhibit a fixed number of proteins. These vary according to the state of development, the tissue type, and the physiological conditions. A proteome nevertheless remains a direct product of a genome. The number of proteins in a proteome can exceed the number of genes expressed in an organism, considering the possibility of protein expressed by alternative splicing or with different posttranslational modifications. The two-dimensional polyacrylamide gel electrophoresis (2D-PAGE) enables separation of similar molecules differing in their isoelectric point (IP) (Wilkins et al. 1996).

Proteomics allows us to find proteins changed by a cell, tissue, or organism's response to internal states, external stimulations, or developmental changes and to profile any differential protein expression (Mus-Veteau 2002; Wang et al. 2010). Proteomics not only measures the amount of a given protein but also whether there are any modifications of a protein as phosphorylation, ubiqutination, palmitoylation, oxidation, and other posttranslational modifications (Alzate 2010). Currently, the technique of proteomics has been widely used in the search for biomarkers associated with diseases (Liu et al. 2010). However, proteomics technology is not only applicable to study disease biomarkers but also in agronomy researchers (i.e., corn, sugarcane, rice, wheat, etc.) or organisms with economic impact (i.e., *Rhizhobium* spp., which set nitrogen to legumes, or *Xanthomonas* spp., which cause diseases in bean or citrus cultivation) (Di Ciero and Bellato 2003).

Proteomic technology applied to understanding the nervous system is called "neuroproteomics" or "neuromics". The neuroproteomics enables to study proteome of brain fragments or single cell, in cultures or isolated, and this is important to determine the dynamics of sub-proteome under different conditions (i.e., oxidative stress, drugs, etc.). In a global analysis, complementary studies could contribute to the understanding of complex biological networks which include protein interactions, and the complexity of signal and metabolic pathways which can be applied to select potential targets for specific drug therapy and to the development of diagnosis or prognosis for neurological disorders (Liu et al. 2010). Proteomics is a multidisciplinary method which is based on principles biochemical, biophysical, and bioinformatics.

8.1.1 Techniques Used in Proteomics

The proteomic analysis has four basic stages, which are extraction, purification, separation, and identification of proteins. The current techniques used to separation of proteins in proteomics are 2D-PAGE, which allows the separation of hundreds to thousands of proteins in a single experiment (Van den Bergh and Arckens 2005;

Kim et al. 2007), and mass spectrometry (MS) to detect either digested peptides or intact proteins (Li and Smit 2008; Zetterberg et al. 2008).

There are five types of mass analyzers commonly used for proteomics research and they vary in their physical principles and analytical performance (see Liu et al. 2010). MALDI-TOF (time-of-flight, TOF) is generally used in proteomics studies to identify protein from in-gel digestion of gel separated protein band by peptide mass fingerprinting, due to its excellent mass accuracy, resolution, and sensitivity (Pappin et al. 1993). Nowadays it is possible to conduct a study of proteomics analysis without the need for two-dimensional electrophoresis. There are different methods which enable the analysis without 2-DE gels, one being accomplished by methodology 2D-LC-MS, in which the proteins are labeled with a probe, trypsinized and then analyzed by LC-MS, which makes the simple and reproducible method, but it is more expensive.

Other protein identification methods, like amino acid composition analysis, N-terminal sequencing, or immunochemistry, as well as column chromatography can be used (Fountoulakis 2001; Fountoulakis and Takács 2002).

8.1.2 *Mass-Spectrometry-Based Proteomics Analysis in Epilepsy*

The neurosciences have benefited greatly from the increased use of the proteomics technique in the last 15 years. However, the application of proteomics in studies of epilepsies is still discrete. Study of brain tissue obtained surgically or by autopsy can be helpful, but it is limited in quantity, quality, and versatility, and control tissue frequently is unavailable. Thus, animal models are used in analogy to the human epilepsy to help identify molecular clues to the clinical conditions (see Buckmaster 2004). In the following sections, we briefly review the results obtained with the technique of proteomics in epilepsy models and patients.

Epilepsy is a common chronic brain disorder characterized by the presence of spontaneous and recurrent seizures that occur in the absence of condition toxic-metabolic or febrile illness (Engel 2001). It is a serious neurological condition affecting approximately 1 % of people worldwide (Li and Sander 2003).

Temporal lobe epilepsy (TLE) represents approximately 40 % of all cases of epilepsy and can be subclassified into mesial temporal lobe epilepsy (MTLE) and lateral temporal neocortical epilepsy (Engel 2001). The MTLE constitutes 60 % of cases of TLE, where seizures originate in limbic structures, particularly in the hippocampus and amygdala complex (Engel 1996; French et al. 1993). The MTLE is characterized by simple or complex focal seizures (loss of consciousness), and seizures with secondary generalization (tonic-clonic seizures) are uncommon (Engel 1996). Seizures in these patients are frequently pharmacoresistant to antiepileptic drugs (Li and Sander 2003). Neuropathological studies indicate that TLE is frequently associated with hippocampal sclerosis (HS) that is routinely detected by imaging studies during the presurgical evaluation of patients with this disorder (Mathern et al. 1995). About 70 % of hippocampi removed from patients with intractable TLE showed HS and the etiology and the pathogenesis of the damage are not known. Although several studies have shown a correlation between severe childhood illness (i.e., febrile seizures, infection, etc.), not all patients exhibiting HS have a history of an initial insult.

The hippocampus is one of the most vulnerable areas in the temporal lobe to damage following seizures. The histological patterns frequently associated with HS include loss of pyramidal cells in the prosubiculum, CA1, CA3, and hilus of dentate gyrus from the hippocampal formation (Mathern et al. 1995). In addition, phenomena of rearrangement synaptic (sprouting of mossy fibers) and dispersion of granule cells of the dentate gyrus are frequently observed in the HS from patients with TLE (Babb et al. 1991; House et al. 1990). Changes can also be found in other regions of the mesial temporal lobe, the entorhinal cortex and white matter (Kasper et al. 1999). Patients who develop TLE demonstrate a progression both in the number of seizures and in the neurological symptoms related to the seizures, such as cognitive and behavioral disorders (Engel 1991; French et al. 2004). The high prevalence and refractoriness to pharmacological treatment make this disease a subject of great interest for researchers in basic and clinical area (Li and Sander 2003).

Despite technological advances applied to neurosciences, little is known about the cellular and molecular phenomena related to the process of epileptogenesis, the process by which a previously asymptomatic brain becomes capable of generating spontaneous seizures (Silva and Cabral 2008). Until now, there is no antiepileptic drug able to prevent seizures in patients with TLE that is efficient in preventing epileptogenesis (Temkin 2009). Thus, the question is whether the epileptogenic process could be explained by common molecular and network events that would be applied in new therapeutics. In this way, proteomics has been a powerful tool for protein profiling because it allows comparing proteomes of cells and tissues in normal and pathological conditions. Since the expression of proteins is determined, the transcriptional level can be examined in order to find the underlying mechanism for reduction or increase of certain gene products. For this reason, proteomics has been widely used in clinical research to identifying biomarkers associated with epileptogenesis.

Few proteomic studies have been done in epilepsy. Some authors employed proteomics analysis to identify proteins that are differentially expressed in hippocampi of patients with MTLE compared to control tissue obtained at autopsy. They found altered expression of several proteins with different roles in the central nervous system (CNS). The cytosolic enzyme acyl-CoA thioester hydrolase known for its role in energy production by B-oxidation in mitochondria and peroxisomes, signal transduction, ion fluxes, and activation of protein kinase C had reduced expression in hippocampus of patients with MTLE (Yang et al. 2004). In subsequent studies, these authors verified a decreased expression of collapsing response-mediated protein-2 (CMRP-2, 55 kDa protein) often involved with axonal outgrowth, path finding, and neuronal polarity (Czech et al. 2004). They also observed a decrease in expression of 18 proteins playing different roles in brain (Yang et al. 2006). Proteins that play a role as chaperone (TCP-1-alpha and HSP70), cell signaling (MAPKK), transcriptional signaling (NAD-dependent deacetylase sirtui-2), or which are

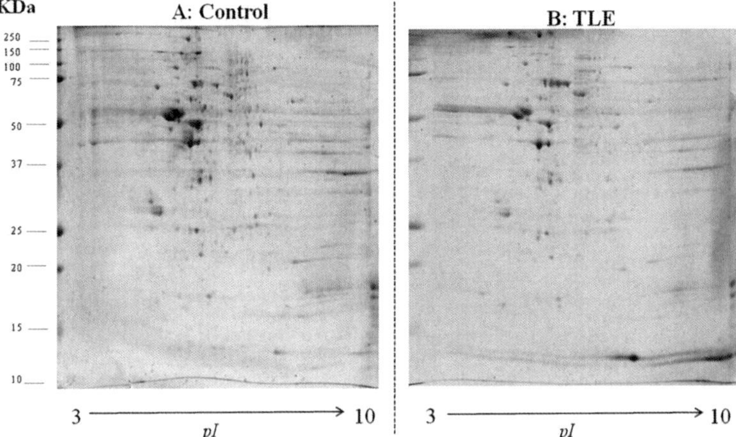

Fig. 8.1 Representative 2D-PAGE image of hippocampal protein extracts from control (**A**) and patients with temporal lobe epilepsy (TLE) (**B**). An amount (0.5 mg) of total protein of each sample was separated by isoelectrofocusing on a pH 3–10 linear gradient followed by the second dimension SDS-PAGE. Gels were stained with Coomassie brilliant blue. The peptides obtained from protein digestion of spots differentially expressed were analyzed by LC-ESI-MS/MS

components of synaptosomes (synaptogmin I, alpha-synuclein) and cytoskeleton (tubulins, vinculin, and profiling) are among them. In the other hand, increased expression of proteins associated with antioxidant function (peroxiredoxin 6), gliosis, and increased microvascular endothelial cells (apo A-I) was also reported by the authors (Yang et al. 2005, 2006).

With the aim of obtaining biomarkers for TLE, Xiao et al. (2009) analyzed cerebrospinal fluid (CSF) of patients by proteomics. The authors found five differentially expressed proteins in TLE patients compared to control, and six proteins expressed only in patients. Vitamin D-binding protein (DBP) was increased, whereas cathepsin D, apolipoprotein J, Fam3c, and superoxide dismutase 1 (SOD1) were decreased in TLE compared to control. The proteins identified only in patients were tetranectin (TN), talin-2, apolipoprotein E, immunoglobulin lambda light chain, immunoglobulin kappa variable light chain 1–5 (IGKV1–5), and procollagen C-endopeptidase enhancer 1 (PCOLCE). Abnormal expression of some of these proteins as cathepsin D and SOD1 for example, has been reported in other proteomics studies employing cerebral cortex of epileptic patients (Eun et al. 2004), indicating that the lower level in CSF may reflects the deficiency in the brain (Xiao et al. 2009).

In a recent study, Persike et al. (2011) using proteomics (2D-PAGE coupled to LC–ESI–MS/MS) showed that the total number of spots was noticeably smaller in the hippocampus of patients with pharmacoresistant TLE than in control tissue (Fig. 8.1). A total of 16 proteins were differentially expressed in the hippocampus of these patients compared to control but only nine proteins were identified as shown in Table 8.1. Among the nine changed proteins, six had increased expression,

Table 8.1 Proteins differentially expressed in the hippocampus of patients with pharmacoresistant TLE

IP	Protein name	MW	Changes
5.92	Isoform 1 ofa serum albumin—ALB	71, 317	↑
5.56	Heat shock-related 70 kDa protein 2—HSPA2	70, 263	↑
8.2	Dihydropyrimidinase-related protein 2—DPYSL2	77, 912	↑
9.79	Isoform 1 of myelin basic protein—MBP	33, 097	↑
5.21	Isoform 3 of spectrin alpha chain, brain—SPTAN1	282, 906	⇩
5.35	V-type proton ATPase catalytic subunit A—ATP6V1A	68, 660	↑
5.43	Glutathione *S*-transferase P—GSTP1	23, 569	+
6.33	Protein DJ-1—PARK7	20, 050	+
7.96	Dihydrolipoyllysine-residue acetyltransferase component of pyruvate dehydrogenase complex, mitochondrial—DLAT	69, 466	↑

Proteins identified by LC-ESI-MS/MS and peptide matched by using Mascot MS/MS ion search and NCBI protein database. (*Filled up arrow*) Up-regulated proteins, (*open down arrow*) down-regulated proteins (TLE versus control), and (+) proteins expressed only in the hippocampus of TLE patients. *MW* molecular weight, *IP* isoelectric point

one had reduced expression in the TLE group compared to control, and two proteins were identified as only present in the 2D-PAGE of epilepsy patients. Through the NCBI database the following proteins were identified: isoform 1 of serum albumin (ALB1), HSP70, dihydropyrimidinase-related protein 2 (DPYSL2), isoforms of myelin basic protein (MBP1), isoform 3 of spectrin alpha chain (SPTAN1), proton ATPase catalytic subunit A (ATP6V1A), glutathione *S*-transferase P (GSTP1), protein DJ-1 (PARK7), and dihydrolipoyllysine-residue acetyltransferase component of pyruvate dehydrogenase complex (DLAT). Glutathione *S*-transferase P and PARK7 were detected only in hippocampus. The expression of spectrin was down-regulated in the hippocampi of patients with pharmacoresistant TLE. All other proteins were up-regulated in epilepsy. The results obtained to HSP-70, ATP6V1A, and GSTP1 were validated by western blot (Persike et al. 2011).

Most of the identified proteins do not possess well-defined function in the epileptic process. However, knowing the role of these proteins in physiologic condition, it is possible to suggest their role in the pathophysiological condition. The increased expression of myelin basic protein and albumin in TLE may be indicative of changes in the permeability of the barrier and the myelination process. Similar results were reported in animal model of epilepsy (Huang et al. 2008; Marchi et al. 2010).

The vacuolar H^+ATPase, an evolutionarily ancient enzyme involved in neurotransmitter release mechanism (Wilkens et al. 2005) and in acidification of synaptic vesicles after exocytosis to be reused (Li et al. 2005), is with its expression increased in patients with TLE. Likewise, the HSP70 expression was also increased in patients with epilepsy and the function of HSP70 appears to be related to the activation of compensatory mechanisms or just reflecting the increase in protein synthesis, since it is a chaperone protein involved in the mechanism of new protein folding (Mayer and Bukau 2005).

The dihydropyrimidinase-related protein 2 (DPYSL2) is a member of cytosolic phosphoproteins which is involved in growth of axons and neurites and in synaptic plasticity. Changes in DPYSL2 have been related with susceptibility to psychiatric disorders such as schizophrenia (Ujike et al. 2006) or with diseases in which the psychiatric disorders appear as comorbidity as in Alzheimer's disease (Castegna et al. 2002). Based on these findings, the increased expression of DPYSL2 may be a marker of psychiatric comorbidity in patients with TLE (Persike et al. 2011).

The spectrin, a protein that showed reduced expression in TLE, has been reported as responsible for anchoring of the NMDA receptor to the membrane. It has been demonstrated that changes in the expression of spectrin can be related to disorders in LTP and cognition (Wechsler and Teichberg 1998).

The glutathione *S*-transferase P (GSTP1) and PARK-7 were expressed only in gels of patients with TLE. This was an interesting find since these proteins play an important role as antioxidant (Sharma et al. 2004). In addition to the antioxidant role for GSTP1, this protein has been associated with inactivation of antiepileptic drugs in the liver (Shang et al. 2008). This protein may represent an important target for studies related to pharmacoresistance frequently present in TLE.

Although these findings are interesting and enables us to obtain clues about the mechanisms involved with intractable epilepsy, we have to bear in mind that these clues refer to mechanisms already established and irreversible, as cell loss, sprouting, cell dispersion, glial scar, metabolic changes, etc. Studies employing human tissue are limited by the low amount obtained by surgical procedures and for ethical reasons. The use of experimental model of epilepsy can expand our knowledge regarding these mechanisms involved in epileptogenesis, allowing interfere or prevent the onset of the spontaneous seizures. An overview about laboratory animal models of TLE is available in the literature (Buckmaster 2004).

Chemical convulsants such as pilocarpine (Cavalheiro et al. 1991; Cavalheiro 1995) and kainic acid (Ben-Ari 1985) can initiate *status epilepticus* in rodents and cause hippocampal sclerosis, memory impairment, and spontaneous and recurrent seizures.

Experimental models of epilepsy have been used in proteomics studies. A preliminary study employing the proteomics technique for studying protein expression in the hippocampus of rats subjected to pilocarpine-induced epilepsy model (90 days after *status epilepticus* induction) revealed 40 proteins with altered expression compared to control animals (see Table 8.2). The protein profile showed that 31 proteins were up-regulated, seven were down-regulated, and two were expressed only in control animals (Persike et al. 2012).

Among the down-regulated proteins there are several enzymes related to the carbohydrate metabolism, ATP production and oxidation, reflecting disturbs in the energetic metabolism. These data are in line with findings obtained in hippocampus (Greenberg et al. 2005; Masino et al. 2009). The gene encoding the malate dehydrogenase was reported as a factor that leads to generalized idiopathic epilepsy (Greenberg et al. 2005). Altered proteins such as phospholipase A2, fructose-bisphosphate aldolase, and enolase have been reported by other authors associated with neuropsychiatric processes (Martins-de-Souza et al. 2009; Ross et al. 1997; Adibhatla and Hatcher 2008). A recent study showed that phospholipase A2 participates in processes of neurogenesis (Talib et al. 2008).

Table 8.2 Proteins differentially expressed in rat hippocampus of pilocarpine-induced epilepsy model

IP	Protein name	MW	Changes
5.5	L-Lactate dehydrogenase A chain	36,874	Ø
5.2	Phosphatidylethanolamine-binding protein 1	20,902	Ø
9.3	Fructose-bisphosphate aldolase A	39,783	⇩
5.2	Cytosolic phospholipase A2 gamma (Fragment)	37,522	⇩
9.3	ATP-binding cassette subfamily B member 6, mitochondrial	93,305	⇩
6.0	Malate dehydrogenase, cytoplasmic	36,631	⇩
5.4	Guanine nucleotide-binding protein G(I)/G(S)/G(T) subunit beta-1	38,151	⇩
5.4	F-actin-capping protein subunit alpha-2	33,118	⇩
5.3	Guanine nucleotide-binding protein G(I)/G(S)/G(T) subunit beta-3	38,125	⇩
5.8	Dihydropyrimidinase-related protein 2	62,638	⬆
5.9	Isoform 1 of dihydropyrimidinase-related protein 3	62,327	⬆
5.4	V-type proton ATPase subunit B, brain isoform	56,857	⬆
5.2	V-type proton ATPase catalytic subunit A	68,564	⬆

Proteins identified by LC-ESI-MS/MS and peptide matched by using Mascot MS/MS ion search and IPI protein database. (*Filled up arrow*) Up-regulated proteins, (*open down arrow*) down-regulated proteins (pilocarpine versus control rats), and (Ø) proteins expressed only in hippocampus of control rats. *MW* molecular weight, *IP* isoelectric point

The guanine nucleotide-binding protein (G proteins) was down-regulated in the hippocampi of the pilocarpine-induced epilepsy. This is an important finding considering the wide role of this protein in the signal transduction by hormones, neurotransmitters, chemokines, and autocrine and paracrine factors (Neves et al. 2002).

Two genetic models of absence epilepsy, GAERS and WAG/Rij, are resistant to progression of partial seizures induced by amygdaloid (Aker et al. 2006; Onat et al. 2007), hippocampal (Akman et al. 2008), or perirhinal cortex electrical kindling (Akman et al. 2010). Because the absence seizures are originated on the thalamocortical circuitry these findings suggest an interaction between thalamocortical loop and limbic circuitry (Danober et al. 1998). Danis et al. (2011) performed a 2D-PAGE study, comparing GAERS to non-epileptic control (NEC) rats. This study showed six proteins differentially expressed, two in the parietal cortex (ATP synthase subunit delta and the 14-3-3 zeta isoform), two in the thalamus (myelin basic protein and macrophage migration inhibitory factor—MIF), and two in the hippocampus (MIF and 0-beta 2 globulin). Almost all proteins were up-regulated in GAERS compared to NEC with the exception of 0-beta globulin. In line with this study, MIF was also found up-regulated in the frontal cortex and in the hippocampus of rats subjected to kainic acid-induced epilepsy (Lo et al. 2010). MIF, a pro-inflammatory cytokine released in response to inflammatory stimuli, is highly expressed in immune and nonimmune cells, including those in the brain. A recent study by Conboy et al. (2011) showed that MIF is important to the process of hippocampal neurogenesis, affecting cell proliferation in the *dentate gyrus*.

8.2 Conclusions

In this chapter, we have revisited some aspects related to TLE and how proteomics has contributed to improve the knowledge about altered mechanisms in the hippocampus (the main area affected in this disease). Patients with TLE frequently present pharmacoresistant seizures and surgery to remove the epileptic focus is the only way to give effective treatment. The proteomics, a powerful methodology that matches ancient techniques (i.e., two-dimensional electrophoresis and amino acids analysis) with advanced technology (mass spectrometry), emerges as a powerful alternative in the search for target proteins for treat or perhaps prevent the occurrence of seizures. Until now we do not have defined biomarkers for TLE, because this disease is very complex and multifactorial and moreover, we still know little about the proteome or the dynamics of proteomes. In the near future, with the progress of biotechnologies (biophysics, bioinformatics, etc.) enabling to determine the complete proteome and how it changes in different tissues and conditions, we believe that will be possible to obtain biomarkers to enable more effective treatments for patients. The use of good experimental model of pharmacoresistant epilepsy is extremely important to achieve this goal. Our group along with others has made great efforts in this area and some data are presented in the text.

Acknowledgements The authors thank Fapesp, CNPq, CAPES, and INNT/MCT for financial support and UNIPETE-UNIFESP.

References

Adibhatla RM, Hatcher JF. Altered lipid metabolism in brain injury and disorders. Subcell Biochem. 2008;49:241–68. doi:10.1007/978-1-4020-8831-5_9.

Aker RG, Yananli HP, Gurbanova AA, Özkaynakça AE, Ates N, Luijtelaar G, et al. Amygdale kindling in the WAG/Rij rat model of absence epilepsy. Epilepsia. 2006;47:33–40. doi:10.1111/j.1528-1167.2006.00367.x.

Akman O, Karson A, Aker EG, Ates N, Onat FY. Hippocampal kindling in rats with absence epilepsy resembles amygdaloid kindling. Epilepsy Res. 2008;81:211–9. doi:10.1016/j.eplepsyres.2008.06.004.

Akman O, Karson A, Aker EG, Ates N, Onat FY. Perirhinal cortical kindling in rats with genetic absence epilepsy. Neurosci Lett. 2010;479:74–8. doi:10.1016/j.neulet.2010.05.034.

Alzate O. Neuroproteomics. In: Alzate O, editor. Neuroproteomics. Boca Raton, FL: CRC Press; 2010.

Babb TL, Kupfer WR, Pretorius JK, Crandall PH, Levesque MF. Synaptic reorganization by mossy fibers in human epileptic fascia dentata. Neuroscience. 1991;42:351–63. doi:10.1016/0306-4522(91)90380-7.

Ben-Ari Y. Limbic seizures and brain damage produced by kainic acid: mechanisms and relevance to human temporal lobe epilepsy. Neuroscience. 1985;14:375–403.

Buckmaster PS. Laboratory animal models of temporal lobe epilepsy. Comp Med. 2004;54:473–85.

Castegna A, Aksenov M, Thongboonkerd V, Pierce WM, Booze R, Markesbery WR, et al. Proteomic identification of oxidatively modified profiles proteins in Alzheimer's disease brain.

Part II: dihydropyrimidinase-related protein 2, alpha-enolase and heat shock cognate 71. J Neurochem. 2002;82:1524–32. doi:10.1046/j.1471-4159.2002.01103.x.

Cavalheiro EA. The pilocarpine model of epilepsy. Italian J Neurol Sci. 1995;16:33–7. doi:10.1007/BF02229072.

Cavalheiro EA, Leite JP, Bortolotto ZA, Turski WA, Ikonomidou C, Turski L. Long-termeffects of pilocarpine in rats: structural damage of the brain triggers kindling and spontaneously recurrent seizures. Epilepsia. 1991;32:778–82. doi:10.1111/j.1528-1157.1991.tb05533.x.

Conboy L, Varea E, Castro JE, Sakaouhi-Ouertatani H, Calandra T, Lashuel HA, et al. Macrophage migration inhibitory factor is critically involved in basal and fluoxetine-stimulated adult hipocampal cell proliferation and in anxiety, depression, and memory-related behaviors. Mol Psychiatry. 2011;16:533–47. doi:10.1038/mp. 2010.15.

Czech T, Yang JW, Csaszar E, Kappler J, Baumgartner C, Lubec G. Reduction of hippocampal collapsin response mediated protein-2 in patients with mesial temporal lobe epilepsy. Neurochem Res. 2004;29:2189–96. doi:0364-3190/04/1200-2189/0.

Danis O, Demir S, Günel A, Aker RG, Gülçebi M, Onat F, et al. Changes in intracellular protein expression in cortex, thalamus and hippocampus in a genetic rat model of absence epilepsy. Brain Res Bull. 2011;84:381–8. doi:10.1016/j.brainresbull.2011.02.002.

Danober L, Deransart C, Depaulis A, Vergnes M, Marescaux C. Pathophysiological mechanisms of genetic absence epilepsy in the rat. Prog Neurobiol. 1998;55:27–57. PII: S0301-0082(97)00091-9.

Di Ciero L, Bellato CM. Proteoma: avanços recentes em técnicas de eletroforese bidimensional e espectrometria de massa. Biotecnol Clin Desenvolv. 2003;29:158–64. http://www.biotecnologia.com.br/revista/bio29/proteoma.pdf. Acessed 24 Aug 2012.

Engel J. Clinical aspects of epilepsy. Epilepsy Res. 1991;10:9–17.

Engel Jr J. Introduction to temporal lobe epilepsy. Epilepsy Res. 1996;26:141–50. doi:10.1016/S0920-1211(96)00043-5.

Engel Jr J. A proposed diagnostic scheme for people with epileptic seizures and with epilepsy: report of the ILAE Task Force on Classification and Terminology. Epilepsia. 2001;42:796–803. doi:10.1046/j.1528-1157.2001.10401.x.

Eun JP, Choi HY, Kwak YG. Proteomic analysis of human cerebral cortex in epileptic patients. Exp Mol Med. 2004;36:185–91.

Fountoulakis M. Proteomics: current technologies and applications in neurological disorders and toxicology. Amino Acids. 2001;21:363–81. doi:10.1007/s007260170002.

Fountoulakis M, Takács B. Enrichment and proteomic analysis of low-abundance bacterial proteins. Methods Enzymol. 2002;358:288–306. doi:10.1016/S0076-6879(02)58096-4.

French JA, Williamson PD, Thadani VM, Darcey TM, Mattson RH, Spencer SS, et al. Characteristics of medial temporal lobe epilepsy: I. Results of history and physical examination. Ann Neurol. 1993;34:774–80. doi:10.1002/ana.410340604.

French JA, Kanner AM, Bautista J, Abou-Khalil B, Browne T, Harden CL, et al. Efficacy and tolerability of the new antiepileptic drugs I: treatment of new onset epilepsy. Neurology. 2004;62:1252–60.

Greenberg DA, Cayanis E, Strug L, Sudhir M, Durner M, Pal DK, et al. Malic Enzyme 2 underline susceptibility to adolescent-onset idiopatic generalized epilepsy. Am J Hum Genet. 2005;76:139–46. doi:10.1086/426735.

House CR, Miyashiro JE, Swartz BE, Walsh GO, Rich JR, Delgado-Escueta AV. Altered patterns of dynorphin immunoreactivity suggest mossy fiber reorganization in human hippocampal epilepsy. J Neurosci. 1990;10:267–82. doi:0270-6474/90/010267-16$02.00/0.

Huang ZL, Zhou Y, Xiao B, Wu J, Wu XM, Yang P, et al. Proteomic screening of postsynaptic density proteins related with temporal lobe epilepsy. Zhonghua Yi Xue Za Zhi. 2008;88:3205–9.

Kasper BS, Stefan H, Buchfelder M, Paulus W. Temporal lobe microdysgenesis in epilepsy versus control brains. J Neuropathol Exp Neurol. 1999;58:22–8. doi:00005072-199901000-00003.

Kim H, Eliuk S, Deshane J, Meleth S, Sanderson T, Pinner A, et al. 2D gel proteomics: an approach to study age-related differences in protein abundance or isoform complexity in biological samples. Methods Mol Biol. 2007;371:349–91. doi:10.1007/978-1-59745-361-5_24.

Li LM, Sander JW. National demonstration project on epilepsy in Brazil. Arq Neuropsiquiatr. 2003;61:153–6. doi:10.1590/S0004-282X2003000100033.

Li KW, Smit AB. Subcellular proteomics in neuroscience. Front Biosci. 2008;13:4416–25. doi:doi.org/10.2741/3014.

Li Z, Burrone J, Tyler WJ, Hartman KN, Albeanu DF, Murthy VN. Synaptic vesicle recycling studied in transgenic mice expressing synaptopHluorin. Proc Natl Acad Sci USA. 2005;102:6131–6. doi:10.1073/pnas.0501145102.

Liu X, Wen F, Yang J, Chen L, Wei YQ. A review of current applications of mass spectrometry for neuroproteomics in epilepsy. Mass Spectrom Rev. 2010;29:197–246. doi:10.1002/mas.20243.

Lo WY, Tsai FJ, Liu CH, Tang NY, Su SY, Lin SZ, et al. Uncaria rhynchophylla upregulates the expression of MIF and cyclophilin A in kainic acid-induced epilepsy rats: a proteomic analysis. Am J Chin Med. 2010;38:745–59. doi:10.1142/S0192415X10008214.

Marchi N, Teng Q, Ghosh C, Fan Q, Nguyen MT, Desai NK, et al. Blood-brain barrier damage, but not parenchymal white blood cells, is a hallmark of seizure activity. Brain Res. 2010;1353:176–86. doi:10.1016/j.brainres.2010.06.051.

Martins-de-Souza D, Gattaz WF, Schmitt A, Novello JC, Marangoni S, Turck CW, et al. Proteome analysis of schizophrenia patients Wernicke's area reveals an energy metabolism dysregulation. BMC Psychiatry. 2009;9:17. doi:10.1186/1471-244X-9-17.

Masino SA, Kawamura M, Wasser CD, Pomeroy LT, Ruskin DN. Adenosine, ketogenic diet and epilepsy: the emerging therapeutic relationship between metabolism and brain activity. Curr Neuropharmacol. 2009;7:257–68. doi:10.2174/157015909789152164.

Mathern GW, Babb TL, Vickrey BG, Melendez M, Pretorius JK. The clinical-pathogenic mechanisms of hippocampal neuron loss and surgical outcomes in temporal lobe epilepsy. Brain J Neurol. 1995;118:105–18. doi:10.1093/brain/118.1.105.

Mayer MP, Bukau B. Hsp70 chaperones: cellular functions and molecular mechanism. Cell Mol Life Sci. 2005;62:670–84. doi:10.1007/s00018-004-4464-6.

Mus-Veteau I. Heterologous expression and purification systems for structural proteomics of mammalian membrane proteins. Comp Funct Genomics. 2002;3:511–7. doi:10.1002/cfg.218.

Neves SR, Ram PT, Iyengar R. G protein pathways. Science. 2002;296:1636–9. doi:10.1126/science.1071550.

Onat FY, Aker RG, Gurbanova AA, Ates N, Luijtelaar G. The effect of generalized absence seizures on the progression of kindling in the rat. Epilepsia. 2007;5:150–6. doi:10.1111/j.1528-1167.2007.01303.x.

Pappin DJ, Hojrup P, Bleasby AJ. Rapid identification of proteins by peptide-mass fingerprinting. Curr Biol. 1993;3:327–32. doi:10.1016/0960-9822(93)90195-T.

Persike DS, Casarini DE, Lima ML, Amorim RP, Yacubian EMT, Centeno R, Canzian M, Fernandes MJS. Differential expression of proteins in the hippocampus of patients with temporal lobe epilepsy. In: 8th Ibro World Congress of Neuroscience. International Brain Research Organization, Florence. 2011. http://www.ibro2011.org.

Persike DS, Lima ML, Amorim RP, Araújo MGL, Sierra LF, Cavalheiro EA, Schenkman S, Fernandes MJS. Proteomics profile of rat hippocampus subjected to the pilocarpine model of epilepsy. In: XXVII Annual FeSBE Meeting. Serviço de Biblioteca e Informação Biomédica do Instituto de Ciências Biomédicas da Universidade de São Paulo, Águas de Lindóia. 2012. http://www.fesbe.org.br/fesbe2012.

Ross BM, Hudson C, Erlich J, Warsh JJ, Kish SJ. Increased phospholipid breakdown in schizophrenia. Evidence for the involvement of a calcium independent phospholipase A2. Arch Gen Psychiatry. 1997;54:487–94. doi:00000756-199705000-00012.

Shang W, Liu WH, Zhao XH, Sun QJ, Bi JZ, Chi ZF. Expressions of glutathione S-transferase alpha, mu, and pi in brains of medically intractable epileptic patients. BMC Neurosci. 2008;9:67. doi:10.1186/1471-2202-9-67.

Sharma R, Yang Y, Sharma A, Awasthi S, Awasthi YC. Antioxidant role of glutathione S-transferases: protection against oxidant toxicity and regulation of stress-mediated apoptosis. Antioxid Redox Signal. 2004;6:289–300. doi:10.1089/152308604322899350.

Silva AV, Cabral FR. Ictogênese, Epileptogênese e Mecanismo de Ação das Drogas na Profilaxia e Tratamento da Epilepsia. J Epilepsy Clin Neurophysiol. 2008;14:39–45.

Talib LL, Yassuda MS, Diniz BSO, Forlenza OV, Gattaz WF. Cognitive training increases platelet PLA2 activity in healthy elderly subjects. Prostaglandins Leukot Essent Fatty Acids. 2008;78:265–9. doi:10.1016/j.plefa.2008.03.002.

Temkin NR. Preventing and treating posttraumatic seizures: the human experience. Epilepsia. 2009;50:10–3. doi:10.1111/j.1528-1167.2008.02005.x.

Ujike H, Sakai A, Tanaka Y, Kodaka T, Okahisa Y, Harano M, et al. Association study of the dihydropyrimidinase-related protein 2 gene and methamphetamine psychosis. Ann N Y Acad Sci. 2006;1074:90–6. doi:10.1196/annals.1369.008.

Van den Bergh G, Arckens L. Recent advances in 2D electrophoresis: an array of possibilities. Expert Rev Proteomics. 2005;2:243–52. doi:10.1586/14789450.2.2.243.

Wang YY, Smith P, Murphy M, Cook M. Global expression profiling in epileptogenesis: does it add to the confusion? Brain Pathol. 2010;20:1–16. doi:10.1111/j.1750-3639.2008.00254.x.

Wechsler A, Teichberg VI. Brain spectrin binding to the NMDA receptor is regulated by phosphorylation, calcium and calmodulin. EMBO J. 1998;17:3931–9. doi:10.1093/emboj/17.14.3931.

Wilkens S, Zhang Z, Zheng Y. A structural model of the vacuolar ATPase from transmission electron microscopy. Micron. 2005;36:109–26. doi:10.1016/j.micron.2004.10.002.

Wilkins MR, Sanchez IC, Gooley AA, Appel RD, Humphery-Smith I, Hochstrasser DF, et al. Progress with proteome projects: why all proteins expressed by a genome should be identified and how to do it. Biotechnol Genet Eng Rev. 1996;13:19–50. doi:0264-8725/94/12/1-38$20.00+$0.00.

Xiao F, Chen D, Lu Y, Xiao Z, Guan LF, Yuan J, et al. Proteomic analysis of cerebrospinal fluid from patients with idiopathic temporal lobe epilepsy. Brain Res. 2009;1255:180–9. doi:10.1016/j.brainres.2008.12.008.

Yang JW, Czech T, Yamada J, Csaszar Z, Baumgartner C, Slavc I, et al. Aberrant cytosolic acyl-CoA thioester hydrolase in hippocampus of patients with mesial temporal lobe epilepsy. Amino Acids. 2004;27:269–75. doi:10.1007/s00726-004-0138-9.

Yang JW, Czech T, Gelpi E, Lubec G. Extravasation of plasma proteins can confound interpretation of proteomic studies of brain: a lesson from apo A-I in mesial temporal lobe epilepsy. Mol Brain Res. 2005;139:348–56. doi:10.1016/j.molbrainres.2005.06.010.

Yang JW, Czech T, Felizardio M, Baumgartner C, Lubec G. Aberrant expression of cytoskeleton proteins in hippocampus from patients with mesial temporal lobe epilepsy. Amino Acids. 2006;30:477–93. doi:10.1007/s00726-005-0281-y.

Zetterberg FL, Ruetschi U, Portelius E, Brinkmalm G, Andreasson U, Blennow K, et al. Clinical proteomics in neurodegenerative disorders. Acta Neurol Scand. 2008;118:1–11. doi: 10.1111/j.1600-0404.2007.00985.x.

Chapter 9
Abnormalities of GABA System and Human Pharmacoresistant Epilepsy

Sandra Orozco-Suárez, David Escalante-Santiago, Iris Angélica Feria-Romero, Monica E. Ureña-Guerrero, Luisa Rocha, Mario A. Alonso-Vanegas, Juana Villeda-Hernandez, and Ana Luisa Velasco

Abstract Despite the availability of various newly developed antiepileptic drugs (AEDs), pharmacoresistance remains a major challenge in epilepsy management. Unraveling the mechanisms underlying AED resistance has been the focus of intense efforts, in order to develop new rationally designed therapies for as yet refractory epilepsies. Based on experimental and clinical studies, one of the major neurobiological theories that has been put forward is the target hypothesis, which suggests that AEDs are not effective because of target alterations in the epileptogenic brain. Several studies have shown that seizure activity results in altered expression of gamma-aminobutyric acid (GABA) components such as GABA

S. Orozco-Suárez, Ph.D. (✉) • D. Escalante-Santiago, M.Sc. • I.A. Feria-Romero, Ph.D.
Medical Research Unit in Neurological Diseases, National Medical Center, "Siglo XXI", IMSS Hospital of Specialities, Cuauhtemoc No. 330-4, Col. Doctores, Mexico City, Mexico DF 06720, Mexico
e-mail: sorozco5@hotmail.com; irisferi@yahoo.com.mx

M.E. Urena-Guerrero, Ph.D.
Departamento de Biología Celular y Molecular, Centro Universitario de Ciencias Biológicas y Agropecuarias, Universidad de Guadalajara, Km. 15.5 Caretera Guadalajara-Nogales, Predio Las Agujas, Zapopan, Jalisco 45110, Mexico
e-mail: murena@cucba.udg.mx; monica.urena.guerrero@gmail.com

L. Rocha, M.D., Ph.D.
Department of Pharmacobiology, Center for Research and Advanced Studies, Bolivar 782-305, Col. Alamos, Del. Benito Juarez, Mexico City 03400, Mexico

M.A. Alonso-Vanegas, M.D.
ABC Hospital, Santa Fé, Neurology Center, and National Institute of Neurology and Neurosurgery "Manuel Velasco Suárez", Mexico City, Mexico

J. Villeda-Hernandez, Ph.D.
Pathology Department, National Institute of Neurology and Neurosurgery "Manuel Velasco Suárez", Mexico City, Mexico

A.L. Velasco, M.D., Ph.D.
Department of Neurology and Neurosurgery, General Hospital of Mexico, Mexico City, Mexico

L. Rocha and E.A. Cavalheiro (eds.), *Pharmacoresistance in Epilepsy: From Genes and Molecules to Promising Therapies*, DOI 10.1007/978-1-4614-6464-8_9,

transporters (GATs) and GABA receptors. Indeed, changes in the composition of subunits expression appear to affect the functioning of GABAergic neurotransmission. Here, we review the current literature on epilepsy-associated changes in the GABA system conducted in experimental models and observations made in patients with treatment-resistant epilepsy, as well as genetic abnormalities in the GABA system in refractory human epilepsy.

Keywords Pharmacoresistant epilepsy • GABA neurotransmission • GABA receptors • Human data • Animal models • GABA subunits • Antiepileptic drugs

9.1 Introduction

Epidemiological data indicate that 20–40 % of patients with epilepsy are refractory to treatment with antiepileptic drugs (AEDs). Based on experimental and clinical studies, two major neurobiological theories have been put forward to explain the mechanisms or factors that result in drug-resistant epilepsy: (a) the multidrug transporter hypothesis, which suggests that increased brain expression of drug efflux transporters such as P-glycoprotein (P-gp) decreases AED levels at certain brain targets, and (b) the target hypothesis, which indicates that AEDs are not effective because of target alterations in epileptogenic brain tissue (Löscher and Schmidt 2001; Löscher and Potchka 2005; Schmidt and Löscher 2005; Remy and Beck 2006).

The main targets of AEDs exert their effects either by modulation of voltage-dependent ion channels or by enhancing the inhibitory action of gamma-aminobutyric acid (GABA) (Rogawski and Löscher 2004). Fast inhibition in the central nervous system (CNS) is governed by the actions of GABA type A receptors ($GABA_A$Rs). $GABA_A$Rs mediate both phasic and tonic inhibition, and are the principle targets of action for numerous classes of drugs including anxiolytics and AEDs, as well as sedative hypnotic agents including benzodiazepines, barbiturates, alcohol, some general anesthetics and neurosteroids. $GABA_A$Rs are ubiquitously expressed throughout the CNS, and, as such, changes in their expression and function are implicated in virtually all aspects of brain function. Deficits in $GABA_A$Rs-mediated neurotransmission are implicated in diverse disorders of the CNS such as epilepsy. This review focuses on the changes that have been detected in the various components of GABAergic neurotransmission, emphasizing clinical studies.

9.2 GABAergic Neurotransmission

The GABA system is a ubiquitous system regulated by a number of different genes, regulating the synthesis of various receptor subunits, interacting proteins, transporters, synthetic and catabolic enzymes. Figure 9.1 illustrates a GABAergic synapse with its main pharmacological components. Pharmacology has focused on the modification of receptors and transmitters of this system.

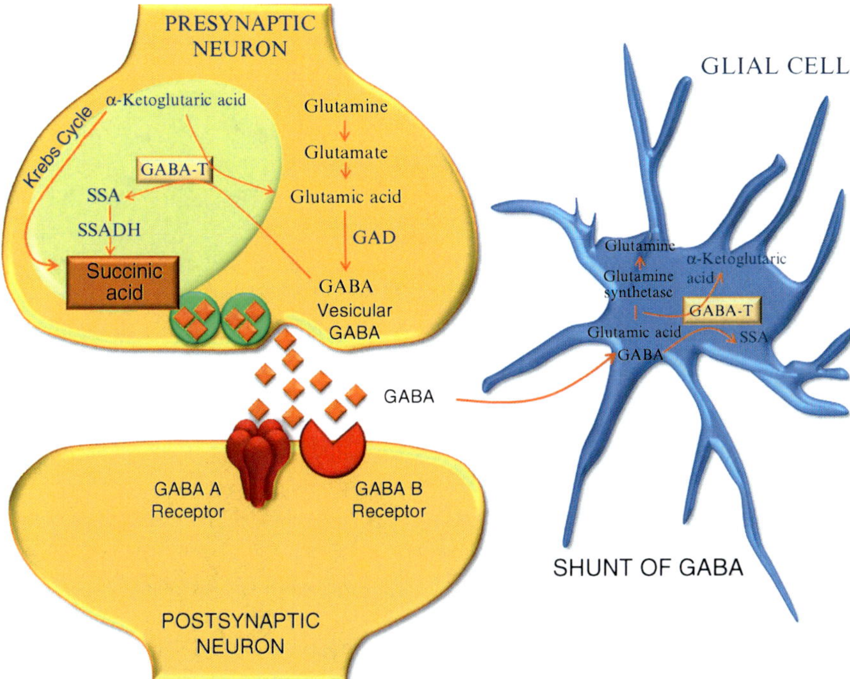

Fig. 9.1 γ-Aminobutyric acid (GABA) is synthesized by decarboxylation of glutamate by glutamic acid decarboxylase (GAD). Upon release into the synaptic cleft, GABA can interact with receptors. To terminate this effect, the neurotransmitter is taken up by high affinity membrane transporters into neurons and surrounding glia, where they can be recycled or metabolized via several enzymes. GABA is converted to glutamine in glial cells. The high activity of glutamine synthase metabolizes glutamic acid to glutamine, and can be recycled to neurons to produce glutamate or GABA. *GABA-T* GABA-transaminase, *GAD* glutamate decarboxylase, *SAS* succinic semialdehyde, *SASDH* SAS-dehydrogenase GABA-A receptor GABA A, *GABA-B* GABAB receptor (modified from McGeer and McGeer 1989)

GABA is synthesized by decarboxylation of glutamate by glutamic acid decarboxylase (GAD). GAD exists in two isoforms, GAD65 and GAD6 7 (Fig. 9.1), which have different molecular weights (65 kDa and 67 kDa, respectively), catalytic and kinetic properties, and subcellular localization (Walls et al. 2010, 2011). As discussed below, this is of importance for seizure control. Degradation of GABA requires GABA-transaminase (GABA-T) to convert GABA to succinic semialdehyde (SSA) by transamination with the co-substrates glutamate and α-ketoglutarate (αKG). SSA is subsequently oxidized by SSA dehydrogenase (SSADH) to succinate, a constituent of the tricarboxylic acid cycle (TCA). Alternatively, SSA can be reduced by c-OH-butyric acid dehydrogenase (GHBDH) to c-OH-butyric acid, which can activate $GABA_B$Rs (Kaupmann et al. 2003). Inhibition of GAD, the GABA-synthesizing enzyme, is known to produce seizures (Tapia and Pasantes 1971). Since GAD is dependent on pyridoxal phosphate as the coenzyme, carbonyl trapping agents like derivatives of hydrazine are generally convulsant in nature (Tapia 1975). Interestingly, aminooxyacetic acid acts as a convulsant at high doses while at lower doses it is an anticonvulsant (Tapia 1975). In the nerve terminals, GABA can be released to the synaptic cleft by two different pathways; i.e., via a Ca^{2+} dependent vesicular release or Ca^{2+} independent release via transporter reversal (Belhage et al. 1993). Upon release to the synaptic cleft, GABA mediates its action via two classes of receptors, ionotropic $GABA_A$Rs and $GABA_C$Rs and metabotropic $GABA_B$Rs. Unlike $GABA_A$Rs and $GABA_C$Rs, which form Cl^- channels and are involved in fast synaptic inhibition, $GABA_B$Rs are guanine nucleotide-binding (G) protein-coupled receptors that modulate calcium (Ca^{2-}) and potassium (K^+) channels and elicit both presynaptic and slow postsynaptic inhibition (Watanabe et al. 2002).

After dissociation from the receptor complex, GABA is transported back into the presynaptic nerve terminal or into surrounding astrocytes via a high-affinity GABA transport system, thereby terminating GABA's inhibitory action (Iversen and Kelly 1975). It has been estimated that the neuronal GABA transport system is three to sixfold more efficient than the astrocytic GABA transport mechanism, which could indicate a reutilization of GABA taken up in the neuron (Hertz and Schousboe 1987). The degradation of GABA is brought about via the enzymes GABA transaminase (GABA-T) and succinic semialdehyde dehydrogenase yielding succinate. GABA-T is located in both neurons and astrocytes, with the highest activity in the latter cell type (Schousboe et al. 1983).

$GABA_A$R are pentameric complexes of subunits, and they form an integral anion channel permeable to chloride and bicarbonate ions (Fig. 9.2). In the brain, $GABA_A$R are composed by two α subunits, which in turn are presented as six isoforms (α1, α2, α3, α4, α5, and α6), two β subunits present as three isoforms (β1, β2S, β2L, and β3) that contribute to the binding site of GABA (Pirker et al. 2003; Scimemi et al. 2005), and one γ subunit with three isoforms (γ1, γ2S, γ2L, and γ3) (Buró and Kamatchi 1991). This diversity of different combinations of isoforms and their assembly determines the properties of $GABA_A$Rs such as affinity for GABA, allosteric modulation, interaction with intracellular proteins, probability of channel opening, kinetics, and conductance. Therefore, changes in the composition of the receptors' subunits appear to affect the function of GABAergic neurotransmission (Wang and Buzsaki 1996; Lambert et al. 2003).

$GABA_B$Rs are broadly expressed in the nervous system, modulating synaptic excitability and plasticity in the cerebral cortex, generating rhythmic activity in cortico-thalamic circuits, relaying primary afferent input to the spinal cord and brainstem, and modulating the activity of dopaminergic and other monoaminergic neurons. These receptors have been implicated in a wide variety of neurologic and psychiatric disorders, including absence seizures, γ-hydroxybutyrate toxicity, and more recently, autoimmune limbic encephalitis. Baclofen is the only clinically available $GABA_B$R agonist and is utilized for treatment of spasticity, dystonia, and some types of neuropathic pain (Bormann 1988; Bowery 1989; Marshall et al. 1999). The $GABA_B$R, like other members of this class, is an obligatory heterodimer in vivo and is formed by two subunits; $GABA_{B1}$ and $GABA_{B2}$ (Fig. 9.3). The $GABA_{B1}$ subunit contains a large extracellular domain that binds GABA or other ligands such

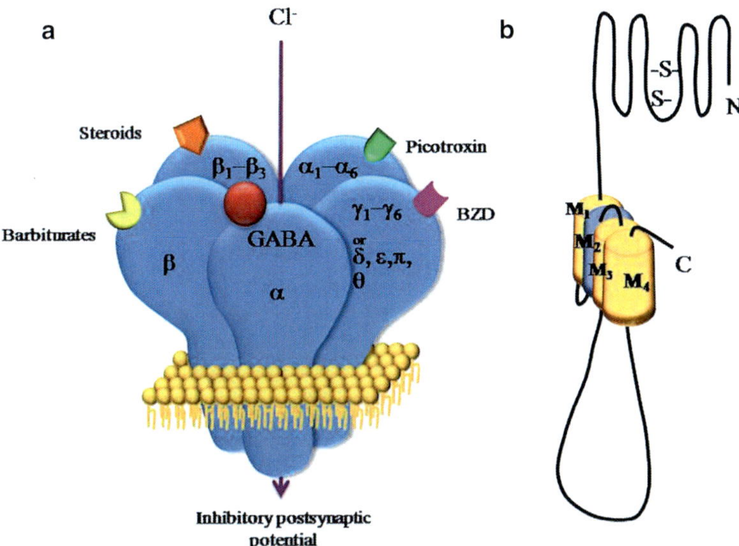

Fig. 9.2 (**a**) $GABA_AR_S$ structure. It is a ionotropic receptor type that comprises different subunits: *α* alpha subunit, *β* beta subunit, *γ* gamma subunit, *δ* delta subunit, *ε* epsilon subunit, *π* subunit phi, *θ* theta subunit. Benzodiazepine-binding site (BZD), *Cl* chlorine ion. (**b**) Each subunit comprises four transmembrane domains (TM1–TM4). The large intracellular loop between TM3 and TM4 contains consensus sites for phosphorylation by protein kinases (P). The amphiphilic TM2 provides the lining of the Cl2 pore intrinsic to the pentameric structure. The most abundant $GABA_AR$ in the brain is the α1β2γ2 isoform

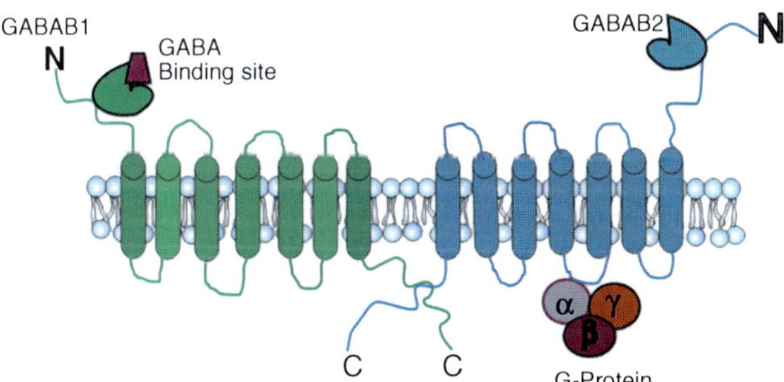

Fig. 9.3 The $GABA_B$ receptor is a metabotropic receptor that acts through second messengers. $GABA_{B1}$ and $GABA_{B2}$ subunits form a functional heterodimer. Agonists bind to the N-terminal of the $GABA_{B1}$ subunit whereas allosteric modulators bind to the $GABA_{B1}$ subunit. *N* amino terminal, *C* carboxyl terminal

as baclofen; the $GABA_{B2}$ subunit couples the receptor with the effector G protein. Activation of $GABA_BRs$ results from successive conformational changes within and across its two subunits. It has been proposed that for the binding of GABA to the extracellular domain, the $GABA_{B1}$ subunit induces a relative movement of the extracellular domains of both $GABA_{B1}$ and $GABA_{B2}$, which elicits a conformational

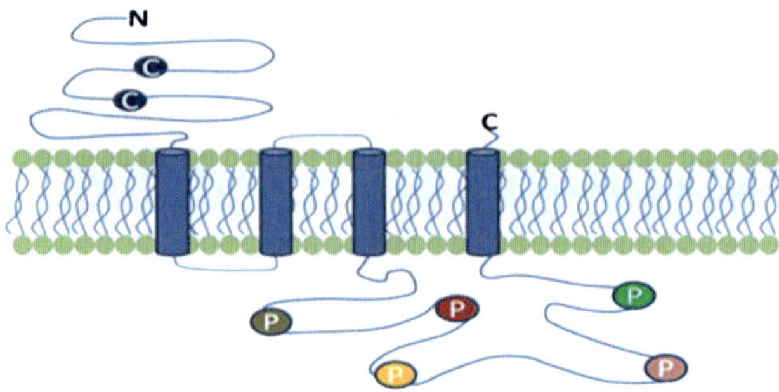

Fig. 9.4 $GABA_C$Rs structure. The structure comprises a long extracellular region, with N-terminal and two cysteine residues. It presents four domains that cross the cell membrane and end with a short C-terminal region. The second domain comprises the ionic channel of the receptor. The extracellular domain includes the GABA binding sites and other modulatory sites. *N* amino terminal, *C* carboxyl terminal; *blue circle* cysteine residues, *P* phosphorylation sites

change of a transmembrane domain that activates the G protein. There are two isoforms of $GABA_{B1}$ subunits, $GABA_{B1a}$ and $GABA_{B1b}$, which differ mainly by the presence in $GABA_{B1a}$ of a tandem pair of extracellular domains, called sushi domains, in their amino (N)-terminal region. These domains are conserved protein-binding motifs that are involved in protein–protein interactions that may determine the different synaptic distribution and functions of these two isoforms (Ulrich and Bettler 2007; Benarroch 2012).

GABA analogue *cis*-4-aminocrotonic acid (CACA) selectively activates a third class of $GABA_A$Rs in the mammalian CNS. These receptors, which were tentatively designated $GABA_C$Rs in 1984, are Cl_2 pores insensitive to both bicuculline and baclofen (Johnston 1996) (Fig. 9.4). Only recently it has been possible to study these novel GABA Rs at the molecular level in clearly defined subpopulations of retinal neurons (Bormann and Feigenspan 1995; Feigenspan and Bormann 1998). Several lines of evidence now indicate that $GABA_C$Rs are composed of ρ-subunits (Bormann and Feigenspan 1995; Enz and Cutting 1998). Heterologously expressed, these subunits form homo-oligomeric channels with the characteristic $GABA_C$Rs (Bormann and Feigenspan 1995; Feigenspan and Bormann 1998; Enz and Cutting 1998, 1999). $GABA_C$Rs comprise the GABAρ1 subunit but eventually grew to a total of three subunits: GABAρ1, GABAρ2, and GABAρ3. Currently, the name $GABA_C$ is in disuse, and the three GABAρ genes are included in the $GABA_A$Rs family ($GABA_A$R, ρ subunits). They are part of the Cys-loop superfamily of neurotransmitter receptors, also called the ligand-gated ion-channel (LGIC), which includes the $GABA_A$Rs, nicotinic acetylcholine receptors (nAChR), glycine receptors, ionotropic 5-HT receptors ($5HT_3$), and a Zn^{2+}-activated ion channel (Olsen and Sieghart 2008).

Fast synaptic GABAergic transmission relies essentially on Cl^- fluxes through $GABA_A$Rs (Farrant and Nusser 2005), for which the maintenance of electrochemical Cl^- gradient is crucial to determine the GABA-mediated neuronal effects (Ben-Ari et al. 2012). Changes in neuronal Cl^- homeostasis affect $GABA_A$Rs-mediated transmission and may contribute to epileptic activities. In this sense, the cation-Cl^- cotransporters (CCC), studied initially for their role in the regulation of cellular volume, are now also considered for their crucial role in the control of the cellular electrochemical Cl^- gradient (Blaesse et al. 2009). The CCC family in mammals consists of nine members encoded by the genes *Slc12a1-9* (Blaesse et al. 2009). The CCCs proteins are glycoproteins of 120–200 kDa, seven of which have been identified as plasmatic proteins (Mercado et al. 2004) with a predicted secondary structure of 12 membrane-spanning segments flanked by carboxy and amino intracellular termini (Gerelsaikhan and Turner 2000). Functionally, CCCs are categorized in three groups: (1) two members cotransport $Na^+/K^+/2Cl^-$ toward the inside of the cell and are named NKCC1 and NKCC2; (2) four members cotransport K^+/Cl^- toward the outside of the cell and are named KCC1-4; and (3) one member cotransports Na^+/Cl^- toward the inside the cell and is named NCC. The physiological roles of proteins encoded by Scl12a8 (CIP1) and Scl1a9 (CCC9) genes remain unknown (Mercado et al. 2004; Blaesse et al. 2009; Briggs and Galanopoulou 2011). Except for NKCC2 and NCC, which are predominantly found in the kidney, all CCCs are expressed in neurons, glial cells, or both, in at least some stage of the CNS development (Mercado et al. 2004; Blaesse et al. 2009). KCC2 is exclusively expressed in the neurons (Payne et al. 1996; Rivera et al. 1999; Gulyas et al. 2001) and linked to NKCC1; both are responsible for maintaining the neuronal electrochemical Cl^- gradient (Ben-Ari et al. 2012). Interestingly, in immature neurons, the expression level of NKCC1 is higher than KCC2, and thus the intracellular Cl^- concentration is higher than the extracellular, and $GABA_AR$ activation induces membrane depolarization and neuronal excitation through Cl^- efflux. In mature neurons, the expression level of KCC2 is higher than NKCC1, and thus $GABA_AR$ activation produces neuronal inhibition (Rivera et al. 1999; Dzhala et al. 2005; Briggs and Galanopoulous 2011; Ben-Ari et al. 2012).

9.3 GABA in Epilepsy

9.3.1 Experimental Evidences

At least in part, pharmacoresistance in epilepsy has been related with modifications in the molecular targets of AEDs, such as voltage-dependent ionic channels, GABA and glutamate receptors, in both experimental epilepsy models and human epilepsy patients (Remy and Beck 2006). In this sense, several AEDs lose their effectiveness when their effect depends on interaction with $GABA_ARs$ (Remy and Beck 2006). Thus, in the pilocarpine model of epilepsy for example, clonazepam effects were significantly reduced in CA1 pyramidal neurons and lightly increased in dentate granule cells (DGCs) of epileptic animals (Gibbs et al. 1997). Moreover, valproate and phenobarbital did not have an effect on spike-like activity of CA3 pyramidal neurons (Klitgaard et al. 2003). Clonazepam ineffectiveness has been associated with a switch between α subunits of $GABA_A$Rs, where the α4 subunit is highly expressed in epileptic animals and substitutes the α1 subunit in the receptors (Brooks-Kayal et al. 1998). In $GABA_A$Rs, the benzodiazepine binding-site is located at the interface between the α and γ subunits, and its pharmacology is thus influenced by these subunits (Fig. 9.2) (Ogris et al. 2004). $GABA_A$Rs with α1–3 or α5 subunits have approximately the same affinity for classical benzodiazepines, but have differential affinity from nonclassical benzodiazepines, such as zolpidem, zaleplon, and abecarnil (Korpi et al. 2002; Ogris et al. 2004). Insensitivity of α4 and α6 subunit-containing $GABA_A$Rs to benzodiazepines is based on the presence of an arginine residue instead of a histidine at a conserved position in its binding site (residue 101) (Wieland et al. 1992). Other significant changes observed in several epilepsy models, including both kainate and pilocarpine models, are related with increments in the γ2 subunit expression in the dentate molecular layer and in CA1 (Fritschy et al. 1999; Peng et al. 2004; Schwarzer et al. 1997), and with pronounced reductions in the α5 subunit (Schwarzer et al. 1997; Fritschy et al. 1999; Houser and Esclapez, 2003) and δ subunit (Schwarzer et al. 1997; Peng et al. 2004) as well as subunits in both the hippocampus and dentate gyrus. These observations suggest that in principal neurons of epileptic hippocampi, γ2 could be substituting for δ subunit in $GABA_A$Rs containing α4 subunit. In this sense, ultrastructural studies have recently demonstrated that in the pilocarpine model, both γ2 and α4 subunits have similar perisynaptic locations (Zhang et al. 2007) but α4 subunit expression is reduced (Lund et al. 2008). On the other hand, the presence of α4βXγ2 $GABA_A$Rs in principal neurons of epileptic hippocampi suggest an increment in tonic inhibition, with less sensitivity to benzodiazepines and zinc, and more sensitivity to the recruitment and trafficking regulation by γ2 subunit phosphorylation (Farrant and Nusser 2005; Jacob et al. 2008; Leidenheimer 2008). In general, $GABA_A$Rs containing α5 subunit are positioned extrasynaptically and modulate NMDA receptors (Li et al. 2005). Thus, reduction of this kind of receptors in epileptic hippocampi could also improve NMDA excitation. The decreased expression of the $GABA_A$R δ subunit, which mediates tonic GABAergic inhibition in DGCs produces an increase in GABAergic inhibition (Nishimura et al. 2005; Zhang et al. 2007; Zhan and Nadler 2009), probably as consequence of a compensatory up-regulation of the extrasynaptic $GABA_A$R α5 subunit in DGCs (Fritschy et al. 1999). Consistent with a role of extrasynaptic $GABA_A$Rs in epilepsy, mice deficient in the $GABA_A$Rs δ subunit and $GABA_A$Rs α5 exhibit increased seizure susceptibility (Mihalek et al. 1999; Glykys et al. 2009). Shifting of subunit location has also been demonstrated in animal models of epilepsy. In addition to a general decrease in the $GABA_A$Rs δ subunit, a more specific decrease in δ subunit labeling at perisynaptic locations on DGCs was detected in pilocarpine-induced status *epilepticus*. However, tonic inhibition was maintained in agreement with previous studies, which was paralleled by a corresponding decrease in the phasic inhibition of granule cells (Zhang et al. 2007). The δ subunit-containing receptors, which mediate tonic inhibition of DGCs, have higher neurosteroid sensitivity (Mihalek et al. 1999; Wohlfarth et al. 2002). Joshi et al. (2011) hypothesize that loss of neurosteroid sensitivity on DGCs increases their excitability. It is proposed that tonic inhibition mediated by

$GABA_A$Rs, primarily the δ and α5 subunit containing receptors, provides powerful shunting inhibition keeping neuronal excitability in check by potentially modulating the offset (threshold) of the I/O curve (Stell et al. 2003; Pavlov et al. 2009). Thus, tonic conductance mediated by these receptors increases the excitatory drive needed to induce action potential firing. The down-regulation of these receptors in temporal lobe epilepsy (TLE) can contribute to enhanced excitability (Glykys and Mody 2006; Mihalek et al. 2001). Thus, in epilepsy models, changes in the subcellular location of $GABA_A$Rs subunits could limit the inhibitory system's ability to respond to excessive excitation. Changes in other $GABA_A$Rs subunits are less consistent, reporting increments or reductions depending of the experimental epilepsy model, brain region, subcellular locations or the methodological approach selected to do the determinations (Brooks-Kayal et al. 1998; Laschet et al. 2007; Schwarzer et al. 1997). For this reason, they are not extensively discussed here.

GABA excitatory signals in early stages of CNS development have trophic effects on neural differentiation and migration, and circuit formation (Manent et al. 2006; Cancedda et al. 2007; Wang and Kriegstein 2010). But at the same time, GABA-mediated excitation could be implicated in high seizure susceptibility (Jensen 2009; Briggs and Galanopoulous, 2011), and could also regulate glutamate-mediated excitotoxicity (Hilton et al. 2005) in early developmental stages of the CNS. Interestingly, the condition of CNS immaturity, where the expression level of NKCC1 is higher than KCC2, an also be observed in pathological conditions such as human epilepsies (Muñoz et al. 2007; Bragin et al. 2009). Therefore, in recent years, blockage of NKCC1 with bumetanide has been employed as coadjutant therapy in the treatment of neonatal seizures (Dzhala et al. 2005; Almeida et al. 2011; Löscher et al. 2012) and in patients with medically intractable TLE with mesial sclerosis or different cortical malformations (Maa et al. 2007; Kahle and Staley 2009). Furthermore, since Brain Derived Neurotrophic Factor (BDNF) down-regulates KCC2 expression, blockage of the neuronal receptor of BDNF (TrkB) could interrupt seizure propagation (Rivera et al. 2002; Ben-Ari et al. 2007, 2012). Finally, the volume/Cl^- sensitive regulatory kinases of CCCs, known as WNK or AK/OSR1 pathways, could be useful in selective functional regulation of NKCC1 and KCC2, although the role of these kinases in the mammalian CNS is still unknown (Kahle and Staley 2009).

9.3.2 *GABA in Pharmacoresistant Epilepsy*

The potential involvement of the GABA system in the pathogenesis of pharmacoresistant human epilepsy has been documented in several studies. Some of them support the hypothesis that changes in the molecular targets can be associated with resistance to drugs acting through the GABAergic system. Most relevant data reveal alterations in numerous $GABA_A$Rs subunits found in biopsies from epileptic patients including changes in extrasynaptic $GABA_A$Rs (for review see Sperk et al. 2009); an increase in extrasynaptic $GABA_A$Rs α5 subunit expression, which mediates tonic GABAergic inhibition in CA1 pyramidal neurons; as well as an increase in $GABA_A$Rs δ subunit expression, which mediates tonic GABAergic inhibition in DGCs (Stell et al. 2003). These data are supported by evidence that tonic GABAergic inhibition is preserved in tissue from epileptic patients and demonstrates a role for extrasynaptic $GABA_A$Rs in epilepsy. Similarly, using immunocytochemistry techniques, other studies have shown alterations in subunit architecture and localization of $GABA_A$Rs subtypes (α1, α2,α3, β2, β3, γ2) in the resected hippocampus from mesial TLE and non-mesial LTE patients compared with control tissues, obtained at autopsy. Consistent with the severe neurodegeneration in the CA1 sector, significant decreases in α1-, α3-, β3-, and γ2-subunit immunoreactivity (IR) were detected in sclerotic, but not in non-sclerotic, specimens. In contrast, pronounced increases in IR of all 3 β-subunits were observed in most sectors of the hippocampal formation both in sclerotic and non-sclerotic specimens, being especially pronounced in the dentate molecular layer and in the subiculum where subunit α3- and γ2-IR were also elevated. Using in situ hybridization for subunits β2 and β3, increased expression of the respective mRNAs was detected in DGCs of patients with and without hippocampal sclerosis. Data from our laboratory revealed an increased expression of the mRNA of the α1, α2, α4, α6, β1, β3, γ1, γ2 subunits in the cerebral cortex of patients with mesial TLE as well as an over-expression of the mRNA of α1, α4, γ2 subunits in the hippocampus (Escalante-Santiago et al. in press). Those data indicate pronounced adaptive changes in the expression of these $GABA_A$Rs subunits related to seizure activity and suggest altered assembly of $GABA_A$Rs in pharmacoresistant TLE.

Likewise, different patterns of $GABA_A$Rs subunit expression have been shown in cortical dysplasia (Crino et al. 2001). The authors observed a decrease in the expression of the β1 subunit in dysplastic neurons compared with pyramidal and heterotopic neurons. They also found reduction in the expression of $GABA_A$Rs α1, α2, and β2 subunits in both dysplastic and heterotrophic neurons. Interestingly, in human TLE most subunits expressed in the hippocampus seem to be up-regulated (notably subunits α2, α3, α5, β1–3, γ2, and δ), indicating little functional change but consistent up-regulation of receptors. However, it is unknown if these changes are associated with alterations in GABAergic transmission.

Human studies have been conducted to evaluate other components of the GABA system. For example, data obtained from patients with epilepsy demonstrate that GABA transport is largely preserved (Mathern et al. 1999; Lee et al. 2006). However, Arellano et al. (2004) showed dramatic morphological and neurochemical reorganizations of chandelier-terminals (Ch) and basket formations in the sclerotic hippocampus of epileptic patients. These changes varied considerably across different hippocampal fields in each patient, and among patients. The changes were not correlated with the clinical characteristics or the degree of histopathological changes, such as granular cell dispersion, neuronal loss and proliferation of mossy fibers (Arellano et al. 2004). However, certain surviving neurons adjacent to areas of neuronal loss were consistently innervated by dense basket formations and complex Ch. In the subicular complex, no apparent alterations were found in epileptic patients with regard to the cytoarchitecture or the distribution of GAT-1.

These results emphasize that, in the epileptic human hippocampus, GABAergic circuits present significant changes that might be important in the pathophysiology of TLE associated with hippocampal sclerosis (Arellano et al. 2004). Similarly, data from our laboratory revealed a significant reduction in mRNA and protein expression of GAT-1 in hippocampus of patients with TLE, a situation that could be associated with cell loss observed in the sclerotic hippocampus (Mathern et al. 2002).

GABA is the inhibitory neurotransmitter used by the majority of interneurons, and thus, the changes observed could represent compensatory plastic mechanisms to enhance inhibition of some pyramidal cells. However, a recent study by Cohen and colleagues raised the intriguing possibility that GABAergic circuits may have excitatory effects in the sclerotic hippocampus of epilepsy patients (Cohen et al. 2002). Their results showed that in the damaged subiculum there is a subpopulation of pyramidal cells in which GABAergic effects result in depolarization instead of hyperpolarization. These cells discharge interictal-like bursts and presumably act as pacemaker cells in generating interictal synchrony (Cohen et al. 2002). Additionally, data obtained from patients with pharmacoresistant epilepsy suggest changes in the relative expression of NKCC1 and KCC2 that may contribute to epileptiform activity in the subicular regions adjacent to sclerotic areas of the hippocampus (Muñoz et al. 2007)

9.4 Genetic Abnormalities in GABA Receptors Associated with Refractory Human Epilepsy

Among the molecules that compose the GABAergic system, changes in $GABA_A$Rs subunits genes (*GABRA1*, *GABRD*, *GABRG2*) and $GABA_B$Rs subunit genes (*GABRB3* and *GABABR2*) have been linked to different types of idiopathic and cryptogenic epilepsies that are resistant to AED control.

9.4.1 Genetic Alterations of $GABA_A$Rs Involved in Epilepsy

Mutations in $GABA_A$Rs genes can be divided into four general classes: (1) coding sequence missense mutations, (2) coding sequence nonsense mutations, (3) coding sequence frameshift mutations, and (4) noncoding sequence mutations (intronic or 5′ upstream). $GABA_A$Rs mutations have been associated with changes in receptor function (impaired channel gating) and/or by impairing receptor biogenesis (impaired subunit mRNA transcription or stability, subunit folding, stability, oligomerization, or receptor trafficking) (Macdonald et al. 2010). Figure 9.5 summarizes mutations in $GABA_A$Rs related to epilepsy.

The most outstanding genetic alterations in $GABA_A$Rs associated with human refractory epilepsy are described below.

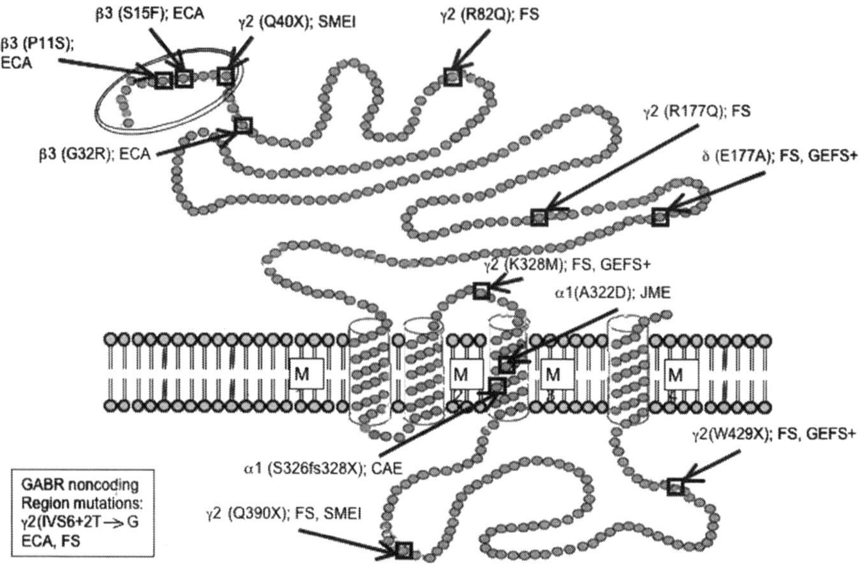

Fig. 9.5 The scheme shows GABA$_A$Rs α1, β3, γ2, and δ subunit mutations (*small squares*) associated with genetic epilepsy syndromes at their appropriate protein domain within the subunit. GABA$_A$ receptor subunits are translated as a precursor protein whose signal sequence (*double circle*) is removed leaving a mature protein consisting of a large extracellular domain at the N-terminus, four transmembrane domains (M1–M4) and a large cytoplasmic domain (modified from Macdonald et al. 2010)

9.4.1.1 Gamma-Aminobutyric Acid A Receptor-α1 Gene or *GABRA1*, NCBI RefSeq NM_000806.5

This gene encodes variant 1 of the α subunit in GABA$_A$R and is located in the chromosomal region 5q34. It is comprised of 9 exons with 1,371 nucleotides to result in a protein of 456 amino acids (aa). There are seven reported variants of *GABRA1* that differ in the 5′ UTR (Garrett et al. 1988).

The relationship between *GABRA1* and susceptibility to juvenile myoclonic epilepsy (EJM5) was studied in four generations of a French Canadian family with an autosomal dominant pedigree pattern. The mutation screen showed a C to A (cytosine to adenine) substitution in this gene, resulting in a change on A322D (ala to asp in 322 aa) (Cossette et al. 2002). This mutant is present in the M3 transmembrane domain, causes misfolding of this protein, and therefore the majority of protein is degraded. In this context, the residual no-degraded mutant A322D reduces the surface expression of GABA$_A$Rs by associating with wild type subunits within the endoplasmic reticulum and preventing them from trafficking to the cell surface. In vitro cellular studies indicated that this mutant reduces surface expression of *GABRA3* by a greater amount than α–1–containing receptors, thus contributing to cortical excitability. So, this mutation allows a modest dominant–negative effect that likely contributes to the epilepsy phenotype (Ding et al. 2010). In this regard, various studies have reported the position of these mutant amino acids in *GABRA1*, *GABRB3*, and *GABRD* in the immature peptide that includes the signal sequence. Further, mutations in *GABRG2* have also been reported in the mature peptide in the same position.

On the other hand, in a German boy with childhood absence epilepsy (ECA4) a de novo heterozygous 975delC in the GABRA1 gene was identified, resulting in a frameshift and premature truncation of the protein at codon 328 within the third transmembrane domain. The mutation was absent in both parents and brother, and in 292 ethnically matched controls (Maljevic et al. 2006).

9.4.1.2 Gamma-Aminobutyric Acid A Receptor-δ Gene or *GABRD*, NCBI RefSeq NM_000816.3

This gene encodes the delta subunit of the $GABA_AR$ and is located in the chromosomal region 1p36.3. It is comprised of 9 exons with 1,404 nucleotides to result in a protein of 467 aa (Sommer et al. 1990).

Generalized epilepsy with febrile seizures plus (GEFS+) was studied in a small family from the South of Australia: a heterozygous A530C (adenine/citocine 530 position) in exon 5 of the GABRD gene was found, resulting in the polymorphism E177A (glu to ala substitution in 177aa) of the N-terminal extracellular domain. However, the unaffected mother also carried the mutation, suggesting that it represents a susceptibility allele (Dibbens et al. 2004). In this study, the authors also identified a heterozygous G659A (guanine/citocine 656 position) polymorphism in exon 6 of the GABRD gene, resulting in an R220H (arg to his in 220aa) substitution in the N-terminal extracellular domain of the protein, with different forms of epilepsy. The polymorphism was found in 8.3 % of patients with idiopathic generalized epilepsy (EIG10), 3.1 % with GEFS+, and 4.2 % of control individuals (Dibbens et al. 2004). However, Lenzen et al. (2005) did not find an association between the R220H variant and idiopathic generalized epilepsy (EIG) or juvenile myoclonic epilepsy (EJM) among 562 German patients and 664 controls (Lenzen et al. 2005).

9.4.1.3 Gamma-Aminobutyric Acid A Receptor-γ2 or *GABRG2*, NCBI RefSeq NM_000806.5

This gene encodes variant two of the α subunit of the $GABA_AR$ located in the chromosomal region 5q34 and shares approximately 40 % sequence identity with the α and β subunits. It is comprised of 9 exons with 1,371 nucleotides to result in a protein of 456 aa. There are three reported isoforms of *GABRG2* (Wilcox et al. 1992).

Childhood absence epilepsy (ECA2) and febrile seizures alone or in combination, were studied in a four–generation family. The authors found a heterozygous G245A resulting in a R43Q (arg to gln in 43aa) substitution in the GABRG2 protein, a situation associated with abolished diazepam sensitivity. In this pedigree there were three individuals with febrile seizure plus and two with myoclonic astatic epilepsy (MAE), confirming that the R43Q mutation in *GABRG2* also contributes to the $GEFS^+$ syndrome. The authors suggest that, even though both syndromes have different ages of seizure onset and the physiology of absences and seizures are distinct, the

R43Q mutation has age-dependent effects on different neuronal networks that influence the expression of these clinically distinct, but genetically related, conditions (Wallace et al. 2001). *In vitro* studies have demonstrated that brief increases in temperature result in impaired trafficking, accelerated endocytosis, and decreased surface expression of the heterozygous R43Q mutant GABA-αR, which could be an explanation for triggering of seizures by fever in patients with this mutation (Kang et al. 2006).

In a screening of 1,200 unrelated patients with various epilepsy phenotypes [GEFS$^+$, febrile seizures, and idiopathic generalized epilepsy (IGE)] by single strand conformation polymorphism (SSCP) analysis, a bilinear family (obtained on 156 family members) initially described as "family G" was identified. In this family a proband was taken, and a C1168T (cytosine/thymine 1,168 position) transition in exon 9 of the GABRG2 gene was detected, resulting in a Q351X (gln to ter in 351aa) substitution, associated with generalized epilepsy with febrile seizures plus type 3 (GEFS$^+$3). Later, the proband developed Dravet syndrome, also known as severe myoclonic epilepsy in infancy (SMEI) (Harkin et al. 2002). As with the R45Q mutation, Kang et al. (2006) showed the same behavior for the Q351X mutant (Kang et al. 2006).

In one screening, 135 unrelated German patients with idiopathic absence epilepsy were compared with 154 unrelated and ethnically matched controls. In this study, a family with childhood absence epilepsy (ECA2) and febrile convulsions seizures (FEB8) was identified. In this family, the affected sister and affected father of the index patient (the first medically identified patient in a family or other group, with a particular condition, often an infection, which triggers a line of investigation) but not the clinically unaffected mother carried the IVS6+2T-G mutation (thymine to guanine substitution occurring at the splice donor site of intron 6) of the GABRG2 gene, suggesting exon skipping, premature truncation, and a nonfunctional protein (Kananura et al. 2002).

In a family with febrile seizures (FEB8) three affected members (two affected sibs and their father) were identified as carrying a heterozygous 529C-G transversion in exon 4 of the GABRG2 gene, resulting in an R139G (arg-to-gly 139 aa substitution) in the second benzodiazepine-binding site of the protein. The mutation was not identified in 368 control chromosomes. The paternal grandfather, who was reportedly unaffected, also carried the mutation, suggesting incomplete penetrance. All patients had normal mental development, and none developed epilepsy later in life. In vitro functional analysis showed that the mutant receptor currents desensitized more rapidly than the wild-type and had significantly decreased sensitivity to diazepam (Audenaert et al. 2006).

9.4.1.4 Gamma-Aminobutyric Acid Receptor-β3 or *GABRB3*, NCBI RefSeq NM_000814.5

This gene encodes variant 1 of the β subunit 3 of the $GABA_A$R located in the chromosomal region 15q12. It is comprised of 9 exons with 1,422 nucleotides to result in a protein of 473 aa. There are four reported variants of *GABRB3* and all have a distinct N-terminus (Wagstaff et al. 1991).

From two promoter regions upstream of the alternative first exons, exon 1a and exon 1 of the human GABRB3 gene, the 5′-untranslated regions (5′-UTRs), the coding region and the 3′-UTR of the GABRB3 gene were screened in 45 childhood absence epilepsy (ECA) Austrian patients by SSCP analysis. After amplification and sequencing 1,400 bp of the genomic DNA upstream of exon 1a and a 650 bp fragment between exon 1a and exon 1 in 11 patients and 9 unrelated control samples, a total of 13 single-nucleotide polymorphisms (SNPs) were found, of which 2 SNPs were novel. The association analysis using a Monte Carlo version of the multiallele Transmission Disequilibrium Test, found that polymorphism −897 °C corresponding to SNP rs4906902 had the most important association ($P=0.007075$). The authors propose that this change could impair the potential binding site of the neuron-specific transcriptional activator POU3F2 (Feucht et al. 1999). The SNP result correlated with the haplotype 2 obtained from a microsatellite DNA marker 155CA2 (Urak et al. 2006). Another microsatellital study to determine allele frequency was performance on 90 ECA patient–mother–father trios of Han ethnicity (China). The allele frequencies with TDT analysis suggested that the microsatellite DNA repeats 85CA, 155CA1, and 155CA2 related with GABRA5 and GABRB3 genes were associated with ECA (Lü et al. 2004).

Others polymorphisms related with ECA patients were found in members of two unrelated Mexican families with ECA5, where a heterozygous C31T transition in exon 1a of the GABRB3 gene was identified, resulting in a P11S (pro to ser in 11aa) substitution in the alternative signal peptide, although three unaffected family members from both families carried the mutation, indicating incomplete penetrance. This research group also identified a Honduran patient with ECA5, a heterozygous C44T transition in exon 1a of the GABRB3 gene, resulting in a S15F (ser to phe in 15aa); the mutation was also present in his unaffected mother and half-brother. A third mutation was identified in two Honduran patients with ECA5, where a heterozygous G32R transition in exon 2 of the GABRB3 gene resulted in a G32R (gly to arg in 32aa). Two additional family members with EEG abnormalities but without absence seizures and one relative who had had a febrile seizure also showed the mutation. Both, Mexican and Honduran patients were compared with 630 controls in which the mutations were not identified. *In vitro* cellular functional expression studies showed that P11S, S15F, and G32R mutants of the GABRB3 protein were hyperglycosylated and had reduced mean current densities compared to the wild type (Tanaka et al. 2008).

9.4.2 Gamma-Aminobutyric Acid B Receptor 2 or **GABBR2**, *NCBI RefSeq NM_005458.7*

This gene encodes the GABBR subunit 2 located in the chromosomal region 9q22.1-q22.3. This gene is comprised of 19 exons with 2,826 nucleotides to result in a protein of 941 aa. There are no reported isoforms (Kaupmann et al. 1998).

Two SNPs of *GABBR1* and four SNPs of *GABBR2*, all in intronic regions, were selected and genotyped in 318 mesial TLE patients and 315 non-epileptic individuals in a Han Chinese population. SNPs rs29259 of *GABBR1*, rs1999501 and rs944688 of *GABBR2* were thought to be associated with mesial TLE; however, after a Bonferroni correction, these associations were not observed and only the rs967932 A-allele of GABBR2 was found to increase the risk of mesial TLE in the dominant model ($P=0.036$). The frequency at which the haplotype G-C-A-C (rs3780428-rs1999501-rs967932-rs944688) of *GABBR2* occurred in mesial TLE patients was significantly higher compared to the controls (12.26 % vs. 6.51 %, $P=0.0004$), and patients carrying this haplotype exhibited an earlier onset of mesial TLE ($P=0.028$) (Wang et al. 2008).

9.5 Concluding Remarks

Modulation of GABAergic function remains as one of the main strategies in epilepsy treatment. There are many data in animal models and in humans that indicate that refractory epilepsy affects $GABA_A$Rs stereochemistry and function. These modifications could produce changes in the sensitivity of recognition of the binding site or alterations in the sites of GABA binding and thereby changes in the action of the agonists. This functional receptor changes could provide some cellular clues to explain drug resistant epilepsy and could support the development of novel therapeutic strategies. For example, tonic $GABA_A$Rs-mediated conductance in various animal models of epilepsy and in neurons from epileptic human tissue suggests that targeting this form of inhibition can be used to suppress network excitability and prevent seizure generation. However, the successful use of this approach requires a better understanding of epilepsy-induced changes in the pharmacology of tonic currents in cell types that comprise the networks involved in generation of pathological activity.

Acknowledgments This study was supported by the Research in Health Found, FIS/IMSS/PROT/548 grant and National Council for Sciences and Technology of Mexico (Grant 98386). We thank Dr. Erika Brust-Mascher for English improvement.

References

Audenaert D, Schwartz E, Claeys KG, Claes L, Deprez L, Suls A. et al. Combined effect of bumetanide, bromide, and GABAergic agonists: an alternative treatment for intractable seizures. Epilepsy Behav. 2011;20:147–9.

Arellano JI, Muñoz A, Ballesteros-Yañez I, Sola RG, DeFelipe J. Histopathology and reorganization of chandelier cells in the human epileptic sclerotic hippocampus. Brain. 2004;127:45–64.

Audenaert D, Schwartz E, Claeys KG, et al. A novel GABRG2 mutation associated with febrile seizures. Neurology. 2006;67:687–90.

Belhage B, Hansen GH, Schousboe A. Depolarization by K+and glutamate activates different neurotransmitter release mechanisms in GABAergic neurons: vesicular versus non-vesicular release of GABA. Neuroscience. 1993;54:1019–34.

Ben-Ari Y, Giarsa JL, Tyzio R, Khazipov R. GABA: a pioneer transmitter that excites immature neurons and generates primitive oscillations. Physiol Rev. 2007;87:1215–84.

Ben-Ari Y, Khalilov I, Kahle KT, Cherubini E. The GABA excitatory/inhibitory shift in brain maturation and neurological disorders. Neuroscientist. 2012;18(5):467–86.

Benarroch E. GABAB receptors structure, functions, and clinical implications. Neurology. 2012;78:578–82.

Blaesse P, Airaksinen MS, Rivera C, Kaila K. Cation-chloride cotransporters and neuronal function. Neuron. 2009;61:820–38.

Bormann J. Electrophysiology of GABAA and GABAB receptor subtypes. Trends Neurosci. 1988;11:112–6.

Bormann J, Feigenspan A. GABAC receptors. Trends Neurosci. 1995;18:515–9.

Bowery NG. GABAB receptors and their significance in mammalian pharmacology. Trends Pharmacol Sci. 1989;10:401–7.

Bragin DE, Sanderson JL, Peterson S, Connor JA, Müller WS. Development of epileptiform excitability in the deep entorhinal cortex after status epilepticus. Eur J Neurosci. 2009;30(4):611–24.

Briggs SW, Galanopoulou AS. Altered GABA signaling in early life epilepsies. Neural Plast. 2011;2011:527605.

Brooks-Kayal AR, Shumate MD, Jin H, Rikhter TY, Coulter DA. Selective changes in single cell GABA(A) receptor subunit expression and function in temporal lobe epilepsy. Nat Med. 1998;4:1166–72.

Buró D, Kamatchi G. GABAA receptor subtypes: from pharmacology to molecular biology. FASEB J. 1991;5:2916–23.

Cancedda L, Fiumelli H, Chen K, Poo MM. Excitatory GABA action is essential for morphological maturation of cortical neurons in vivo. J Neurosci. 2007;27:5224–35.

Cohen I, Navarro V, Clemenceau S, Baulac M, Miles R. On the origin of interictal activity in human temporal lobe epilepsy in vitro. Science. 2002;298:1418–21.

Cossett P, Liu L, Brisebois K,Dong H, Lortie A, Vannase M, et al. Mutation of GABRA1 in an autosomal dominant form of juvenile myoclonic epilepsy. Nat Genet. 2002;31:184–9.

Crino PB, Duhaime AC, Baltuch G, White R. Differential expression of glutamate and GABA-A receptor subunit mRNA in cortical dysplasia. Neurology. 2001;56:906–13.

Dibbens LM, Feng HJ, Richards MC,Harkin LA,Hudqson BL, Scott D, et al. GABRD encoding a protein for extra- or peri-synaptic GABA-A receptors is a susceptibility locus for generalized epilepsies. Hum Mol Genet. 2004;13:1315–9.

Ding L, Feng HJ, Macdonald RL, Botzolakis EJ, Hu N, Gallagher MJ. GABA(A) receptor alpha−1 subunit mutation A322D associated with autosomal dominant juvenile myoclonic epilepsy reduces the expression and alters the composition of wild type GABA(A) receptors. J Biol Chem. 2010;285:26390–405.

Dzhala VI, Talos DM, Sdrulla DA, Brumback AC, Mathews GC, Benke TA, et al. NKCC1 transporter facilitates seizures in the developing brain. Nat Med. 2005;11:1205–13.

Enz R, Cutting GR. Molecular composition of GABAC receptors. Vision Res. 1998;38:1431–41.

Enz R, Cutting GR. GABAC receptor r subunits are heterogeneously expressed in the human CNS and form homo- and heterooligomers with distinct properties. Eur J Neurosci. 1999;11:41–50.

Escalante-Santiago E, Feria-Romero I, Rocha L, Alonso M, Villeda J, Ureña-Guerrero ME, Munguia J, Nicolini-Sánchez H, Velasco AL, Chávez L, Orozco-Suárez S (in press) Changes in the expression of mRNA and protein of the GABA system in pharmacoresistant temporal lobe epilepsy Posgrado en Ciencias Genómicas, Universidad Autónoma de la Ciudad de México, 2010

Farrant M, Nusser Z. Variations on an inhibitory theme: phasic and tonic activation of GABAA receptors. Nat Rev Neurosci. 2005;6:215–29.

Feigenspan A, Bormann J. GABA-gated Cl2 channels in the rat retina. Prog Retinal Eye Res. 1998;17:99–126.

Feucht M, Fuchs K, Pichlbauer E, Hornik K, Scharfetter J, Goessler R, et al. Possible association between childhood absence epilepsy and the gene encoding GABRB3. Biol Psychiatry. 1999;46:997–1002.

Fritschy JM, Kiener T, Bouilleret V, Loup F. GABAergic neurons and GABAA-receptors in temporal lobe epilepsy. Neurochem Int. 1999;34:435–45.

Garrett KM, Duman RS, Saito N,Blume AJ, Vitek MP, Tallman JF, et al. Isolation of a cDNA clone for the alpha subunit of the human GABA-A receptor. Biochem Biophys Res Commun. 1988;156:1039–45.

Gerelsaikhan T, Turner RJ. Transmembrane topology of the secretory Na^{+}-K^{+}-$2Cl^{-}$ cotransporter NKCC1 studied by in vitro translation. J Biol Chem. 2000;275:40471–7.

Gibbs III JW, Shumate M, Coulter D. Differential epilepsy-associated alterations in postsynaptic GABAA receptor function in dentate granule and CA1 neurons. J Neurophysiol. 1997;77: 1924–38.

Glykys J, Mody I. Hippocampal network hyperactivity after selective reduction of tonic inhibition in GABA A receptor alpha5 subunit-deficient mice. J Neurophysiol. 2006;95:2796–807.

Glykys J, Dzhala VI, Kuchibhotla KV, Feng G, Kuner T, Augustine G, et al. Differences in cortical versus subcortical GABAergic signaling a candidate mechanism of electroclinical uncoupling of neonatal seizures. Neuron. 2009;63:657–72.

Gulyas AI, Sik A, Payne JA, Kaila K, Freund TF. The KCI cotransporter, KCC2, is highly expressed in the vicinity of excitatory synapses in the rat hippocampus. Eur J Neurosci. 2001;13:2205–17.

Harkin LA, Bowser DN, Dibbens LM, Singh R., Phillips F, Wallace RH, et al. Truncation of the GABA-A-receptor gamma-2 subunit in a family with generalized epilepsy with febrile seizures plus. Am J Hum Genet. 2002;70:530–6.

Hertz L, Schousboe A. Primary cultures of GABAergic and glutamatergic neurons as model systems to study neurotransmitter functions. Differentiated cells. In: Vernadakis A, Privat A, Lauder JM, Timiras PS, Giacobini E, editors. Model systems of development and aging of the nervous system. Boston: Martinus Nijhoff Publishing; 1987.

Hilton GD, Ndubuizu A, Nunez JL, McCarthy MM. Simultaneous glutamate and GABA(A) receptor agonist administration increases calbindin levels and prevents hippocampal damage induced by either agent alone in a model of perinatal brain injury. Brain Res Dev Brain Res. 2005;159: 99–111.

Houser CR, Esclapez M. Downregulation of the α5 subunit of the $GABA_A$ receptor in the pilocarpine model of temporal lobe epilepsy. Hippocampus. 2003;13:633–45.

Iversen LL, Kelly JS. Uptake and metabolism of gamma-aminobutyric acid by neurones and glial cells. Biochem Pharmacol. 1975;24:933–8.

Jacob TC, Moss SJ, Jurd R. GABA(A) receptor trafficking and its role in the dynamic modulation of neuronal inhibition. Nat Rev Neurosci. 2008;9:331–43.

Jensen FE. Neonatal seizures: an update on mechanisms and management. Clin Perinatol. 2009;36:881–900.

Johnston GA. GABAC receptors: relatively simple transmitter gated ion channels? Trends Pharmacol Sci. 1996;17:319–23.

Joshi S, Rajasekaran, K Kapur J (2011) GABAergic transmission in temporal lobe epilepsy: The role of neurosteroids. Exp Neurol

Kahle KT, Staley KJ. Cation-chloride cotransporters as pharmacological targets in the treatment of epilepsy. In: Alvarez-Leefmans F, Delpire E, editors. Physiology and pathology of chloride transporters and channels in the nervous system. New York: Academic; 2009.

Kananura C, Haug K, Sander T, Runge u, Gu W, Hallmann K, et al. A splice-site mutation in GABRG2 associated with childhood absence epilepsy and febrile convulsions. Arch Neurol. 2002;59:1137–41.

Kang JQ, Shen W, Macdonald RL. Why does fever trigger febrile seizures? GABAA receptor gamma2 subunit mutations associated with idiopathic generalized epilepsies have temperature-dependent trafficking deficiencies. J Neurosci. 2006;6:2590–7.

Kaupmann K, Malitschek B, Schuler V. GABA(B)-receptor subtypes assemble into functional heteromeric complexes. Nature. 1998;396:683–7.
Kaupmann K, Cryan JF, Wellendorph P, Mombereau C, Sansig G, Klebs K, et al. Specific gamma-hydroxybutyrate-binding sites but loss of pharmacological effects of gamma-hydroxybutyrate in GABA(B)(1)- deficient mice. Eur J Neurosci. 2003;18:2722–30.
Klitgaard H, Matagne A, Grimee R, Vanneste-Goemaere J, Margineanu DG. Electrophysiological, neurochemical and regional effects of levetiracetam in the rat pilocarpine model of temporal lobe epilepsy. Seizure. 2003;12:92–100.
Korpi ER, Gründer G, Lüddens H. Drug interactions at GABAA receptors. Prog Neurobiol. 2002;67:113–59.
Lambert JJ, Belelli D, Peden DR, Vardy AW, Peters JA. Neurosteroid modulation of GABAA receptors. Prog Neurobiol. 2003;71:67–80.
Laschet JJ, Kurcewicz I, Minier F, Trottier S, Khallov-Laschet J, Louvel J.et al. Dysfunction of GABAA receptor glycolysis-dependent modulation in human partial epilepsy. Proc Natl Acad Sci U S A. 2007;104:3472–7.
Lee TS, Bjørnsen LP, Paz C, Kim JH, Spencer SS, Spencer DD, et al. GAT1 and GAT3 expression are differently localized in the human epileptogenic hippocampus. Acta Neuropathol. 2006;111:351e363.
Leidenheimer NJ. Regulation of excitation by GABA(A) receptor internalization. Results Probl Cell Differ. 2008;44:1–28.
Lenzen KP, Heils A, Lorenz S,Hempelman A, Sander T. Association analysis of the arg220-to-his variation of the human gene encoding the GABA delta subunit with idiopathic generalized epilepsy. Epilepsy Res. 2005;65:53–7.
Li RW, Yu W, Christie S, Miralles CP, Bai J, Loturco JJ, et al. Disruption of postsynaptic GABA receptor clusters leads to decreased GABAergic innervation of pyramidal neurons. J Neurochem. 2005;95:756–70.
Löscher W, Potchka H. Drug resistance in brain diseases and the role of drug efflux transporters. Nat Rev Neurosci. 2005;6(8):591–602.
Löscher W, Schmidt D. New horizons in the development of antiepileptic drugs: the search for new targets. Epilepsy Res. 2001;60:77–159.
Löscher W, Puskarjov, M, Kaila K (2012) Cation-chloride cotransporters NKCC1 and KCC2 as potential targets for novel antiepileptic and antiepileptogenic treatments. Neuropharmacology. 2012; http://dx.doi.org/10.1016/j.neuropharmacol.2012.05.045
Lü JJ, Zhang YH, Pan H, Chen YC, Liu XY, Jiang YW, et al. Case-control study and transmission/disequilibrium tests of the genes encoding GABRA5 and GABRB3 in a Chinese population affected by childhood absence epilepsy. Chin Med J (Engl). 2004;117:1497–14501.
Lund IV, Hu Y, Raol YH, Benham RS, Faris R, Russek SJ, et al. BDNF selectively regulates $GABA_A$ receptor transcription by activation of the JAK/STAT pathway. Sci Signal. 2008;1(41):ra9.
Maa E, Bainbridge J, Spitz MC, Staley KJ. Oral bumetanide add-on therapy in refractory temporal lobe epilepsy. Epilepsia. 2007;48(Suppl. 6) [abstract # 3.222]
Macdonald RL, Kang JQ, Gallagher MJ. Mutations in GABAA receptor subunits associated with genetic epilepsies. J Physiol. 2010;588:1861–9.
Maljevic S, Krampfl K, Cobilanschi J, Filgen N, Beyer S. Weber YG, et al. A mutation in the GABA-A receptor alpha-1-subunit is associated with absence epilepsy. Ann Neurol. 2006;59:983–7.
Manent JB, Jorquera I, Ben Ari Y, Aniksztejn L, Represa A. Glutamate acting on AMPA but not NMDA receptors modulates the migration of hippocampal interneurons. J Neurosci. 2006;26:5901–9.
Marshall FH, Jones KA, Kaupmann K, Bettler B. GABAB receptors—the first 7TM heterodimers. Trends Pharmacol Sci. 1999;20:396–9.
Mathern GW, Mendoza D, Lozada A, Pretorius JK, Danbolt NV, Nelson N, et al. Hippocampal GABA and glutamate transporter immunoreactivity in patients with temporal lobe epilepsy. Neurology. 1999;52:453e–72e.
Mathern GW, Adelson PD, Cahan LD, Leite JP. Hippocampal neuron damage in human epilepsy. Meyer's hypothesis revisited. Prog Brain Res. 2002;135:237–51.

McGeer PL, McGeer EG. Amino acid neurotransmitters. In: Siegel GJ, Agranoff BW, Albers RW, Molinoff PB, editors. Basic neurochemistry: molecular, cellular and medical aspects. 4th ed. New York: Raven; 1989.
Mercado A, Mount DB, Gamba G. Electroneutral cation-chloride cotransporters in the central nervous system. Neurochem Res. 2004;29:17–25.
Mihalek RM, Banerjee PK, Korpi ER, et al. Attenuated sensitivity to neuroactive steroids in gamma-aminobutyrate type A receptor delta subunit knockout mice. Proc Natl Acad Sci U S A. 1999;96:12905–10.
Mihalek RM, Bowers BJ, Wehner JM, Kralic JE, VanDoren MJ, Morrow AL. Homanics GE. GABA(A)-receptor delta subunit knockout mice have multiple defects in behavioral responses to ethanol. Alcohol Clin Exp Res. 2001;25:1708–18.
Muñoz A, Mendez P, DeFelipe J, Alvarez-Leefmans FJ. Cation-chloride cotransporters and GABA-ergic innervation in the human epileptic hippocampus. Epilepsia. 2007;48:663–73.
Nishimura T, Schwarzer C, Gasser E, Kato N, Vezzani A, Sperk G. Altered expression of GABA(A) and GABA(B) receptor subunit mRNAs in the hippocampus after kindling and electrically induced status epilepticus. Neuroscience. 2005;134:691–704.
Ogris W, Poltl A, Hauer B, Ernst M, Oberto A, Wulff P, et al. Affinity of various benzodiazepine site ligands in mice with a point mutation in the GABAA receptor $\gamma 2$ subunit. Biochem Pharmacol. 2004;68:1621–9.
Olsen RW, Sieghart W. International Union of Pharmacology. LXX. Subtypes of gamma-aminobutyric acid (A) receptors: classification on the basis of subunit composition, pharmacology, and function. Update. Pharmacol Rev. 2008;60:243–60.
Pavlov I, Savtchenko LP, Kullmann DM, Semyanov A, Walker MC. Outwardly rectifying tonically active GABAA receptors in pyramidal cells modulate neuronal offset, not gain. J Neurosci. 2009;29:15341–50.
Payne JA, Stevenson TJ, Donaldson LF. Molecular characterization of a putative K-Cl cotransporter in rat brain. A neuronal-specific isoform. J Biol Chem. 1996;271:16245–52.
Peng Z, Huang CS, Stell BM, Mody I, Houser CR. Altered expression of the d subunit of the $GABA_A$ receptor in a mouse model of temporal lobe epilepsy. J Neurosci. 2004;24:8629–39.
Pirker S, Schwarzer C, Czech T, Baungartner C, Pockberg H, Maier H et al. Increased expression of $GABA_A$ receptor β-subunits in the hippocampus of patients with temporal lobe epilepsy. J Neuropathol Exp Neurol. 2003;62:820–34.
Remy S, Beck H. Molecular and cellular mechanisms of pharmacoresistance in epilepsy. Brain. 2006;129:18–35.
Rivera C, Voipio J, Payne JA, Rusuvuori E, Lahtinen H, Lamsa K, et al. The K^+/Cl^- co-transporter KCC2 renders GABA hyperpolarizing during neuronal maturation. Nature. 1999;397:251–5.
Rivera C, Li H, Thomas-Crusells J, Lahtinen H,Viitanen T, Nanobashuili A, et al. BDNF-induced TrkB activation down-regulates the K^+-Cl^+ cotransporter KCC2 and impairs neuronal Cl^- extrusion. J Cell Biol. 2002;159:747–52.
Rogawski MA, Löscher W. The neurobiology of antiepileptic drugs. Nat Rev Neurosci. 2004;5:553–64.
Schmidt D, Löscher W. Drug resistance in epilepsy: putative neurobiologic and clinical mechanisms. Epilepsia. 2005;46(6):858–77.
Schousboe A, Larsson OM, Wood JD, Krogsgaard-Larsen P. Transport and metabolism of gamma-aminobutyric acid in neurons and glia: implications for epilepsy. Epilepsia. 1983;24:531–8.
Schwarzer C, Tsunashima K, Wanzenböck C, Fuchs K, Sieghart W, Sperk G. $GABA_A$ receptor subunits in the rat hippocampus II: altered distribution in kainic acid-induced temporal lobe epilepsy. Neuroscience. 1997;80:1001–17.
Scimemi A, Semyanov A, Sperk G, Kullmann DM, Walker MC. Multiple and plastic receptors mediate tonic GABAA receptor currents in the hippocampus. J Neurosci. 2005;25:10016–24.
Sommer B, Poustka A, Spurr NK, Seeburg PH, et al. The murine GABAA receptor delta-subunit gene: structure and assignment to human chromosome 1. DNA Cell Biol. 1990;9:561–8.
Sperk G, Drexel M, Pirker S. Neuronal plasticity in animal models and the epileptic human hippocampus. Epilepsia. 2009;50:29–31.

Stell BM, Brickley SG, Tang CY, Farrant M, Mody I. Neuroactive steroids reduce neuronal excitability by selectively enhancing tonic inhibition mediated by delta subunit-containing GABAA receptors. Proc Natl Acad Sci U S A. 2003;100:14439–44.

Tanaka M, Olsen RW, Medina MT, Schwartz E, Alonso ME, Duron RM, et al. Hyperglycosylation and reduced GABA currents of mutated GABRB3 polypeptide in remitting childhood absence epilepsy. Am J Hum Genet. 2008;82:1249–61.

Tapia R. Biochemical pharmacology of GABA in CNS. In: Iversen LL, Iversen SD, Snyder SH, editors. Handbook of psychopharmacology. New York: Plenum Publishing Corporation; 1975.

Tapia R, Pasantes H. Relationships between pyridoxal phosphate availability, activity of vitamin B 6 -dependent enzymes and convulsions. Brain Res. 1971;29:111–22.

Ulrich D, Bettler B. GABA(B) receptors: synaptic functions and mechanisms of diversity. Curr Opin Neurobiol. 2007;17:298–303.

Urak L, Feucht M, Fathi N, Hornik K, Fuchs K, et al. A GABRB3 promoter haplotype associated with childhood absence epilepsy impairs transcriptional activity. Hum Mol Genet. 2006;15:2533–41.

Wagstaff J, Chaillet JR, Lalande M. The GABAA receptor beta 3 subunit gene: characterization of a human cDNA from chromosome 15q11q13 and mapping to a region of conserved synteny on mouse chromosome 7. Genomics. 1991;11:1071–8.

Wallace RH, Marini C, Petrou S, Harkin LA, Bowser DN, Panchai RG, et al. Mutant GABA(A) receptor gamma-2-subunit in childhood absence epilepsy and febrile seizures. Nat Genet. 2001;28:49–52.

Walls AB, Nilsen LH, Eyjolfsson EM, et al. GAD65 is essential for synthesis of GABA destined for tonic inhibition regulating epileptiform activity. J Neurochem. 2010;115:1398–408.

Walls AB, Eyjolfsson EM, Smeland OB,Vestergaard HT, Hansen SL, Schousboe, et al. Knockout of GAD65 has major impact on synaptic GABA synthesized from astrocyte-derived glutamine. J Cereb Blood Flow Metab. 2011;31:494–503.

Wang XJ, Buzsaki G. Gamma oscillation by synaptic inhibition in hippocampal interneuronal network model. J Neurosci. 1996;16:6402–13.

Wang DD, Kriegstein AR. Blocking early GABA depolarization with bumetanide results in permanent alterations in cortical circuits and sensorimotor gating deficits. Cereb Cortex. 2010;21:574–87.

Wang X, Sun W, Zhu X, Li L, Wu X, Lin H, et al. Association between the gamma-aminobutyric acid type B receptor 1 and 2 gene polymorphisms and mesial temporal lobe epilepsy in a Han Chinese population. Epilepsy Res. 2008;81:198–203.

Watanabe M, Maemura K, Kanbara K, Tamayama T, Hayasaki H. GABA and GABA receptors in the central nervous system and other organs. In: Jeon KW, editor. A survey of cell biology. San Diego, CA: Academic; 2002.

Wieland HA, Luddens H, Seeburg PH. A single histidine in $GABA_A$ receptors is essential for benzodiazepine agonist binding. J Biol Chem. 1992;267:1426–9.

Wilcox AS, Warrington JA, Gardiner K, et al. Human chromosomal localization of genes encoding the gamma 1 and gamma 2 subunits of the gamma-aminobutyric acid receptor indicates that members of this gene family are often clustered in the genome. Proc Natl Acad Sci U S A. 1992;89:5857–61.

Wohlfarth KM, Bianchi MT, Macdonald RL. Enhanced neurosteroid potentiation of ternary GABAA receptors containing the δ subunit. J Neurosci. 2002;22:1541–9.

Zhan RZ, Nadler JV. Enhanced tonic GABA current in normotopic and hilar ectopic dentate granule cells after pilocarpine-induced status epilepticus. J Neurophysiol. 2009;102:670–81.

Zhang N, Wei W, Mody I, Houser CR. Altered localization of $GABA_A$ receptor subunits on dentate granule cell dendrites influences tonic and phasic inhibition in a mouse model of epilepsy. J Neurosci. 2007;27:7520–31.

Chapter 10
Pharmacoresistant Epilepsy and Immune System

Lourdes Lorigados Pedre, Lilia Maria Morales Chacón, Sandra Orozco-Suárez, and Luisa Rocha

Abstract The concept that the immune system plays a role in the epileptogenic process of some epileptic syndromes was first proposed more than 20 years ago. Numerous studies have reported the existence of a variety of immunological alterations in epileptic patients, favorable responses of refractory epilepsy syndromes to immune modulator treatment and the association of certain immune-mediated disease states with epilepsy. All common contributing factors to epilepsy such as trauma, malignancies, and infections are accompanied by different levels of central nervous system (CNS) inflammation, which, in turn, have been associated with the occurrence of seizures. In this chapter we provide an overview of the current knowledge on the relationship between the immune system and epilepsy. Recent knowledge suggesting the involvement of specific inflammatory pathways in the pathogenesis of seizures in patients with pharmacoresistant temporal lobe epilepsy (TLE) highlights the potential for new therapeutic strategies. We describe experimental and clinical evidences of immunological dysfunctions with special emphasis

L. Lorigados Pedre, Ph.D. (✉)
Neuroimmunology Department, International Center for Neurological Restoration,
Ave 25 No 15805 e/158 y160, Playa, Habana 11300, Cuba
e-mail: lourdes.lorigados@infomed.sld.cu

L.M. Morales Chacón, Ph.D.
Clinical Neurophysiology Department, International Center for Neurological Restoration,
Habana, Cuba

S. Orozco-Suárez, Ph.D.
Medical Research Unit in Neurological Diseases, National Medical Center "Siglo XXI",
IMSS, Hospital of Specialities, Cuauhtemoc No. 330-4, Col. Doctores, Mexico City,
Mexico DF 06720, Mexico

L. Rocha, M.D., Ph.D.
Department of Pharmacobiology, Center for Research and Advanced Studies,
Mexico City, Mexico

L. Rocha and E.A. Cavalheiro (eds.), *Pharmacoresistance in Epilepsy: From Genes and Molecules to Promising Therapies*, DOI 10.1007/978-1-4614-6464-8_10,

on clinical aspects, once the epileptogenic focus is resected. Further insight into the complex role of cellular immunity and inflammation in epileptogenesis should lead to new treatment options.

Keywords Cytokine • Inflammation • Temporal lobe epilepsy • Immune system • Pharmacoresistance

10.1 Introduction

Epilepsy, characterized by spontaneous repeated unprovoked seizures, may be caused by any process that alters the structure or function of neurons and, possibly, glial cells. The molecular mechanisms that lead to seizures and epilepsy are not well understood. Normal function of the central nervous system (CNS) is achieved through a balance of excitation and inhibition, and the initiation of a seizure is the result of increased neuronal excitation, decreased inhibition or both. Seizures can be provoked by a number of factors including acute metabolic abnormalities or acute neurologic insults such as infections, stroke, head trauma and fever.

Several authors have suggested the possible relationship between epilepsy and specific immunological changes associated with anti-epileptic treatment (Schwartz et al. 1989b; Illum et al. 1990; Pacifici et al. 1995b; Duse et al. 1996; Aarli 2000). In addition, inmmunological alterations have been associated with different types of epilepsy (Bostantjopoulou et al. 1994; Aarli 2000; Mantegazza et al. 2002; Lorigados-Pedre et al. 2004). The role played by humoral and cellular immunity in the pathogenesis of epilepsy has been more clearly defined in some syndromes such as Rasmussen's encephalitis (RE), where more information about the immunological reactions involved in the disease process is available (Andrews and McNamara 1996).

This chapter provides a brief overview of the evidence linking brain inflammation to epilepsy, the experimental and clinical evidence of immunological alterations in pharmacoresistant temporal lobe epilepsy (TLE) and the timeline of clinical changes in immunological parameters 1 year after surgery.

10.2 Immune System and Brain

The brain has a special relationship with the immune system. The CNS is extremely well protected from invading microorganisms, and the elements of the immune system so well represented in most other organs, are almost conspicuously absent in the intact brain.

The major function of the immune system is the protection of the host against invasion by pathogenic material. The brain has long been regarded as an immune-privileged organ with no immunological activity due to relatively low levels of monocytes and lymphocytes, presence of the blood–brain barrier (BBB), lack of conventional lymphatic drainage and lack of major histocompatibility complex

(MHC) I and II antigens (Barker and Billingham 1977). However, immune and inflammatory reactions do occur in the CNS, originated from either the brain itself or from the systemic circulation through a damaged BBB (Vezzani and Granata 2005; Vezzani et al. 2011a). Thus, the brain is now considered an immunologically specialized site with both innate and acquired immunity (Wekerle et al. 1986; Becher et al. 2000; Ransohoff et al. 2003; Nguyen et al. 2002). The connection between innate and adaptive immunity is mediated by a large variety of inflammatory mediators, among which cytokines and toll-like receptors (TLRs) play a key role (Akira et al. 2001; Vezzani and Granata 2005).

Microglial cells, considered to be the macrophages of the CNS, participate in the innate response in the brain through the expression of TLRs, production of cytokines [interleukin (IL)-1, IL-6 and IL-12, interferon type I] and tumoral necrosis factor (TNF) α (Olson and Miller 2004) as well as expression of chemokin (small cytokines or proteins secreted by cells) receptors (Cartier et al. 2005). The microglia is also involved in specific immune response of the CNS through the expression of MHC molecules and molecules regulated by the presence of the cytokine interferon-γ (IFN-γ) (Streit et al. 2005) and receptors that mediate phagocytosis. In addition, microglia produces inflammatory cytokines such as transforming growth factor (TGF-β1) and IL-10 whose secretion is increased in vitro after phagocytosis of apoptotic bodies (Jack et al. 2005). In summary, in some conditions, microglia cells invade the brain and take on a resting "protective" role as sentinels, scattered uniformly throughout the CNS and forming a network of potential effector cells.

Astrocytes are another cell population with immunological functions in the CNS. Astrocytes suppress T helper 1 and T helper 2 cells activation, proliferation and effector functions of activated T cells, and possess a wide variety of molecular mechanisms to induce apoptosis in activated T cells. The function of astrocytes in CNS defense is based on two key issues: secretion of soluble factors (cytokines and chemokines) and antigen presentation in the context of molecules of the MHC (Dong and Benveniste 2001). Also, astrocytes play an important role in the formation and maintenance of the BBB.

Contrary to the idea that neurons only play a passive role in the immune system, findings indicate that they actively participate in immune regulation by controlling glial cells and infiltrated T cells through both, contact-dependent and contact-independent mechanisms, and by promoting apoptosis of activated microglia and T cells (for more information see Tian et al. 2009).

Bellow, we discuss the main features that characterize the brain as a site presenting a particular immune response: presence of BBB, lack of lymphatic drainage and lack of expression of MHC antigens.

10.2.1 Blood–Brain Barrier

Immune reactions occurring within the CNS take on a distinctive character given the ability of the BBB to control passage of leukocytes from the peripheral blood (de Vries et al. 1997; Pachter et al. 2003). The BBB is a highly specialized structural and biochemical barrier that regulates the entry of blood molecules into brain, and preserves ionic homeostasis within the brain microenvironment. The cellular basis of the BBB is at the level of the CNS microvasculature and consists morphologically of non-fenestrated endothelial cells with inter-endothelial tight junctions. In addition, maintenance of BBB function depends on normal functioning of pericytes, perivascular microglia, astrocytes, and the basal lamina, which are annexed to the capillary and post-capillary venules in the CNS.

Under normal conditions, the BBB limits access to the brain of small nonpolar molecules by passive diffusion, or catalyzed transport of large and/or polar molecules (Pardridge et al. 1975) prevents extravasation of large and small solutes as well as migration of any type of blood cell into the extracellular space. However, this situation is changed in many pathological conditions such as brain trauma, stroke, tumor, infection, and seizures (Lawrence 1990; Zucker et al. 1983; Lossinsky and Shivers 2004). Hence, BBB disruption can lead to increased cellular permeability, allowing entry of leukocytes into brain tissue, and contributing to inflammation. During inflammation, enhanced production of cytokines by the endothelial cells of the BBB, the circulating immune cells, and brain parenchymal microglia and astrocytes result in up-regulation of adhesion molecules, activation of metalloproteinases and catabolism of arachidonic acid at the level of the brain microvasculature (Webb and Muir 2000; Pachter et al. 2003).

One of the mechanisms for cytokines to contribute to the inflammatory response at the level of the BBB and blood–cerebrospinal fluid (CSF) barrier is by increasing the expression of selectins and adhesion molecules, chemokines, and their receptors on endothelial and epithelial cells. These molecules are responsible for leukocyte recruitment from the bloodstream promoting their adhesion and eventual entry into the perivascular space, CSF, and CNS parenchyma by interacting with integrins (adhesion receptors that exchange signals between the extracellular and intracellular compartments) on the leukocyte membrane surface (Ransohoff et al. 2003).

10.2.2 Lack of Lymphatic Drainage

The CNS does not possess defined lymphatic channels that are comparable to lymphatic vessels in organs elsewhere in the body, but this does not mean that the brain is devoid of lymphatic drainage. Lymphatic drainage of the CNS has implications for neuroimmunology and for the homeostasis of the neuronal environment (Abbott 2004).

Both, CSF and interstitial fluid drain to regional lymph nodes. CSF drains to lymph nodes mainly via lymphatics in the nasal mucosa, while lymphatic drainage of interstitial fluid from the brain is along perivascular routes and is separate from the drainage of CSF (Abbott 2004). In adults, the majority of CSF appears to drain directly into the blood through arachnoid villi and granulations (Johanson et al. 2008).

Normally there is a constant traffic of white cells in the perivascular space, while in inflammatory processes such traffic increases considerably, and activated T cells are able to pass from the blood to the brain (Hickey et al. 1991). In general, immune cell invasion across the BBB is highly restricted and carefully regulated. A florid invasion of activated white blood cells can create a predominantly pro-inflammatory local environment in the CNS, leading to immune-mediated diseases of the nervous tissue (de Vries et al. 1997; Pachter et al. 2003; Ballabh et al. 2004).

In summary, there are no conventional lymphatics in the brain but physiological studies have actually revealed substantial significant drainage from the brain to cervical lymph nodes.

10.2.3 Lack of Major Histocompatibility Complex Antigens

MHC antigens count among the classical immune molecules. They act as platforms presenting antigenic peptides to specific receptors on T cells. MHC class I molecules interact with the CD8 T cell lineage, whereas class II molecules present antigens to CD4 T cells.

If there is a disruption of the BBB, microorganisms and viruses invade and attack the brain. Circulating antibodies neutralize viruses, but these might escape and enter brain cells. Due to the presence of MHC class I antigens on infected cells, T cells can recognize them and then attack. Since neurons are post-mitotic irreplaceable cells, this situation has deleterious consequences for the brain.

Although expression of MHC antigens in the brain is low (Brent 1990), MHC products along with many other immune genes, are readily inducible in CNS tissues under various pathological conditions, including autoimmune inflammation, microbial infection and neuronal degeneration (Moran and Graeber 2004).

MHC class I molecules are detected in neurons; however, their expression in the brain differs in many ways from that seen in most other nucleated cells. The principal differences are as follows:

1. Low concentration of MHC class I in neurons in comparison with other cell types (Huh et al. 2000).
2. MHC class I is expressed in most tissues at relatively constant levels in the absence of infection and other challenges (Janeway 2001) whereas MHC class I levels in the brain are highly dynamic and change dramatically during normal development.
3. Some "nonclassical" MHC class I proteins are not detected in other tissues but are strongly or exclusively expressed in specific regions of the CNS. For example, the M10 family of the nonclassical MHC has been detected only in the vomeronasal organ (Ishii et al. 2003; Loconto et al. 2003).

In parallel, it has been shown that the immune privilege of the brain is likely to result of modified responses to MHC class I-peptide complexes in the CNS, rather than a lack of MHC class I proteins on neurons (Streilein 1993; Boulanger 2004).

During inflammatory processes in the CNS, there are several cells expressing MHC class I and II: microglia and macrophages, endothelial cells of the BBB, and epithelial cells of the choroid plexus (Becher et al. 2000; Engelhardt et al. 2001; Williams et al. 2001). The endothelial cells, unlike perivascular microglia, do not constitutively express MHC class II molecules. However, they can be induced to express these molecules by a variety of cytokines. The role of MHC class II in astroglia remains elusive, and a prevailing view is that these cells exert a negative immunoregulatory function by favoring the induction of a nonresponsive state in T cells (Aloisi et al. 2000a, b).

10.3 Inflammation in the CNS

Inflammation is a dynamic process consisting in the production of a cascade of inflammatory mediators, anti-inflammatory molecules and other molecules induced to solve inflammation. Inflammation is a response to noxious stimuli or immune stimulation and helps in the defense against pathogenic threats. It is characterized by the production of an array of inflammatory mediators by tissue-resident or blood-circulating immune competent cells, and involves activation of innate and adaptive immunity. It is recognized that the CNS shows a robust inflammatory response not only to infectious agents but also to a large spectrum of injuries, such as those occurring after ischemic, traumatic or excitotoxic brain damage, or during seizures (Allan and Rothwell 2001; Jankowsky and Patterson 2001). The regional and cellular patterns of induction of inflammatory molecules and their time course of activation and persistence in brain tissue appear to depend on the nature of CNS injury.

The inflammatory mediators in the CNS are produced by microglia, astrocytes, and neurons and by cells of the BBB and choroid plexus. These molecules are not detectable or are barely detectable in physiological conditions. Specially, microglia, astrocytes and neurons are believed to contribute to the innate immune processes that cause inflammation of the brain (Vezzani et al. 2011a, c).

TLRs are transmembrane proteins expressed by immunocompetent cells such as antigen presenting cells (APCs) and share common cytoplasmic domains with the IL-1 receptor family. Mammalian TLRs comprise a large family consisting at least of 11 members, and their activation initiates innate immune responses and inflammation during infection, or in response to tissue injury. Stimulation of TLRs, specifically TLR 2 and TLR 4 in the CNS, leads to release of cytokines, which are involved in the transition between innate and adaptive immunity (Akira et al. 2001).

TLR activation results in induction of transcriptional factors such as nuclear factor kappa-light-chain-enhancer of activated B cells (NFκB), which has the ability to trigger various proinflammatory genes such as those encoding cytokines, chemokines, proteins of the complement system, cyclooxygenase-2 (COX-2), and inducible nitric oxide synthase (Nguyen et al. 2002; Rivest 2003). These receptors are rapidly increased in the brain after lipopolysaccharide injection, suggesting that a systemic immune challenge induces inflammation in the CNS by a direct action on brain cells and not only by increasing cytokines and inflammatory mediators in blood (Rivest et al. 2000).

TLR stimulation activates downstream events in APCs that are in part shared by IL-1-receptor type I intracellular signaling. An immune response in the CNS may also be triggered by endogenous ligands that stimulate TLRs. (For more information on inflammation and nervous system see Vezzani and Granata 2005; Vezzani 2005).

10.4 Inflammation and Epilepsy

Epilepsy is a common neurological disorder which affects around 50 million people worldwide. Seizures are caused by abnormal, high-frequency discharges of a group of neurons. The underlying neurochemical mechanisms are unknown, although increasing evidence implicates proinflammatory factors (Vezzani and Baram 2007; Vezzani et al. 1999; Vezzani and Granata 2005; Vezzani 2008; Ravizza et al. 2011; Aronica and Crino 2011). The first remark on the production of inflammatory mediators was described by Rasmussen in 1958 when he evaluated focal seizures in patients with chronic encephalitis (Rasmussen et al. 1958). Later, it was found that epilepsy is more common in some patients with autoimmune diseases than in the general population (Mackworth-Young and Hughes 1985). Concerning this issue, it is described that inflammation in either neonatal or adult animals may be associated with altered brain excitability and increased sensitivity to seizures (Rodgers et al. 2009; Riazi et al. 2010; Aronica and Crino 2011; Maroso et al. 2010).

Clinical evidences supporting the idea that the immune system is involved in the pathogenesis of certain types of epilepsy are as follows: the existence of immunological alterations in patients with epilepsy (Eeg-Olofsson et al. 1988; Montelli et al. 2003; Lorigados-Pedre et al. 2004; Bauer et al. 2008; Iyer et al. 2010; Li et al. 2011); the high incidence of seizures in autoimmune diseases (Aarli 2000; Choi and Koh 2008; Irani et al. 2011); the discovery of limbic encephalitis as a cause of epilepsy (Bien et al. 2007); and the favorable response of seizure activity to treatment with certain immunomodulatory agents (Duse et al. 1996; Seager et al. 1975; Nieto et al. 2000; Fois and Vascotto 1990).

The notion that inflammatory processes in the brain may constitute a mechanism underlying the pathophysiology of seizures and epilepsy (Vezzani and Granata 2005; Vezzani and Baram 2007; Vezzani et al. 2011a; Choi et al. 2009; Riazi et al. 2010) is supported by the observation that steroids and other anti-inflammatory treatments display anticonvulsant effects in some drug-resistant epilepsies (Schwartz et al. 1989b; Illum et al. 1990; Duse et al. 1996; Riikonen 2004; Wheless et al. 2007; Wirrell et al. 2005; Schwartz et al. 1989a) and the detection of elevated levels of proinflammatory mediators in patients with febrile seizures (Heida et al. 2009). In addition, several reports show increased markers of inflammation in serum, CSF, and brain resident cells in patients with epilepsy. For example, epileptic patients who have recently experienced tonic–clonic seizures display a specific proinflammatory profile of cytokines in plasma and CSF (Pacifici et al. 1995a, b;

Peltola et al. 1998; Sinha et al. 2008). Moreover, complex febrile seizures in childhood have long been associated with the later development of TLE; febrile illnesses in people with otherwise well-controlled epilepsy can trigger seizures; and immunomodulatory agents such as steroids and adrenocorticotrophic hormone have shown efficacy in some epileptic encephalopathies and, occasionally, in refractory status epilepticus (Hart et al. 1994; Snead 2001).

Several studies indicate immunosuppressive side effects of antiepileptic drugs, such as IgA deficiency (Sorrell et al. 1971; Aarli 1976). However, epileptic patients are found to present disorders of the immune system that are not explained by the use of antiepileptic drugs alone (Bassanini et al. 1982; Bostantjopoulou et al. 1994; Lorigados-Pedre et al. 2004).

The inflammatory response detected in rodents with seizure activity includes the following molecular cascade: rapid increase of proinflammatory cytokines (IL-1β, IL-6, TNF-α), up-regulation of TLRs, activation of NFκB, chemokine production, complement system activation and increased expression of adhesion molecules (Ravizza et al. 2011; Fabene et al. 2008; Librizzi et al. 2007; Turrin and Rivest 2004; Vezzani and Granata 2005; Vezzani et al. 2008; Aronica et al. 2007; Maroso et al. 2010). Below we analyze some experimental and clinical evidences of inflammatory responses in epilepsy.

The kindled model in rats induces a significant up-regulation of IL-1 β, IL-1RI, TNF-α and TGF-β1 mRNAs in several limbic brain regions. The overall profile of mRNA changes shows specificity of transcriptional modulation induced by amygdala kindling. The data support a role for cytokines and neuropeptide Y in the adaptive mechanisms associated with generalized seizure activity (Vezzani et al. 2002; Plata-Salaman et al. 2000). Indeed, increased COX-2 levels are detected in mouse rapid kindling (Takemiya et al. 2003).

Experimental models of status epilepticus have mostly been used to study the temporal evolution of inflammatory processes, which occur by activation of microglia and astrocytes and, subsequently, endothelial cells of the BBB (Bernard 2011; Friedman and Dingledine 2011; Ravizza et al. 2008a). Indeed, microglia is activated within the same time course that is observed for neuronal degeneration (Hosokawa et al. 2003; Xiong et al. 2003). Increased synthesis of inflammatory mediators in the brain during status epilepticus-induced seizures was corroborated by microarray analysis (Ravizza et al. 2011).

The inflammatory activity is affected in different ways depending on the severity of the seizures (Minami et al. 1990, 1991; Jankowsky and Patterson 2001; Kubera et al. 2001; Oprica et al. 2003; Turrin and Rivest 2004; Gahring et al. 2001). In particular, analysis of IL-1β and IL-1Ra mRNAs after systemic injection of kainic acid in rats has shown that these transcripts are significantly induced in microglial cells in the hippocampus as well as in other areas of the limbic system (Yabuuchi et al. 1993; Eriksson et al. 1998; Minami et al. 1990, 1991). Indeed, Vezzani et al. provided direct evidence that the rapid increase in the levels of IL-1β in the hippocampus subsequent to kainic acid-induced seizures presumably results from activation of microglia cells (Vezzani et al. 1999). In chronic epileptic tissue, when animals develop spontaneous recurrent seizures, TNF-α and IL-6 also increase in glial cells, similarly to IL-1 (Ravizza et al. 2008b; Ravizza and Vezzani 2006), although their regulation is transient (De Simoni et al. 2000). It appears, therefore, that the increase in IL-1β outlasts the acute inciting event while the increase in the other cytokines is time-locked to ongoing epileptic activity (Vezzani et al. 2008).

The increase in IL-1β, IL-6 and TNF-α in microglia and astrocytes is followed by a cascade of downstream inflammatory events, which may recruit cells of the adaptive immune system (Vezzani and Granata 2005). In contrast, production of proinflammatory molecules is typically accompanied by the concomitant synthesis of anti-inflammatory mediators and binding proteins apt to modulate the inflammatory response, thus avoiding the occurrence of deleterious induction of genes that mediate inflammatory effects (Dinarello 2000). In this respect, up-regulation of IL-1-receptor antagonist (IL-1Ra), a naturally occurring antagonist of IL-1β, has been described after acute seizures, status epilepticus and in kindling (Avignone et al. 2008; Gasque et al. 1997; Gorter et al. 2006). In contrast with classic inflammatory reactions in which IL-1Ra is produced at 100- to 1,000-fold excess and concomitant with IL-1β production, IL-1Ra is produced with a delayed time course when compared to seizure induced-IL-1β production (Dinarello 1996). Thus, the brain is less effective than the periphery in inducing a crucial mechanism for rapidly terminating the actions of a sustained increase in endogenous IL-1β.

Another important component of the immune response is a prominent activation of the complement cascade during epileptogenesis in experimental models and in the sclerotic hippocampus from human patients with TLE (Aronica et al. 2007). Although complement factors might invade the brain via a leaky BBB, part of the increased expression is likely to originate from activated glial cells (Ravizza et al. 2006; Vezzani et al. 2008). Interestingly, sequential infusion of individual proteins of the membrane attack pathway (C5b6, C7, C8, and C9) into the hippocampus of awake, freely moving rats induces both behavioral and electrographic seizures as well as cytotoxicity, suggesting a role for the complement system in epileptogenesis (Xiong et al. 2003). In addition, there is selective expression of clusterin (SGP-2) and complement C1qB and C4 during responses to kainic acid administration in vivo and in vitro, an effect associated with prolonged exposure to glutamate. Interestingly, expression of CD59 is increased in microglia, but only modestly in neurons, suggesting that complement activation may be poorly controlled in this cell population (Rozovsky et al. 1994).

Experimental seizures are associated with changes in the function of the peripheral immune system. For example, during kainate-induced seizures the thymus shows reduced weight, probably due to elevated corticosterone plasma levels, as well as an increase in the metabolic activity of splenocytes, an effect that may be associated with enhanced phagocytic activity of macrophages (Kubera et al. 2001).

10.4.1 Rasmussen Encephalitis

The presence of inflammation in the brain of patients with RE is interpreted as an indication of specific immune reactions that occur during the course of the disease. Thus, RE is considered the prototype of inflammatory epilepsy. RE is a very rare chronic progressive neurological disorder affecting mostly children and associated with hemispheric atrophy, focal epilepsy, intellectual decline and progressive neurological deficits (Rasmussen et al. 1958; Bien and Elger 2005; Dubeau et al. 2007).

Histopathological findings in RE comprise lymphocytic infiltrates, microglial nodules, neuronal and astrocytic loss, and gliosis of the affected hemisphere (Farrell et al. 1995). Active brain inflammatory lesions contain large numbers of T lymphocytes, which are recruited early within the lesions suggesting that a T cell dependent immune response contributes to the onset and evolution of the disease (Li et al. 1997; Farrell et al. 1995). Moreover, the histopathological observation of granzyme B-containing CD8+ T cells in direct apposition to MHC class I positive neurons raised the hypothesis of a CD8+ T cell-mediated neuronal attack as a key pathogenetic mechanism underlying RE (Bauer et al. 2002; Bien et al. 2002). In addition to neuronal cell death, CD8 cells may also be responsible for the degeneration of astrocytes found in RE lesions (Bauer et al. 2007). Another important immunological finding in RE is the presence of autoantibodies against GluR3 (Mantegazza et al. 2002). However, these autoantibodies have also been found in focal epilepsy (Wiendl et al. 2001).

Considering all of the above information, RE represents a formidable challenge for specialists interested in epilepsy and immunology. From the immunological point of view, some of the most significant findings are a pathological CSF, an increase in lymphocyte numbers and/or protein concentration, and low levels of IgA in serum (Aarli 2000). Andrews et al. described high titers of antinuclear antibodies in serum, presence of oligoclonal bands in CSF, elevated IgG index, and deposits of IgA and C3 (Andrews and McNamara 1996). For all these reasons, it is evident that immunological mechanisms play an important role in the pathophysiology of RE and support the notion that epileptogenic properties in this disease might be caused by an immunologically mediated cortical injury.

10.5 Inflammation and Immune Response in Human Pharmacoresistant Epilepsy

Data collected using tissue of patients with TLE suggest that specific inflammatory pathways are chronically activated during epileptogenesis and that they persist in chronic epileptic tissue, contributing to the etiopathogenesis of TLE (Ravizza et al. 2008a; van Gassen et al. 2008). Hippocampus obtained from patients with hippocampal sclerosis (HS) shows microglial activation (Sheng et al. 1994; Beach et al. 1995; Aronica et al. 2007; Ravizza et al. 2008a). Expression of proinflammatory molecules (IL-1, IL-6 and TNF) as well as IL-1α, IL-1β and IL-1 receptor type I, NFκB and complex is augmented in surgically resected epileptic tissue from patients with pharmacoresistant epilepsy (Aronica et al. 2007; Crespel et al. 2002; Maldonado et al. 2003). Systemic IL-6 levels in peripheral blood are increased immediately after seizures and long lasting during the post-ictal period (24 h after ictal event) in patients with TLE, an effect not detected in patients with HS (Bauer et al. 2009). Expression of C1q, C3c, and C3d is augmented within regions where neuronal cell loss occurs (Crespel et al. 2002).

The activation of inflammatory pathways in human TLE is supported by gene expression profile analysis (Aronica et al. 2007; van Gassen et al. 2008; De Simoni et al. 2000). Other studies indicate activation of the complement pathway, involving both reactive astrocytes and cells of the microglia/macrophage lineage in human HS specimens (Aronica et al. 2007). These observations suggest the existence of a feedback loop between the pro-inflammatory cytokine system and components of the complement cascade, which may be critical for the propagation of the inflammatory response in human TLE with HS.

Resected tissue of patients with pharmacoresistant epilepsy demonstrates increased β-amyloid immunoreactive protein and augmented expression of IL-1α in microglia adjacent to neuronal cells immunoreactive to precursor protein β-amyloid (PP-β-amyloid) (Sheng et al. 1994; Aronica et al. 2004; Bernardino et al. 2005). Since IL-1α is synthesized and released by activated microglia in the periphery as an acute phase response protein (Dinarello and Wolff 1993), its augmentation in damaged brain (Griffin et al. 1994) may contribute to epileptic neuronal dysfunction by up-regulation of the expression of PPβ-amyloid or by astrogliosis (Giulian et al. 1988). These proteins may also be involved in neuronal dysfunction as a consequence of neurotoxicity (Brenneman et al. 1992).

In patients with pharmacoresistant epilepsy, an increase in serum proinflammatory cytokine concentrations and a decrease in IL-1Ra level and IL-1Rα/IL-1β ratio have been confirmed (Peltola et al. 2001a, b). IL-1Ra is an endogenous protein, which by binding with IL-1, can inhibit seizures (Ravizza and Vezzani 2006). Thus, appropriate IL-1/IL-1Ra ratio represents a natural mechanism to control seizures (Haspolat et al. 2005; Vezzani et al. 2002).

The cellular immune response in patients with pharmacoresistant epilepsy is another issue that has been investigated. Patients with pharmacoresistant TLE show an increased expression of HLA-DR immunoreactive microglia in the hippocampus (Beach et al. 1995) and peripheral expression of lymphocyte activation markers (CD25 and HLA-DR) as well as of CD8+T cells, this last effect limited to patients with temporal and lateralized epileptogenic focus localization (Lorigados-Pedre et al. 2004). The functional implications of these findings are unknown, but support the idea that inflammation might be intrinsic to, and perhaps a biomarker of the epileptogenic process (Vezzani et al. 2011b; Vezzani and Friedman 2011). At present there are multiple research groups assessing the involvement of the immune system and inflammatory processes in the pathogenesis of epilepsy with special emphasis on drug resistant TLE. They attempt to address two basic questions: Do seizures cause inflammation? or does inflammation cause seizures?

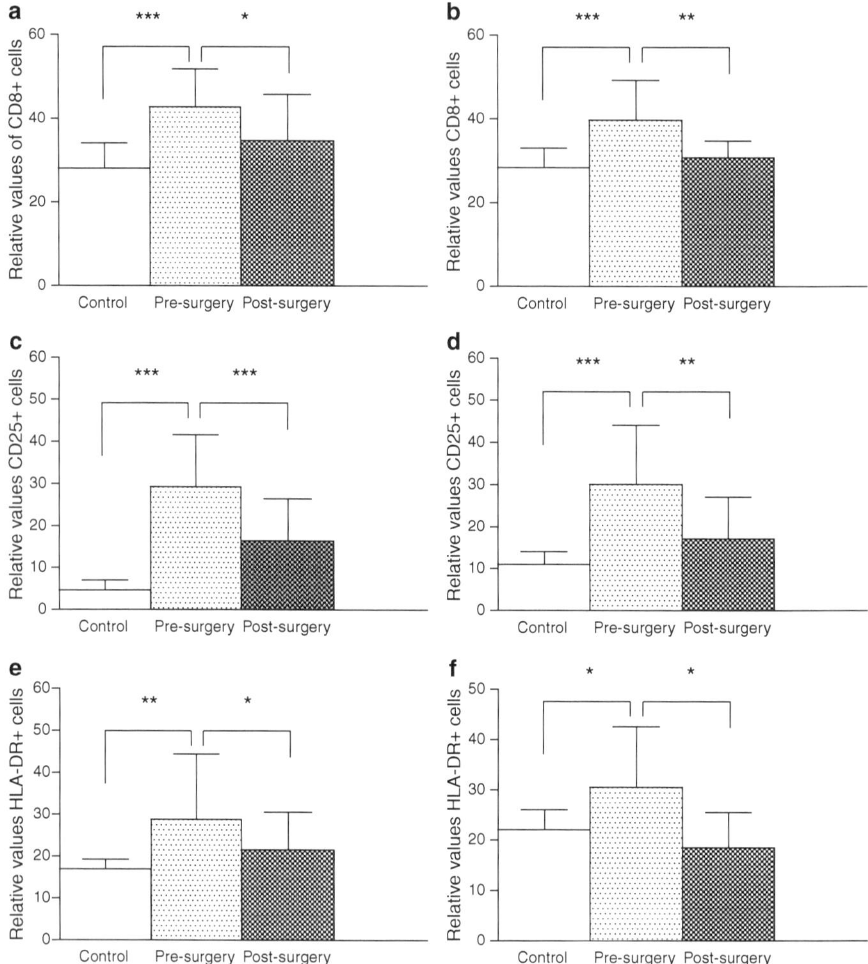

Fig. 10.1 Levels of CD8+ (A and B), CD25+ (C and D) and HLA-DR (E and F) lymphocytes in pheripheral blood (A, C and E) and cerebrospinal fluid (B, D and F) of patients with pharmacoresistant temporal lobe epilepsy before and one year after epilepsy surgery (n = 20). Values were compared with a control group (n = 30). Data are represented as mean±SD of relative values of positive cells. Statistical analysis was performed using Student´s-t test (control vs patient groups) and paried-t test (pre-surgical vs post- surgical patient groups). $^*p \leq 0.05$, $^{**}p \leq 0.005$, $^{***}p \leq 0.0005$

Recently, we evaluated cellular immunity in both, peripheral blood and CSF from patients with pharmacoresistant epilepsy before and after surgical treatment. We found a significant increase in CD8+ lymphocytes, CD25+ and HLA-DR + cells in peripheral samples as well as in CSF before surgery, an effect not detected 1 year after resection, when 75 % of the patients were seizure free (Fig. 10.1). We also

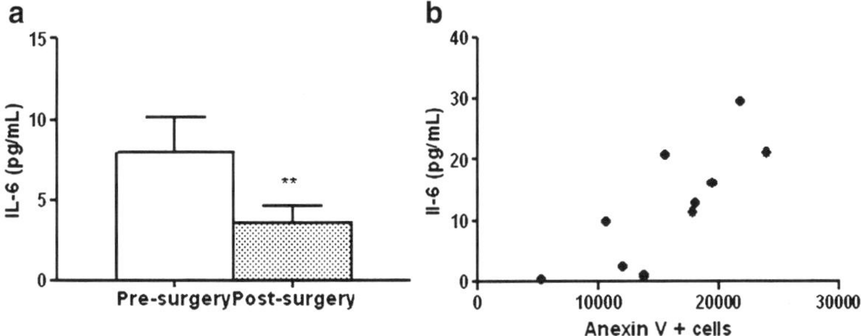

Fig. 10.2 (**a**) IL-6 serum levels in pharmacoresistant lobe temporal epileptic patients ($n=20$) before and 1 year after surgical treatment and, (**b**) correlation study of IL-6 levels and immunoreactive Annexin-V cells in tissue from some of these patients ($n=10$). Data are represented as mean ± SD. Statistical analysis was performed using paired t-test, $p \leq 0.001$ (**a**); and Pearson correlation, $r=0.7771$ (**b**), $p \leq 0.005$

detected a decrease in proinflammatory cytokines (Il-1β, IL-6) in serum from patients with pharmacoresistant TLE 1 year after surgical treatment when compared to presurgical evaluation levels (Fig. 10.2). The decreased IL-6 showed a positive correlation with the expression of Annexin-V (early apoptotic marker) (Lorigados et al. 2008), a finding that supports a relationship between the inflammatory process in epilepsy and the neuronal loss observed in these patients. Our results indicate that once the epileptogenic zone is resected and seizure activity is decreased, there is a restoration of cellular immunity and reduction of proinflammatory cytokines. These findings support the idea that seizures are the cause of the immune and inflammatory disorders observed in patients with drug-resistant epilepsy. However, additional studies should be carried out in experimental models of pharmacoresistant epilepsy to support this idea.

10.6 Conclusions

Clinical and preclinical data support the participation of inflammation and immune responses in the epileptic process, suggesting that specific inflammatory pathways are chronically activated in the epileptogenic brain tissue. These results highlight the need for research that enables us to understand the role of the immune system in the pathogenesis of pharmacoresistant epilepsy and particularly, to clarify whether the immunological abnormalities described above result from the epileptic seizures or induce them. It is also necessary to evaluate new immunomodulatory therapies that reduce the consequences of seizures in these patients. In this regard, there are several groups investigating the potential clinical application of anti-inflammatory treatments (Vezzani et al. 2011b; Aronica and Crino 2011; Ozkara and Vigevano 2011).

Further investigations into the role of inflammation and the immune response in the CNS, particularly in pharmacoresistant epilepsy may add important insights into the understanding of epileptogenic mechanisms and open new ways of neuromodulatory treatment of epilepsy.

Acknowledgments This work was sponsored by CONACYT (Proyect 98386). We thank Leticia Neri Bazán and Héctor Vázquez Espinosa for their useful cooperation, and Lic. Odalys Morales Chacón and Dr. Erika Brust-Mascher for the linguistic revision.

References

Aarli JA. Drug-induced IgA deficiency in epileptic patients. Arch Neurol. 1976;33:296–9.
Aarli JA. Epilepsy and the immune system. Arch Neurol. 2000;57:1689–92.
Abbott NJ. Evidence for bulk flow of brain interstitial fluid: significance for physiology and pathology. Neurochem Int. 2004;45:545–52.
Akira S, Takeda K, Kaisho T. Toll-like receptors: critical proteins linking innate and acquired immunity. Nat Immunol. 2001;2:675–80.
Allan SM, Rothwell NJ. Cytokines and acute neurodegeneration. Nat Rev Neurosci. 2001;2: 734–44.
Aloisi F, De SR, Columba-Cabezas S, Penna G, Adorini L. Functional maturation of adult mouse resting microglia into an APC is promoted by granulocyte-macrophage colony-stimulating factor and interaction with Th1 cells. J Immunol. 2000a;164:1705–12.
Aloisi F, Ria F, Adorini L. Regulation of T-cell responses by CNS antigen-presenting cells: different roles for microglia and astrocytes. Immunol Today. 2000b;21:141–7.
Andrews PI, McNamara JO. Rasmussen's encephalitis: an autoimmune disorder? Curr Opin Neurobiol. 1996;6:673–8.
Aronica E, Crino PB. Inflammation in epilepsy: clinical observations. Epilepsia. 2011;52 Suppl 3:26–32.
Aronica E, Gorter JA, Ramkema M, Redeker S, Ozbas-Gerceker F, van Vliet EA, et al. Expression and cellular distribution of multidrug resistance-related proteins in the hippocampus of patients with mesial temporal lobe epilepsy. Epilepsia. 2004;45:441–51.
Aronica E, Boer K, van Vliet EA, Redeker S, Baayen JC, Spliet WG, et al. Complement activation in experimental and human temporal lobe epilepsy. Neurobiol Dis. 2007;26:497–511.
Avignone E, Ulmann L, Levavasseur F, Rassendren F, Audinat E. Status epilepticus induces a particular microglial activation state characterized by enhanced purinergic signaling. J Neurosci. 2008;28:9133–44.
Ballabh P, Braun A, Nedergaard M. The blood–brain barrier: an overview: structure, regulation, and clinical implications. Neurobiol Dis. 2004;16:1–13.
Barker CF, Billingham RE. Immunologically privileged sites. Adv Immunol. 1977;25:1–54.
Bassanini M, Baez A, Sotelo J. Immunoglobulins in epilepsy. J Neurol Sci. 1982;56:275–81.
Bauer J, Bien CG, Lassmann H. Rasmussen's encephalitis: a role for autoimmune cytotoxic T lymphocytes. Curr Opin Neurol. 2002;15:197–200.
Bauer J, Elger CE, Hans VH, Schramm J, Urbach H, Lassmann H, et al. Astrocytes are a specific immunological target in Rasmussen's encephalitis. Ann Neurol. 2007;62:67–80.
Bauer S, Koller M, Cepok S, Todorova-Rudolph A, Nowak M, Nockher WA, et al. NK and CD4+ T cell changes in blood after seizures in temporal lobe epilepsy. Exp Neurol. 2008;211:370–7.
Bauer S, Cepok S, Todorova-Rudolph A, Nowak M, Koller M, Lorenz R, et al. Etiology and site of temporal lobe epilepsy influence postictal cytokine release. Epilepsy Res. 2009;86:82–8.
Beach T, Woodhurst W, MacDonald D, Jones M. Reactive microglia in hippocampal sclerosis associated with human temporal lobe epilepsy. Neurosci Lett. 1995;191:27.

Becher B, Prat A, Antel JP. Brain-immune conection: immunoregulatory properties of CNS-resident cells. Glia. 2000;29:293–304.
Bernard C. Pathophysiology of epilepsies: recent progresses. Presse Med. 2011;40:256–64.
Bernardino L, Ferreira R, Cristovao AJ, Sales F, Malva JO. Inflammation and neurogenesis in temporal lobe epilepsy. Curr Drug Targets CNS Neurol Disord. 2005;4:349–60.
Bien CG, Elger CE. Recent insights into Rasmussen encephalitis. Nervenarzt. 2005;76:1470. 1472–1480, 1484.
Bien CG, Bauer J, Deckwerth TL, Wiendl H, Deckert M, Wiestler OD, et al. Destruction of neurons by cytotoxic T cells: a new pathogenic mechanism in Rasmussen's encephalitis. Ann Neurol. 2002;51:311–8.
Bien CG, Urbach H, Schramm J, Soeder BM, Becker AJ, Voltz R, et al. Limbic encephalitis as a precipitating event in adult-onset temporal lobe epilepsy. Neurology. 2007;69:1236–44.
Bostantjopoulou S, Hatzizisi O, Argyropoulou O, Andreadis S, Deligiannis K, Kantaropoulou M, et al. Immunological parameters in patients with epilepsy. Funct Neurol. 1994;9:11–5.
Boulanger LM. MHC class I in activity-dependent structural and functional plasticity. Neuron Glia Biol. 2004;1:283–9.
Brenneman D, Schultzberg M, Bartfai T, Gozes I. Cytokine regulation of neuronal survival. J Neurochem. 1992;58:454.
Brent L. Immunologically privileged sites. In: Johansson B, Owman C, Widner H, editors. Pathophysiology of the BBB. New York: Elsevier; 1990. p. 385–453.
Cartier L, Hartley O, Dubois-Dauphin M, Krause KH. Chemokine receptors in the central nervous system: role in brain inflammation and neurodegenerative diseases. Brain Res Brain Res Rev. 2005;48:16–42.
Choi J, Koh S. Role of brain inflammation in epileptogenesis. Yonsei Med J. 2008;49:1–18.
Choi J, Nordli Jr DR, Alden TD, DiPatri Jr A, Laux L, Kelley K, et al. Cellular injury and neuroinflammation in children with chronic intractable epilepsy. J Neuroinflammation. 2009;6:38.
Crespel A, Coubes P, Rousset MC, Brana C, Rougier A, Rondouin G, et al. Inflammatory reactions in human medial temporal lobe epilepsy with hippocampal sclerosis. Brain Res. 2002;952:159–69.
De Simoni MG, Perego C, Ravizza T, Moneta D, Conti M, Marchesi F, et al. Inflammatory cytokines and related genes are induced in the rat hippocampus by limbic status epilepticus. Eur J Neurosci. 2000;12:2623–33.
de Vries HE, Kuiper J, de Boer AG, Van Berkel TJ, Breimer DD. The blood–brain barrier in neuroinflammatory diseases. Pharmacol Rev. 1997;49:143–55.
Dinarello CA. Biologic basis for interleukin-1 in disease. Blood. 1996;87:2095–147.
Dinarello CA. Proinflammatory cytokines. Chest. 2000;118:503–8.
Dinarello C, Wolff S. The role of IL-1 in disease. N Engl J Med. 1993;328:106–13.
Dong Y, Benveniste EN. Immune function of astrocytes. Glia. 2001;36:180–90.
Dubeau F, Andermann F, Wiendl H, Bar-Or A. Rasmussen's encephalitis (chronic focal encephalitis). In: Engel J, Pedley TA, Aicardi J, Dichter MA, Moshe SL, editors. Epilepsy: a comprehensive texbook. Philadelphia: Lippincott Williams and Wilkins; 2007. p. 2439–54.
Duse M, Notarangelo L, Tiberti S, Menegat E, Plebani A, Ugazio A. Intravenous immune globuline in the treatment of intractable childhood epilepsy. Clin Exp Immunol. 1996;104:71–6.
Eeg-Olofsson O, Osterland CK, Guttmann RD, Andermann F, Prchal JF, Andermann E, et al. Immunological studies in focal epilepsy. Acta Neurol Scand. 1988;78:358–68.
Engelhardt B, Wolburg-Buchholz K, Wolburg H. Involvement of the choroid plexus in central nervous system inflammation. Microsc Res Tech. 2001;52:112–29.
Eriksson C, Winblad B, Schultzberg M. Kainic acid induced expression of interleukin-1 receptor antagonist mRNA in the rat brain. Brain Res Mol Brain Res. 1998;58:195–208.
Fabene PF, Navarro MG, Martinello M, Rossi B, Merigo F, Ottoboni L, et al. A role for leukocyte-endothelial adhesion mechanisms in epilepsy. Nat Med. 2008;14:1377–83.
Farrell MA, Droogan O, Secor DL, Poukens V, Quinn B, Vinters HV. Chronic encephalitis associated with epilepsy: immunohistochemical and ultrastructural studies. Acta Neuropathol. 1995;89:313–21.

Fois A, Vascotto M. Use of intravenous immunoglobulins in drug-resistant epilepsy. Childs Nerv Syst. 1990;6:400–5.

Friedman A, Dingledine R. Molecular cascades that mediate the influence of inflammation on epilepsy. Epilepsia. 2011;52 Suppl 3:33–9.

Gahring L, Carlson NG, Meyer EL, Rogers SW. Granzyme B proteolysis of a neuronal glutamate receptor generates an autoantigen and is modulated by glycosylation. J Immunol. 2001;166: 1433–8.

Gasque P, Singhrao SK, Neal JW, Gotze O, Morgan BP. Expression of the receptor for complement C5a (CD88) is up-regulated on reactive astrocytes, microglia, and endothelial cells in the inflamed human central nervous system. Am J Pathol. 1997;150:31–41.

Giulian D, Young D, Woodward J, Brown D, Lachman L. IL-1 is an astroglial growth factor in development brain. J Neurosci. 1988;8:700–14.

Gorter JA, van Vliet EA, Aronica E, Breit T, Rauwerda H, Lopes da Silva FH, et al. Potential new antiepileptogenic targets indicated by microarray analysis in a rat model for temporal lobe epilepsy. J Neurosci. 2006;26:11083–110.

Griffin W, Sheng J, Gentleman S, Graham D, Mrak R, Roberts G. Microglial IL-1alpha expression in human head injury: correlations with neuronal and neuritic β-amiloid precursor protein expression. Neurosci Lett. 1994;136:75–8.

Hart Y, Cotez M, Andermann F, Hwang P, Fish D, Dulac O, et al. Medical treatment of Rasmussen's syndrome (chronic encephalitis and epilepsy): effect of high-dose steroids or immunoglobulins in 19 patients. Neurology. 1994;44:1030.

Haspolat S, Baysal Y, Duman O, Coskun M, Tosun O, Yegin O. Interleukin-1alpha, interleukin-1beta, and interleukin-1Ra polymorphisms in febrile seizures. J Child Neurol. 2005;20: 565–8.

Heida JG, Moshe SL, Pittman QJ. The role of interleukin-1beta in febrile seizures. Brain Dev. 2009;31:388–93.

Hickey W, Hsu B, Kimura H. T-lymphocyte entry into the central nervous system. J Neurosci Res. 1991;28:254–60.

Hosokawa M, Klegeris A, Maguire J, McGeer PL. Expression of complement messenger RNAs and proteins by human oligodendroglial cells. Glia. 2003;42:417–23.

Huh GS, Boulanger LM, Du H, Riquelme PA, Brotz TM, Shatz CJ. Functional requirement for class I MHC in CNS development and plasticity. Science. 2000;290:2155–9.

Illum N, Taudorf K, Heilmann C, Smith T, Wulff K, Mansa B. Intravenous immunoglobulin: a single-blind trial in children with Lennox-Gastaut syndrome. Neuropediatrics. 1990;21:87–90.

Irani SR, Bien CG, Lang B. Autoimmune epilepsies. Curr Opin Neurol. 2011;24:146–53.

Ishii T, Hirota J, Mombaerts P. Combinatorial coexpression of neural and immune multigene families in mouse vomeronasal sensory neurons. Curr Biol. 2003;13:394–400.

Iyer A, Zurolo E, Spliet WG, van Rijen PC, Baayen JC, Gorter JA, et al. Evaluation of the innate and adaptive immunity in type I and type II focal cortical dysplasias. Epilepsia. 2010;51: 1763–73.

Jack CS, Arbour N, Manusow J, Montgrain V, Blain M, McCrea E, et al. TLR signaling tailors innate immune responses in human microglia and astrocytes. J Immunol. 2005;175:4320–30.

Janeway Jr CA. How the immune system works to protect the host from infection: a personal view. Proc Natl Acad Sci U S A. 2001;98:7461–8.

Jankowsky JL, Patterson PH. The role of cytokines and growth factors in seizures and their sequelae. Prog Neurobiol. 2001;63:125–49.

Johanson CE, Duncan III JA, Klinge PM, Brinker T, Stopa EG, Silverberg GD. Multiplicity of cerebrospinal fluid functions: new challenges in health and disease. Cerebrospinal Fluid Res. 2008;5:10.

Kubera M, Budziszewska B, Basta-Kaiml A, Zajicova A, Holan V, Lason W. Immunoreactivity in kainate model of epilepsy. Pol J Pharmacol. 2001;53:541–5.

Lawrence F. Lymphocyte homming to the central nervous system. In: Johansson B, Owman C, Widner H, editors. Pathophysiology of the BBB. New York: Elsevier; 1990. p. 453–64.

Li Y, Uccelli A, Laxer KD, Jeong MC, Vinters HV, Tourtellotte WW, et al. Local-clonal expansion of infiltrating T lymphocytes in chronic encephalitis of Rasmussen. J Immunol. 1997;158: 1428–37.
Li C, Ma WN, Wang H. Changes of regulatory T cells in the peripheral blood of children with epilepsy. Zhongguo Dang Dai Er Ke Za Zhi. 2011;13:889–92.
Librizzi L, Regondi MC, Pastori C, Frigerio S, Frassoni C, De CM. Expression of adhesion factors induced by epileptiform activity in the endothelium of the isolated guinea pig brain in vitro. Epilepsia. 2007;48:743–51.
Loconto J, Papes F, Chang E, Stowers L, Jones EP, Takada T, et al. Functional expression of murine V2R pheromone receptors involves selective association with the M10 and M1 families of MHC class Ib molecules. Cell. 2003;112:607–18.
Lorigados PL, Orozco SS, Morales CL, Garcia MI, Estupinan DB, Bender del Busto JE, et al. Neuronal death in the neocortex of drug resistant temporal lobe epilepsy patients. Neurologia. 2008;23:555–65.
Lorigados-Pedre L, Morales-Chacon L, Pavon-Fuentes N, Serrano-Sanchez T, Robinson-Agramonte MA, Garcia-Navarro ME, et al. Immunological disorders in epileptic patients are associated to the epileptogenic focus localization. Rev Neurol. 2004;39(2):101–4.
Lossinsky AS, Shivers RR. Structural pathways for macromolecular and cellular transport across the blood–brain barrier during inflammatory conditions. Review. Histol Histopathol. 2004;19:535–64.
Mackworth-Young CG, Hughes GR. Epilepsy: an early symptom of systemic lupus erythematosus. J Neurol Neurosurg Psychiatry. 1985;48:185.
Maldonado M, Baybis M, Newman D, Kolson DL, Chen W, McKhann G, et al. Expression of ICAM-1, TNF-alpha, NF kappa B, and MAP kinase in tubers of the tuberous sclerosis complex. Neurobiol Dis. 2003;14:279–90.
Mantegazza R, Bernasconi P, Baggi F, Spreafico R, Ragona F, Antozzi C, et al. Antibodies against GluR3 peptides are not specific for Rasmussen's encephalitis but are also present in epilepsy patients with severe, early onset disease and intractable seizures. J Neuroimmunol. 2002;131:179–85.
Maroso M, Balosso S, Ravizza T, Liu J, Aronica E, Iyer AM, et al. Toll-like receptor 4 and high-mobility group box-1 are involved in ictogenesis and can be targeted to reduce seizures. Nat Med. 2010;16:413–9.
Minami M, Kuraishi Y, Yamaguchi T, Nakai S, Hirai Y, Satoh M. Convulsants induce interleukin-1 beta messenger RNA in rat brain. Biochem Biophys Res Commun. 1990;171:832–7.
Minami M, Kuraishi Y, Satoh M. Effects of kainic acid on messenger RNA levels of IL-1 beta, IL-6, TNF alpha and LIF in the rat brain. Biochem Biophys Res Commun. 1991;176:593–8.
Montelli TC, Soares AM, Peracoli MT. Immunologic aspects of West syndrome and evidence of plasma inhibitory effects on T cell function. Arq Neuropsiquiatr. 2003;61:731–7.
Moran LB, Graeber MB. The facial nerve axotomy model. Brain Res Brain Res Rev. 2004;44: 154–78.
Nguyen MD, Julien JP, Rivest S. Innate immunity: the missing llink in neuroprotection and neurodegeneration? Nat Rev Neurosci. 2002;3:216–27.
Nieto M, Roldan S, Sanchez B, Candau R, Rodriguez R. Immunological study in patients with severe myoclonic epilepsy in childhood. Rev Neurol. 2000;30:412–4.
Olson JK, Miller SD. Microglia initiate central nervous system innate and adaptive immune responses through multiple TLRs. J Immunol. 2004;173:3916–24.
Oprica M, Eriksson C, Schultzberg M. Inflammatory mechanisms associated with brain damage induced by kainic acid with special reference to the interleukin-1 system. J Cell Mol Med. 2003;7:127–40.
Ozkara C, Vigevano F. Immuno- and antiinflammatory therapies in epileptic disorders. Epilepsia. 2011;52 Suppl 3:45–51.
Pachter JS, de Vries HE, Fabry Z. The blood–brain barrier and its role in immune privilege in the central nervous system. J Neuropathol Exp Neurol. 2003;62:593–604.

Pacifici R, Paris L, Di CS, Bacosi A, Pichini S, Zuccaro P. Cytokine production in blood mononuclear cells from epileptic patients. Epilepsia. 1995a;36:384–7.
Pacifici R, Zuccaro P, Iannetti P, Raucci U, Imperato C. Immunologic aspects of vigabatrin treatment in epileptic children. Epilepsia. 1995b;36:423–6.
Pardridge WM, Connor JD, Crawford IL. Permeability changes in the blood–brain barrier: causes and consequences. CRC Crit Rev Toxicol. 1975;3:159–99.
Peltola J, Hurme M, Miettinen A, Keranen T. Elevated levels of interleukin-6 may occur in cerebrospinal fluid from patients with recent epileptic seizures. Epilepsy Res. 1998;31:129–33.
Peltola J, Eriksson K, Keranen T. Cytokines and seizures. Arch Neurol. 2001a;58:1168–9.
Peltola J, Keranen T, Rainesalo S, Hurme M. Polymorphism of the interleukin-1 gene complex in localization-related epilepsy. Ann Neurol. 2001b;50:275–6.
Plata-Salaman CR, Ilyin SE, Turrin NP, Gayle D, Flynn MC, Romanovitch AE, et al. Kindling modulates the IL-1beta system, TNF-alpha, TGF-beta1, and neuropeptide mRNAs in specific brain regions. Brain Res Mol Brain Res. 2000;75:248–58.
Ransohoff RM, Kivisakk P, Kidd G. Three or more routes for leukocyte migration into the central nervous system. Nat Rev Immunol. 2003;3:569–81.
Rasmussen T, Olsewski J, Lloyd-Smith D. Focal seizures due to chronic localized encephalitis. Neurology. 1958;8:435–45.
Ravizza T, Vezzani A. Status epilepticus induces time-dependent neuronal and astrocytic expression of interleukin-1 receptor type I in the rat limbic system. Neuroscience. 2006;137:301–8.
Ravizza T, Boer K, Redeker S, Spliet WG, van Rijen PC, Troost D, et al. The IL-1beta system in epilepsy-associated malformations of cortical development. Neurobiol Dis. 2006;24:128–43.
Ravizza T, Gagliardi B, Noe F, Boer K, Aronica E, Vezzani A. Innate and adaptive immunity during epileptogenesis and spontaneous seizures: evidence from experimental models and human temporal lobe epilepsy. Neurobiol Dis. 2008a;29:142–60.
Ravizza T, Noe F, Zardoni D, Vaghi V, Sifringer M, Vezzani A. Interleukin converting enzyme inhibition impairs kindling epileptogenesis in rats by blocking astrocytic IL-1beta production. Neurobiol Dis. 2008b;31:327–33.
Ravizza T, Balosso S, Vezzani A. Inflammation and prevention of epileptogenesis. Neurosci Lett. 2011;497:223–30.
Riazi K, Galic MA, Pittman QJ. Contributions of peripheral inflammation to seizure susceptibility: cytokines and brain excitability. Epilepsy Res. 2010;89:34–42.
Riikonen R. Infantile spasms: therapy and outcome. J Child Neurol. 2004;19:401–4.
Rivest S. Molecular insights on the cerebral innate immune system. Brain Behav Immun. 2003;17:13–9.
Rivest S, Lacroix S, Vallieres L, Nadeau S, Zhang J, Laflamme N. How the blood talks to the brain parenchyma and the paraventricular nucleus of the hypothalamus during systemic inflammatory and infectious stimuli. Proc Soc Exp Biol Med. 2000;223:22–38.
Rodgers KM, Hutchinson MR, Northcutt A, Maier SF, Watkins LR, Barth DS. The cortical innate immune response increases local neuronal excitability leading to seizures. Brain. 2009;132:2478–86.
Rozovsky I, Morgan TE, Willoughby DA, Dugichi-Djordjevich MM, Pasinetti GM, Johnson SA, et al. Selective expression of clusterin (SGP-2) and complement C1qB and C4 during responses to neurotoxins in vivo and in vitro. Neuroscience. 1994;62:741–58.
Schwartz SA, Gordon KE, Johnston MV, Goldstein GW. Use of intravenous immune globulin in the treatment of seizure disorders. J Allergy Clin Immunol. 1989;84:603–6.
Seager J, Jamison D, Wilson J, Hayward A, Soothill J. IgA deficiency, peilepsy, and phenytoin treatment. Lancet. 1975;10:632–5.
Sheng JG, Boop FA, Mrak RE, Griffin WS. Increased neuronal beta-amyloid precursor protein expression in human temporal lobe epilepsy: association with interleukin-1 alpha immunoreactivity. J Neurochem. 1994;63:1872–9.
Sinha S, Patil SA, Jayalekshmy V, Satishchandra P. Do cytokines have any role in epilepsy? Epilepsy Res. 2008;82:171–6.
Snead III OC. How does ACTH work against infantile spasms? Bedside to bench. Ann Neurol. 2001;49:288–9.

Sorrell TC, Forbes IJ, Burness FR, Rischbieth RH. Depression of immunological function in patients treated with phenytoin sodium (sodium diphenylhydantoin). Lancet. 1971;2:1233–5.
Streilein JW. Immune privilege as the result of local tissue barriers and immunosuppressive microenvironments. Curr Opin Immunol. 1993;5:428–32.
Streit WJ, Conde JR, Fendrick SE, Flanary BE, Mariani CL. Role of microglia in the central nervous system's immune response. Neurol Res. 2005;27:685–91.
Takemiya T, Suzuki K, Sugiura H, Yasuda S, Yamagata K, Kawakami Y, et al. Inducible brain COX-2 facilitates the recurrence of hippocampal seizures in mouse rapid kindling. Prostaglandins Other Lipid Mediat. 2003;71:205–16.
Tian L, Rauvala H, Gahmberg CG. Neuronal regulation of immune responses in the central nervous system. Trends Immunol. 2009;30:91–9.
Turrin NP, Rivest S. Innate immune reaction in response to seizures: implications for the neuropathology associated with epilepsy. Neurobiol Dis. 2004;16:321–34.
van Gassen KL, de Wit WM, Koerkamp MJ, Rensen MG, van Rijen PC, Holstege FC, et al. Possible role of the innate immunity in temporal lobe epilepsy. Epilepsia. 2008;49:1055–65.
Vezzani A. Inflammation and epilepsy. Epilepsy Curr. 2005;5:1–6.
Vezzani A. Innate immunity and inflammation in temporal lobe epilepsy: new emphasis on the role of complement activation. Epilepsy Curr. 2008;8:75–7.
Vezzani A, Baram TZ. New roles for interleukin-1 beta in the mechanisms of epilepsy. Epilepsy Curr. 2007;7:45–50.
Vezzani A, Friedman A. Brain inflammation as a biomarker in epilepsy. Biomark Med. 2011;5:607–14.
Vezzani A, Granata T. Brain inflammation in epilepsy: experimental and clinical evidence. Epilepsia. 2005;46:1724–43.
Vezzani A, Conti M, De LA, Ravizza T, Moneta D, Marchesi F, et al. Interleukin-1beta immunoreactivity and microglia are enhanced in the rat hippocampus by focal kainate application: functional evidence for enhancement of electrographic seizures. J Neurosci. 1999;19:5054–65.
Vezzani A, Moneta D, Richichi C, Aliprandi M, Burrows SJ, Ravizza T, et al. Functional role of inflammatory cytokines and antiinflammatory molecules in seizures and epileptogenesis. Epilepsia. 2002;43 Suppl 5:30–5.
Vezzani A, Balosso S, Ravizza T. The role of cytokines in the pathophysiology of epilepsy. Brain Behav Immun. 2008;22:797–803.
Vezzani A, Aronica E, Mazarati A, Pittman QJ. Epilepsy and brain inflammation. Exp Neurol. (2011a) (Epub ahead of print).
Vezzani A, Bartfai T, Bianchi M, Rossetti C, French J. Therapeutic potential of new antiinflammatory drugs. Epilepsia. 2011b;52 Suppl 8:67–9.
Vezzani A, French J, Bartfai T, Baram TZ. The role of inflammation in epilepsy. Nat Rev Neurol. 2011c;7:31–40.
Webb AA, Muir GD. The blood–brain barrier and its role in inflammation. J Vet Intern Med. 2000;14:399–411.
Wekerle H, Linington H, Lassmann H, Meyerman R. Celular immune reactivity within the CNS. Trends Neurosci. 1986;9:271–7.
Wheless JW, Clarke DF, Arzimanoglou A, Carpenter D. Treatment of pediatric epilepsy: European expert opinion, 2007. Epileptic Disord. 2007;9:353–412.
Wiendl H, Bien CG, Bernasconi P, Fleckenstein B, Elger CE, Dichgans J, et al. GluR3 antibodies: prevalence in focal epilepsy but no specificity for Rasmussen's encephalitis. Neurology. 2001;57:1511–4.
Williams K, Alvarez X, Lackner AA. Central nervous system perivascular cells are immunoregulatory cells that connect the CNS with the peripheral immune system. Glia. 2001;36:156–64.
Wirrell E, Farrell K, Whiting S. The epileptic encephalopathies of infancy and childhood. Can J Neurol Sci. 2005;32:409–18.

Xiong ZQ, Qian W, Suzuki K, McNamara JO. Formation of complement membrane attack complex in mammalian cerebral cortex evokes seizures and neurodegeneration. J Neurosci. 2003;23:955–60.
Yabuuchi K, Minami M, Katsumata S, Satoh M. In situ hybridization study of interleukin-1 beta mRNA induced by kainic acid in the rat brain. Brain Res Mol Brain Res. 1993;20:153–61.
Zucker DK, Wooten GF, Lothman EW. Blood–brain barrier changes with kainic acid-induced limbic seizures. Exp Neurol. 1983;79:422–33.

Chapter 11
Contribution of the Antiepileptic Drug Administration Regime in the Development and/or Establishment of Pharmacoresistant Epilepsy

Pietro Fagiolino, Marta Vázquez, Sandra Orozco-Suárez, Cecilia Maldonado, Silvana Alvariza, Iris Angélica Feria-Romero, Manuel Ibarra, and Luisa Rocha

Abstract Overexpression of membrane transporters is one of the main pharmacokinetic reasons that lead to the lack of response of antiepileptics in drug refractory treatments. The present chapter deals with the difficulty anticonvulsant agents have in reaching the brain receptor sites.

An inducer and substrate of efflux transporter drug, when it is continuously administered so as to maintain constant levels in body fluids could become noneffective throughout time, even it was especially effective for a certain type of epilepsy.

In spite of the fact phenytoin (PHT) is a well-known effective antiepileptic drug with characteristic nonlinear pharmacokinetics; resistance could be developed in epileptic patients during chronic treatments. Some new approaches that challenge conventional assumptions about its peculiar pharmacokinetics were consistent with the mechanism involved in refractory epilepsy.

Salivary drug monitoring was a useful tool for understanding the mechanism of both pharmacokinetics and pharmacoresistance developed by PHT as inducer and substrate of efflux transporters.

P. Fagiolino (✉) • M. Vázquez • C. Maldonado • S. Alvariza • M. Ibarra
Pharmaceutical Sciences Department, Universidad de la República, Av. General Flores 2124, Montevideo 11800, Uruguay
e-mail: pfagioli@fq.edu.uy; mvazquez@fq.edu.uy; cmaldonado@fq.edu.uy; salvariza@fq.edu.uy; mibarra@fq.edu.uy

S. Orozco-Suárez, Ph.D. • I.A. Feria-Romero, Ph.D.
Medical Research Unit in Neurological Diseases, National Medical Center "Siglo XXI", IMSS, Hospital of Specialties, Cuauhtemoc No. 330-4, Col. Doctores, Mexico City, Mexico DF 06720, Mexico

L. Rocha
Department of Pharmacobiology, Center for Research and Advanced Studies, Mexico City, Mexico
e-mail: lrocha@cinvestav.mx

L. Rocha and E.A. Cavalheiro (eds.), *Pharmacoresistance in Epilepsy: From Genes and Molecules to Promising Therapies*, DOI 10.1007/978-1-4614-6464-8_11,

Keywords Phenytoin • Pharmacokinetics • Nonlinear response • Inducer drugs • Efflux transporters • Refractory epilepsy • Arteriovenous drug plasma concentration ratio • Salivary drug monitoring

11.1 Pharmacokinetics and Pharmacodynamics of Drug Treatments

Refractory epilepsy has recently been explained (Remy and Beck 2006; Löscher and Potschka 2005) by two main mechanisms: (a) molecular alterations of drug receptor sites that could reduce drug effectiveness or make antiepileptic agents currently used in therapeutics ineffective; and (b) over-expression of multidrug transporters proteins either because of genetics or of inducing agents causing impairment of drug penetration into the brain and therefore to the sites where drug receptors are located.

Both causes are part of the two classical phases involved in the response to drug treatments (Meibohm and Derendorf 1997; Levy 1998; Eichler and Müller 1998): (1) pharmacodynamic (PD) response; and (2) pharmacokinetic (PK) response. The former refers to the effects, and is the consequence of the action exerted by drugs on individuals, while the latter refers to the concentrations of active ingredients in different body tissues, and is the result of the action exerted by the body on the administered molecules.

There is a lack of precision and several misunderstandings in defining each of the responses and in establishing relations between the two, particularly because PK response is usually quantified by measuring blood levels of the active ingredient, and in general because the measured effect is more a consequence of the reaction of the individual to this action than the immediate result of a pharmacological action. Therefore, PK/PD relations traditionally studied in scientific research simply refer to a relationship between blood drug levels and the clinical response of the individual.

Another issue that obscures PK/PD analysis is the uncertain concentrations of active molecules in the different action sites, which may not only differ among them, but they can also differ significantly from blood or plasma drug concentration (Fagiolino et al. 2006a). For this reason, the same plasma concentration of a drug associated with two different clinical responses is usually treated as pharmacodynamic variability. However, it may be due to pharmacokinetic variability in the corresponding site of action, as a consequence of a change in the biophase/plasma drug concentrations ratio (Eichler and Müller 1998).

Thus, over-expression of membrane transporters could be the PK cause that leads to the lack of response of antiepileptics in drug refractory treatments. The present chapter deals with this PK cause, in other words, with the difficulty anticonvulsant agents have in reaching the brain biophase.

11.2 Pharmacokinetics Modulation of the Clinical Response

It is well known the important pharmaceutical and drug therapy development made through PK modeling. So, the development of controlled release products marked a milestone in the search for greater efficacy and safety of drug treatments, due to reduced drug levels oscillations over time, avoiding toxic effects and therapeutic failures (Dutta et al. 2002). This technological advance modifies the release, and consequently the absorption, of active ingredients. With regards to the distribution phase, new molecules have been developed in order to direct their entry into specific organs, reducing systemic toxicity notoriously and achieving the therapeutic goal in the target organ (Ariens 1971). Drug elimination has also been modulated so that the new chemical entity can stay longer in the body, allowing more comfortable treatments with less frequent dosing and a better patient compliance (Ariens 1971). Other strategies involved new entities that avoided metabolic processes that could lead to reactive specimens, thus diminishing their toxicity (Bodor 1984). Although synthetic approaches were useful for accomplishing the goal, new molecules imply risks not yet fully evaluated. Therefore, maintaining the same therapeutic agent with proved effectiveness upon its long clinical use, but modulating its release-absorption process has the important advantage of increasing efficacy and safety at a cost that can benefit a great number of patients.

11.3 Modulation of the Pharmacokinetic Response Through the Patient Clinical Status

Clinical evolution during the course of drug treatment is in many cases an important determinant of the PK response of the drug used to resolve the disease. Antibiotic treatment of sepsis and septic shock is an extreme case of highly variable pharmacokinetics, which is due to the fast and enormous hemodynamic and circulatory changes in the patient in a very short period of time (Vázquez et al. 2012). In this context, daily monitoring of serum levels of vancomycin has proved to be a good indicator of the clinical course of sepsis, leading to dosage adjustments and a continuous infusion administration of the antibiotic that helped to resolve this clinical situation (Vázquez et al. 2008). Seizures can be observed in critically ill patients and in many cases, sepsis can coexist. The reduction of serum albumin due to the systemic inflammatory response often leads to an erroneous increase in dose as total drug concentration in blood, commonly monitored, is reduced, when in fact the free plasma antiepileptic measurements should be the right choice as they represent drug concentration at its receptor site (Ibarra et al. 2010).

Cardiovascular diseases can also condition PK drug response because any change in cardiac output and its distribution among different organs impact on drug disposition significantly (Fagiolino 2002, 2004; Fagiolino et al. 2003, 2006a).

Uncontrolled seizures can induce over-expression of drug transporters at the epileptogenic focus, at the blood brain barrier (BBB), and even at remote areas of the body (Hoffmann et al. 2006; Lazarowski et al. 2006, 2007; Hoffmann and Löscher 2007). This may lead to refractoriness to drugs that are substrate of these transporters. Refractoriness caused by a reduced access of the active agent to the brain or to the zones where the anticonvulsant action sites are located, or also by the lower concentrations after activation of the elimination processes, both presystemic (reducing oral bioavailability) and systemic (increasing the clearance).

11.4 Modulation of the Pharmacokinetic Response Conditioned by the Pharmacodynamic Response

This section deals with the modulation that the action of a drug can cause of its own pharmacokinetics. The definition of "drug action" must be precise and as it was previously mentioned, it can be defined as the biological process triggered by the drug at the receptors of the individuals. For example, a beta-blocking action of propranolol may be responsible for both reduction in cardiac output and vasoconstriction of the hepatic artery, leading therefore to a reduction in hepatic blood flow (and also in the fraction of cardiac output directed to the liver), decreasing drug clearance and consequently increasing systemic drug concentrations (Stargel and Shand 1981). This is an easy example to illustrate how pharmacodynamics modulates pharmacokinetic response.

Many other actions are much more frequent, although they are not typically classified as PD responses. For example, enzymes and/or transporters induction, or even sub-expression of enzymes or other drug transference mechanisms, are part of the action of the drug and can impact either on other drug kinetics or on its own kinetics.

In this context, administration of some inducer antiepileptic drugs can be the cause of the development of refractory epilepsy, or the consolidation of an existing process of drug resistance provoked by a prolonged therapeutic failure. The crucial point that defines resistance to a certain drug is the fact that dosing adjustments are incapable of seizures control without risk of toxicity. Consequently, there is poor access of drug to the neurons in order to exert the therapeutic action, access that perhaps was previously limited to the body by progressive loss of systemic bioavailability for drugs extravascularly administered.

Among the most common drugs used to treat certain types of epilepsy, carbamazepine (CBZ) is a well-known inducer of both enzymes (Klotz 2007) and membrane transporters (Giessmann et al. 2004), and as such, it acts inducing its own presystemic and systemic metabolism (Fagiolino et al. 2006b), leading to a progressive decrease in oral bioavailability, a progressive increase in its clearance, and a gradual decrease in brain penetration, being a substrate of efflux pumps located at the BBB as well (Potschka et al. 2003).

Phenytoin (PHT), an effective agent used in the treatment of partial, tonic-clonic, and secondarily generalized seizures, is also a well-known enzyme and membrane transporter inducer and substrate showing high affinity for MRP2 (multidrug resistance-associated protein 2) and lower affinity for Pgp (P-glycoprotein). This fact could lead to resistance to the antiepileptic treatment. Due to its particular nonlinear pharmacokinetic a deeper description of the processes involved in drug resistance, of the research methods employed, and of the bibliographic reports that account for its pharmacokinetic properties will be given.

11.5 Nonlinear Pharmacokinetics of Phenytoin

In spite of the fact PHT is a well-known drug with nonlinear PK response to the administered dose, in chronic treatments, and that the most common explanation for this behavior is the enzymatic saturation with clearance restriction, there are some new approaches that challenge conventional assumptions (Fagiolino et al. 2011). Although Michaelis–Menten equation correctly applies to the kinetic description of this drug, and has been successfully used in dose adjustment, with invaluable clinical utility, the traditional mechanistic justifications are questionable.

Single oral doses (range 100–300 mg) of PHT showed a linear pharmacokinetic response, with a reduction in the rate, but not the extent of absorption, as dose increased (Rojanasthien et al. 2007). In other words, the areas under the plasma concentration–time curve (AUC) were proportional to the doses administered. The elimination half-life remained constant and independent of doses (12–13 h).

Administration of single doses between 400 and 1,600 mg showed a progressive loss of bioavailability due to incomplete dissolution of the drug in the gastrointestinal tract, even more evident with increasing doses (Jung et al. 1980). It seemed to be clear the progressive delay in reaching maximum plasma concentrations (C_{max}) at high single doses due to solubility saturation in the intestinal fluid that changed the absorption kinetic pattern (dissolution dependent) from first-order to zero order. When the dose of 1,600 mg was divided into three smaller doses (400 mg every 3 h), the registered bioavailability for low doses was recovered and a C_{max} value was in accordance with a linear behavior.

Paradoxically, the authors of the above mentioned research (Jung et al. 1980) reaffirmed after single doses the classical Michaelis–Menten kinetics reported for PHT during chronic treatment. A change in the declination of plasma concentrations after a single intravenous dose of 15 mg/kg (approximately 1,200 mg) was observed. A concentration-dependent clearance was reported by the authors in light of the progressive increase in the elimination rate observed over time, with the typical parameters values of this kinetic behavior: $K_m = 9.43$ mg/L, $V_{max} = 8.25$ mg/kg/day.

An alternative explanation for the increase in the elimination rate after an intravenous dose of PHT could be given taking into account the enzymatic auto and hetero induction capacity of the drug, a phenomenon seen some time after the activation of the biosynthesis of messenger RNA encoding the corresponding protein (Gerk and Vore 2002). However, this hypothesis is not in agreement with drug dose (concentration)-dependent accumulation observed in chronic treatments, as the opposite effect should be seen if enzymatic induction was the cause of the nonlinear pharmacokinetics of the drug.

Michaelis–Menten kinetics has been explained on the basis of a limited metabolizing capacity of the enzymes involved in PHT clearance (CYP2C9 and CYP2C19), which would lead to an almost enzyme saturation by the drug itself when its concentrations were close to Km value, as it was observed in the aforementioned single intravenous dose and during the clinical practice of antiepileptic treatment (Lin 1994). This phenomenon would result in a non-proportional increase in PHT concentrations (more than expected) when dose adjustments are carried out.

There is strong evidence of a significant PHT secretion from the blood into the digestive tract, after which the drug may reenter the body from the intestinal lumen. Observations of second plasma peaks after intravenous doses of PHT (Handley 1970; Glick et al. 2004) are strong arguments for assuming an important contribution of enterohepatic circulation to the pharmacokinetics of the drug. Furthermore, oral administration of activated charcoal (Howard et al. 1994) has successfully been used to resolve PHT intoxication, proving to be an efficient mechanism to reduce plasma exposure to the drug and to increase its systemic clearance (Mauro et al. 1987).

The role efflux transporters could play in the concentration-dependent kinetics of PHT is based on research results, where reduced plasma concentrations of PHT were obtained after co administration of ciprofloxacin, a well-known transporter inhibitor (Pollack and Slayter 1997; Brouwers et al. 1997).

All these evidences put in doubt the increased elimination rate obtained after a single intravenous dose of 1,200 mg of PHT, since it is likely that the plasma concentration profile of PHT had masked less intense PHT re absorptions throughout time resulting from the lower concentrations that remain in the body after gradual biotransformation.

Due to this inconsistency, a hypothesis has been proposed (Fagiolino et al. 2011) that questions the concentration-dependent kinetics of PHT as a result of the enzymatic auto inhibition of the drug. This new approach focuses on efflux transporters induction at the hepatobiliary membrane and at the enterocytes, which drives molecules from the liver or from the enterocytes to the intestinal lumen. The transporter involved could be the MRP2 (Potschka et al. 2003). Through these efflux pumps the drug would be secreted to the digestive tract significantly, thereby facilitating the appearance of second peaks even after intravenous administration. The concentration-dependent induction of their expression would slow the oral absorption of PHT. This fact is observed when analyzing plasma profiles of the drug in multiple dose regimens, which are much less acute than the ones observed after single doses. Moreover, the deviation of the drug from the liver to the gallbladder, and from there to the internal medium, by reabsorption through the gallbladder wall, or into the intestine via the bile duct, would prevent the majority biotransformation which takes place in the hepatocytes. Because of the greater abundance of CYP2C9 and

CYP2C19 in the liver in comparison to the enterocytes (Läpple et al. 2003), PHT clearance could be reduced in a concentration-dependent way as traditionally verified during chronic treatments.

11.6 Phenytoin as Inducing Agent of Efflux Transporters

Different studies in rats have shown the inductive capacity of PHT over Pgp and MRP2 expression (Wen et al. 2008). In order to test this hypothesis we carried out a treatment regimen in adult female Sprague-Dawley rats, to which were administered oral increasing doses of 25, 50, and 100 mg every 6 h for three consecutive days. We confirmed the above mentioned inductive effect on MRP2 but mainly on Pgp expression in different tissues, having the following order of intensity: enterocyte, salivary gland, hepatocytes, and finally in BBB (unpublished data). This induction was dose dependent, and consequently dependent on the concentration achieved at different sites where expression of transporters was observed. The greatest expression in the intestine and salivary glands was probably due to the highest concentrations of PHT at these sites during the administration of drug suspension. The over expression was mainly seen with Pgp and at higher doses also MRP2 was overexpressed. Interestingly, 1 week after dose discontinuation, the expression of transporters returned to baseline levels in the area with the greatest induction, with a shorter recovery time in less induced organs such as the brain.

Transporter expression was detected in humans after CBZ administration (Giessmann et al. 2004) and, according to our results, only 48 h were required on average to noticed the result of such expression in saliva (Maldonado et al. 2011; Gerk and Vore 2002). A significant impact of the sex of the individuals was observed on both salivary concentrations and saliva/plasma ratio after chronic administration in patients (Maldonado 2011). As several efflux transporters were identified in the acinar and ductal cells of the salivary gland (Uematsu et al. 2001, 2003), saliva has become an interesting tool for the phenotyping of efflux transporters in patients. The specific methodology will be discussed later in this chapter.

11.7 Impact of PHT Transporter Induction on Its Own Pharmacokinetics Response

Oral administration of PHT in rats did not allow to connect efflux transporters induction with the nonlinear kinetics of this drug after multiple doses; however, intraperitoneal administration of 30, 50, and 100 mg/kg/day (Lolin et al. 1994) showed a non-proportional increase in plasma concentrations in response to the administered doses. Comparing the oral and intraperitoneal doses of 25 mg/kg every 6 h, a higher apparent clearance after oral administration was observed (unpublished data).

This could be due to reduced bioavailability, increased systemic clearance, or both reasons when the drug is given orally, because of the stronger inductive effect of both transporters and enzymes in the intestine with this route of administration in relation to the intraperitoneal one.

The interspecies difference between rat and man may be contributing to the different PK response in plasma detected after oral administration of PHT. Rats do not have a gallbladder, but produce bile. The bile flows directly from the liver through the bile duct into the small intestine, so once the PHT is at the enterocyte and due to a high enzymatic expression there, intestinal clearance could contribute significantly to the total clearance of the drug. This could be different in humans due to the eventual absorption of PHT from the gallbladder itself.

The experience in rats has been, however, relevant to appreciate the lack of correlation between PK response in plasma and PK response in cerebrospinal fluid (CSF) when PHT was administered intraperitoneally (Lolin et al. 1994). A more pronounced increase in plasma PHT concentrations in comparison to CSF concentrations with increasing daily doses were observed due to a lower drug passage to the brain as a result of the autoinduction exerted by PHT. This is the key for understanding drug resistance after the administration of PHT or any other efflux transporter inducer in the treatment of epilepsy.

11.8 Monitoring of Salivary Drug Concentrations

Saliva is not only an inexpensive, easy, and less risky way of drug monitoring in clinical practice (Ritschel and Thompson 1983; Fagiolino 1999), but also, in this context, takes a special relevance as it would give information about efflux transporters induction. Among the therapeutic attributes that saliva has, this monitoring fluid closely correlates with free plasma levels of drug present in the arterial circulation (Posti 1982), which makes it a more useful tool to study PK/PD response, since the arterial blood concentration has had an excellent performance in the PK/PD correlation of several drugs with rapid transference to the sites of action (Galeazzi et al. 1976; Gourlay and Benowitz 1997).

The privilege traditionally assigned to plasma drug monitoring becomes irrelevant as it is regularly done on a venous blood sample, and therefore in a section of the circulatory system that transports solutes leaving organs where the action sites are not located. On the contrary, arterial blood carries solutes to all organs of the body in the same concentration. Hence, this is the importance of arterial plasma monitoring, or otherwise saliva.

In order to actually be a good surrogate of arterial plasma, saliva samples should be taken by stimulation (chewing parafilm®, or placing small crystals of citric acid over the tongue). Discarding intermediate collected samples, a final fraction of saliva could be obtained, with a concentration very close to that in the initial portion of the salivary duct (acini) and therefore practically the same as that flowing free within the arterial vessels. Figure 11.1 (Fagiolino 1999) shows schematically the

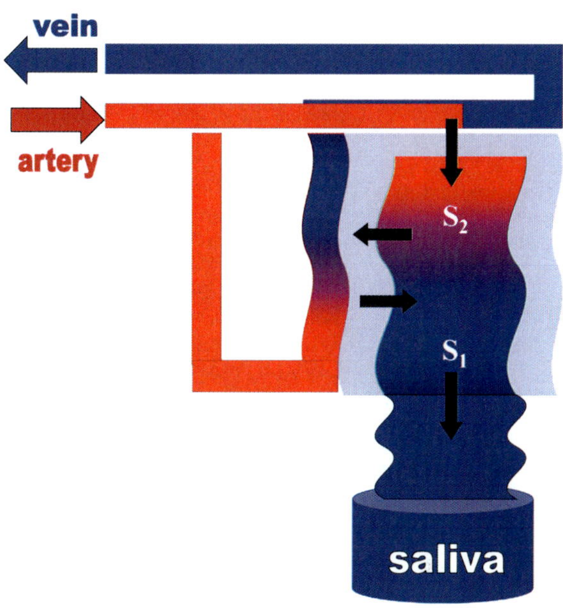

Fig. 11.1 Saliva production in the salivary glands. S1 and S2: first and second fractions of saliva collections, respectively

Table 11.1 Saliva pharmacokinetic parameter means (or medians) of phenytoin after a single oral dose of 100 mg

	Male ($n=10$)	Female ($n=14$)	Significance
T_{max} (h)	4 [2–8]	4 [2–7]	NS
C_{max} (mg/L)	0.188 (0.020)	0.220 (0.020)	$p<0.05$
$AUC_{0-\infty}$ (mg h/L)	3.63 (0.52)	4.42 (1.04)	$p<0.05$
AUC × W (mg h kg/L)	278 (25)	261 (25)	$p<0.05$
$t_{1/2}$ (h)	12.6 (1.3)	13.0 (3.3)	NS

T_{max}, time-to-peak drug concentration; C_{max}, peak concentration of drug; $AUC_{0-\infty}$ (or AUC), area under drug concentration–time curve from zero to infinite; $t_{1/2}$, elimination half life; W, body weight; [ ], range; ( ), standard deviation; NS, no significant

process by which saliva is produced in the glands and the blood irrigating the salivary gland. This portion of saliva, called S2 in the figure, is the basis of therapeutic drug monitoring in saliva.

Recent research has shown that salivary PHT concentrations in samples obtained by stimulation were similar between men and women after a 100-mg single dose bioequivalence study (Ruiz et al. 2011). This similarity is achieved when the concentration obtained is multiplied by the weight of the individual, so that the final outcome refers to the concentration that both sexes would have if the same doses per kilogram of body weight were administered. Table 11.1 shows the most relevant data obtained from the bioequivalence study (Ruiz et al. 2011).

In patients under chronic PHT monotherapy, different S2 levels between genders (see Table 11.2) were obtained, even when they received similar daily doses per

Table 11.2 Phenytoin (PHT) salivary mean exposure after multiple dose administration

	Male ($n=11$)	Female ($n=11$)	Significance
Daily dose (mg/kg)	4.58 (1.20)	4.87 (0.83)	NS
$[S2]_{PHT}$ (mg/L)	0.90 (0.39)	1.91 (1.04)	$p<0.01$
S1/S2 ratio PHT	1.09 (0.08)	1.01 (0.08)	$p<0.05$

[S2], saliva drug concentration in the collected second sample (see on the text); S1/S2, first-to-second-sample ratio of saliva drug concentrations (see on the text); ( ), standard deviation; NS, no significant

kilogram of body weight. Venous plasma concentrations (P) in patients enable us to report S2/P ratios of 0.067 for men and 0.14 for women. One hypothesis is the important PHT induction of efflux transporters, exacerbating the natural difference between men and women in the MRP2 expression (Suzuki et al. 2006). This had very little impact after the first dose since a previous exposure time, a couple of days or so, is required for induction.

11.9 Salivary Monitoring of Drug Absorption and Elimination

Figure 11.1 divides saliva composition in salivary ducts into two fractions: (1) the first fraction collected after salivation coming from the lower part of ducts; and (2) the second fraction coming from the upper part of the ducts if saliva stimulation is maintained. Given the reduced residence time of the fluid flowing by the duct cells, the exchange of solutes could be impeded and therefore the second fraction would have a composition closer to that of arterial blood.

This collection procedure could be designed so as to achieve a small initial volume, more representative of what is in the duct prior its discharge into the oral cavity (S1). Discarding intermediate collected samples a final fraction of saliva could be obtained (S2), with a concentration practically the same as that flowing free within the arterial vessels. If we consider that S1 comes into equilibrium with the capillaries that irrigate the ductal cells, one might assume that this first small portion of saliva would contain a drug concentration that resembles the venous one. Therefore, S1/S2 drug concentration ratio would be directly related to the vein/artery (V/A) plasma free drug concentration ratio.

Drug concentration is not homogeneous in arteries and veins, showing different arteriovenous profiles throughout time as it is shown in Fig. 11.2 (Lam and Chiou 1982). As it can be observed, during the input of a drug the arteries have higher plasma drug concentrations than those veins not involved in the route of entrance, while during the elimination phase the veins exhibit higher concentrations than the arteries. The same behavior was observed for S1 and S2 concentrations, with smaller S1/S2 ratios during the absorption in comparison with the elimination phase (Fagiolino et al. 2000).

An interesting recent finding (Maldonado 2011), showed that the increase in the daily dose of CBZ in patients correlated with an increase in S1/S2 predose drug

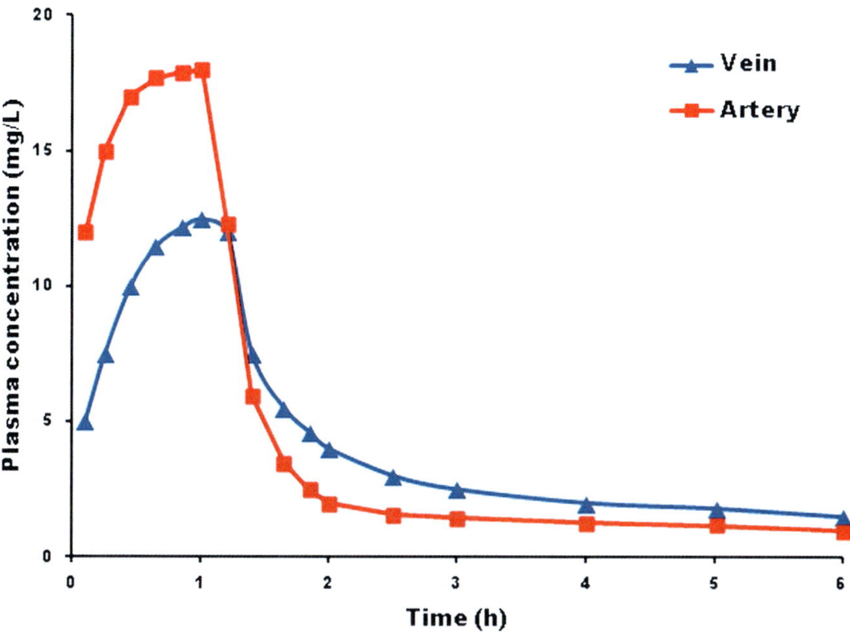

Fig. 11.2 Arterial and venous plasma concentration profiles in rabbit after intravenous infusion of procainamide (adapted from Lam and Chiou 1982)

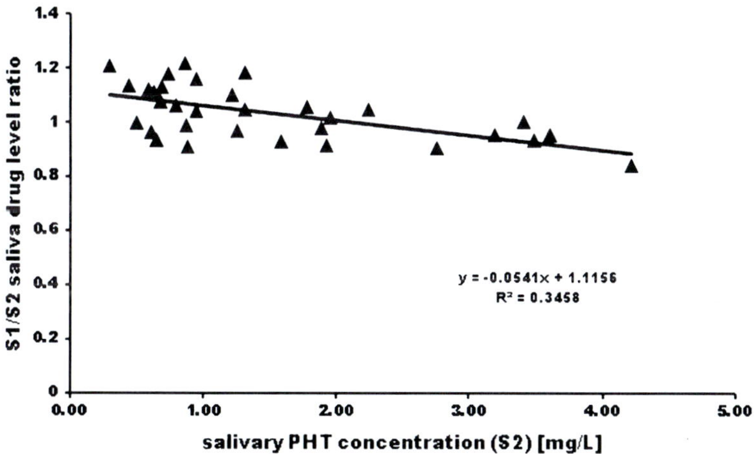

Fig. 11.3 S1/S2 saliva phenytoin (PHT) concentration ratio in relation with its salivary levels (or daily dose)

concentration ratio. However, for PHT, the increase in the daily dose (systemic levels) was associated with a decrease in the respective S1/S2 ratio (see Fig. 11.3). Bearing in mind that CBZ induces its own elimination and PHT, on the contrary, reduces its elimination with increasing daily doses, we could have a clear demonstration of the significant contribution of S1/S2 drug concentration ratio in the assessment of the change in clearance after dosage adjustments.

Interestingly, significant differences in S1/S2 salivary concentration ratio between genders (lower in women) were observed in patients under PHT monotherapy (see Table 11.2). This could reveal a lower clearance in women, as daily doses were similar for both sexes. However, plasma concentrations in women were lower than in men. Therefore, one possible hypothesis is that absorption may be prolonged and possibly more intense in women, due to an increased enterocyte/hepatocyte—intestinal lumen circulation. Other authors (Ratanakorn et al. 1997) have reported a greater distribution volume (V_d) of PHT in women, which could now be explained by an increased shedding of the drug into the intestinal lumen as a storage site of the drug.

Differences in human MDR1 gene lead to different activities of P-gp protein. Lower plasma concentrations of PHT in individuals carrying the high-activity genotype (Kerb et al. 2001) were observed, when single doses of 300 mg of the drug were administered, revealing a possible greater distribution of the drug into the intestinal lumen.

Therefore, several observations come together to demonstrate efflux transporters induction in humans after chronic administration of PHT. Such an induction would be different, either at the salivary gland or at organs of the splanchnic region (gut and liver), regarding the sex of the individual. It seems likely that this induction will also operate at the efflux transporters expressed at the BBB, limiting therefore drug delivery to the target brain sites.

11.10 Pharmacokinetics Paradox of Efflux Transporters Inducers

As the dose rate of a drug increases, higher steady-state concentrations are expected, becoming this paradigm the basis of dosage adjustments. However, for some drugs, the plasma drug concentration changes either more (e.g., PHT inhibiting its elimination), or less (e.g., CBZ inducing its own elimination) than would be expected from a change in dose rate. If a drug does not modify its elimination, the concentration at steady state will increase proportionately. But as it has been discussed in this chapter, even for a drug like PHT, which causes a very important increase in plasma concentrations with a small increase in daily dose, induction of membrane transporters at the BBB, or at the vicinity of the neurons (astrocytes), will provoke a smaller increase in brain levels to the point that perhaps their values could drop below the minimum effective concentration. This could result in pharmacoresistance to this antiepileptic drug and thus in treatment failure.

The condition shown by several efflux transporter substrates of inducing its own expression is of great concern, as pharmacoresistance is not only seen in epilepsy but it is also present in cancer and HIV treatments (Harmsen et al. 2009; Perloff et al. 2001). Although the development of specific inhibitors of efflux transporters is an interesting strategy to enhance drug delivery to its target action site, this down-modulation could affect endogenous agent disposition, altering important function of living systems. Besides, the inhibition of efflux transporter could also allow the entrance of other non-desirable substances. Thus, their long-term use may not be advisable or possible.

11.11 Controlling the Exposure Time to the Inducing Agent

Not only the concentration of an inducing agent, but also the exposure time to it, can cause the expression of transporter proteins (Gerk and Vore 2002). Low concentrations of the inducing agent may return the transporters expression to baseline values (unpublished data, Maldonado et al. 2011), thus strategies for finding a new mode of administration of the antiepileptic drug, both substrate and inducer of the efflux transporter, have been developed. Contrary to what was proposed as a paradigm of therapy, the minimizing of peak-trough oscillations of the active ingredient with frequent administrations of low doses, or with extended-release formulation, high doses spaced enough in time could be an strategy to take in the future for highly effective drugs such as PHT, but efflux pumps substrates and inducers.

The association of an antiepileptic drug working against almost every type of epilepsy and that is not an efflux transporter inducer, such as the case of valproic acid, administered through extended-release formulations (Fagiolino et al. 2007) could be an ideal adjunctive treatment of intermittent administration of PHT. Thus, there would be a basal control of epileptogenic discharges reinforced at spaced intervals with one of the most effective agents in blocking the axonal conduction of action potentials.

11.12 Conclusions

Overexpression of membrane transporters is one of the mechanisms that promotes drug resistance in the treatment of epilepsy. This process of overexpression occurs spontaneously in response to seizure activity when seizures are poorly controlled. The administration of antiepileptic agents, which are substrates of efflux transporters, is prone to eventual therapeutic failure if seizures are not controlled. But the usage of such agents, which also posses the ability to induce the expression of these transporters, leads to the consolidation of refractory epilepsy, as the increase in transporters expression is such that turns the antiepileptic agent into a real shield against resolution of the seizures.

Transporter hypothesis of drug resistance has triggered efforts to develop approaches to overcome enhanced BBB efflux transport. These approaches include: modulation of transport function, blocking the signaling pathway that up-regulated the transporters in response to seizure activity, bypassing BBB transporters by encapsulation of antiepileptic drugs in nano-sized carrier systems, or intracerebral administration. But none of these novel approaches has focused on avoiding the inducing capacity of the antiepileptic agent.

On the assumption that a drug is especially effective for a certain type of epilepsy, its continuous administration so as to maintain constant levels of active ingredient, as a therapeutic agent and as an efflux transporter inducer, is a therapeutic problem. Consequently, a less frequent dosing regimen in time is proposed in order to obtain therefore, lower drug concentrations during treatment that would allow a down regulation of the over expression of efflux transporters and in this way the following dose of the antiepileptic drug is once again effective.

References

Ariens EJ. Modulation of pharmacokinetics by molecular manipulation. In: Ariens EJ, editor. Drug design, vol. 2. New York: Academic; 1971.

Bodor N. Soft drugs: principles and methods for the design of safe drugs. Med Res Rev. 1984;4:449–69.

Brouwers PJ, de Boer LE, Guchelaar HJ. Ciprofloxacin–phenytoin interaction. Ann Pharmacother. 1997;31:498.

Dutta S, Zhang Y, Selness DS, Lee LL, Williams LA, Sommerville KW. Comparison of the bioavailability of unequal doses of divalproex sodium extended-release formulation relative to the delayed-release formulation in healthy volunteers. Epilepsy Res. 2002;49:1–10.

Eichler HG, Müller M. Drug distribution: the forgotten relative in clinical pharmacokinetics. Clin Pharmacokinet. 1998;34:95–9.

Fagiolino P. Salivary drug monitoring: biopharmaceutic, pharmacokinetic and therapeutic applications [in spanish]. Montevideo, Uruguay: Comisión Sectorial de Investigación Científica. Universidad de la República; 1999.

Fagiolino P. The influence of cardiac output distribution on the tissue/plasma drug concentration ratio. Eur J Drug Metab Pharmacokinet. 2002;27:79–81.

Fagiolino P. Multiplicative dependence of the first order rate constant and its impact on clinical pharmacokinetics and bioequivalence. Eur J Drug Metab Pharmacokinet. 2004;29:43–9.

Fagiolino P, Duré C, Vázquez M. Sympathetic tone evaluation in patients treated with phenytoin and carbamazepine [in Spanish]. Acta Farm Bonaerense. 2000;19:119–24.

Fagiolino P, Wilson F, Samaniego E, Vázquez M. In vitro approach to study the influence of the cardiac output distribution on drug concentration. Eur J Drug Metab Pharmacokinet. 2003;28:147–53.

Fagiolino P, Eiraldi R, Vázquez M. The influence of cardiovascular physiology on dose-pharmacokinetic and pharmacokinetic-pharmacodynamic relationships. Clin Pharmacokinet. 2006a;45:433–48.

Fagiolino P, Vázquez M, Olano I, Delfino A. Systemic and presystemic conversion of carbamazepine to carbamazepine-10,11-epoxide during long term treatment. J Epilepsy Clin Neurophysiol. 2006b;12:13–6.

Fagiolino P, Martín O, González N, Malanga A. Actual bioavailability of divalproex sodium extended-release tablets and its clinical implications. J Epilepsy Clin Neurophysiol. 2007; 13:75–8.

Fagiolino P, Vázquez M, Eiraldi R, Maldonado C, Scaramelli A. Efflux transporter influence on drug metabolism: theoretical approach for bioavailability and clearance prediction. Clin Pharmacokinet. 2011;50:75–80.

Galeazzi RL, Benet LZ, Sheiner LB. Relationship between the pharmacokinetics and pharmacodynamics of procainamide. Clin Pharmacol Ther. 1976;20:278–89.
Gerk PM, Vore M. Regulation of the multidrug resistance-associated protein 2 (MRP2) and its role in drug disposition. J Pharmacol Exp Ther. 2002;302:407–15.
Giessmann T, May K, Modess C, Wegner D, Hecker U, Zschiesche M, et al. Carbamazepine regulates intestinal P-glycoprotein and multidrug resistance protein MRP2 and influences disposition of talinolol in humans. Clin Pharmacol Ther. 2004;76:192–200.
Glick TH, Workman TP, Gaufberg SV. Preventing phenytoin intoxication: safer use of a familiar anticonvulsant. J Fam Pract. 2004;53:197–202.
Gourlay SG, Benowitz NL. Arteriovenous differences in plasma concentration of nicotine and catecholamines and related cardiovascular effects after smoking, nicotine nasal spray, and intravenous nicotine. Clin Pharmacol Ther. 1997;62:453–63.
Handley AJ. Phenytoin tolerance tests. Br Med J. 1970;3:203–4.
Harmsen S, Meijerman I, Febus CL, Maas-Bakker RF, Beijnen JH, Schellens JH. PXR-mediated induction of P-glycoprotein by anticancer drugs in a human colon adenocarcinoma-derived cell line. Cancer Chemother Pharmacol. 2009;66:765–71.
Hoffmann K, Löscher W. Upregulation of brain expression of P-glycoprotein in MRP2-deficient TR^- rats resembles seizure-induced up-regulation of this drug efflux transporter in normal rats. Epilepsia. 2007;48:631–45.
Hoffmann K, Gastens AM, Volk HA, Löscher W. Expression o the multidrug transporter MRP2 in the blood-brain barrier after pilocarpine-induced seizures in rats. Epilepsy Res. 2006;69:1–14.
Howard CE, Roberts RS, Ely DS, Moye RA. Use of multiple-dose activated charcoal in phenytoin toxicity. Ann Pharmacother. 1994;28:201–3.
Ibarra M, Vázquez M, Fagiolino P, Mutilva F, Canale A. Total, unbound plasma and salivary phenytoin levels in critically ill patients. J Epilepsy Clin Neurophysiol. 2010;16:69–73.
Jung D, Powell JR, Walson P, Perrier D. Effect of dose on phenytoin absorption. Clin Pharmacol Ther. 1980;28:479–85.
Kerb R, Aynacioglu AS, Brockmöller J, Schlagenhaufer R, Bauer S, Szekeres T, et al. The predictive value of MDR1, CYP2C9 and CYP2C19 polymorphisms for phenytoin plasma levels. Pharmacogenomics J. 2001;1:204–10.
Klotz U. The role of pharmacogenetics in the metabolism of antiepileptic drugs: pharmacokinetic and therapeutic implications. Clin Pharmacokinet. 2007;46:271–9.
Lam G, Chiou WL. Determination of the steady-state volume of distribution using arterial and venous plasma data from constant infusion studies with procainamide. J Pharm Pharmacol. 1982;34:132–4.
Läpple F, von Richter O, Fromm MF, Richter T, Thon KP, Wisser H, et al. Differential expression and function of CYP2C isoforms in human intestine and liver. Pharmacogenetics. 2003;13:565–75.
Lazarowski A, Czornyj L, Lubieniecki F, Vázquez S, D'Giano C, Sevlever G, et al. Multidrug-resistance (MDR) proteins develops refractory epilepsy phenotype: clinical and experimental evidences. Curr Drug Ther. 2006;1:291–309.
Lazarowski A, Czornyj L, Lubieniecki F, Girardi E, Vázquez S, D'Giano C. ABC transporters during epilepsy and mechanisms underlying multidrug resistance in refractory epilepsy. Epilepsia. 2007;48:140–9.
Levy G. Predicting effective drug concentrations for individual patients: determinants of pharmacodynamics variability. Clin Pharmacokinet. 1998;34:323–33.
Lin JH. Dose-dependent pharmacokinetics: experimental observations and theoretical considerations. Biopharm Drug Dispos. 1994;15:1–31.
Lolin YI, Ratnaraj N, Hjelm M, Patsalos PN. Antiepileptic drug pharmacokinetics ad neuropharmacokinetics in individual rats by repetitive withdrawal of blood and cerebrospinal fluid: phenytoin. Epilepsy Res. 1994;19:99–110.
Löscher W, Potschka H. Drug resistance in brain diseases and the role of drug efflux transporters. Nat Rev Neurosci. 2005;6:591–602.

Maldonado C. Understanding the role of membrane transporters in the therapeutics of epilepsy [in Spanish] [Dissertation]. Uruguay: Faculty of Chemistry, University of the Republic; 2011

Maldonado C, Fagiolino P, Vázquez M, Eiraldi R, Alvariza S, Bentancur C, et al. Time-dependent and concentration-dependent upregulation of carbamazepine efflux transporter. A preliminary assessment from salivary drug monitoring. Lat Am J Pharm. 2011;30:908–12.

Mauro LS, Mauro VF, Brown DL, Somani P. Enhancement of phenytoin elimination by multiple-dose activated charcoal. Ann Emerg Med. 1987;16:1132–5.

Meibohm B, Derendorf H. Basic concepts of pharmacokinetic/pharmacodynamic (PK/PD) modelling. Int J Clin Pharmacol Ther. 1997;35:401–13.

Perloff MD, Von Moltke LL, Marchand JE, Greenblatt DJ. Ritonavir induces P-glycoprotein expression, multidrug resistance-associated protein (MRP1) expression, and drug transporter-mediated activity in a human intestinal cell line. J Pharm Sci. 2001;90:1829–37.

Pollack PT, Slayter KL. Hazards of doubling phenytoin dose in the face of an unrecognized interaction with ciprofloxacin. Ann Pharmacother. 1997;31:61–4.

Posti J. Saliva-plasma drug concentration ratios during absorption: theoretical considerations and pharmacokinetic implications. Pharm Acta Helv. 1982;57:83–92.

Potschka H, Fedrowitz M, Löscher W. Multidrug resistance protein MRP2 contributes to blood-brain barrier function and restricts antiepileptic drug activity. J Pharmacol Exp Ther. 2003;306:124–31.

Ratanakorn D, Kaojarern S, Phuapradit P, Mokkhavesa C. Single oral loading dose of phenytoin: a pharmacokinetics study. J Neurol Sci. 1997;147:89–92.

Remy S, Beck H. Molecular and cellular mechanism of pharmacoresistance in epilepsy. Brain. 2006;129:18–35.

Ritschel WA, Thompson GA. Monitoring of drug concentration in saliva: a non-invasive pharmacokinetic procedure. Methods Find Exp Clin Pharmacol. 1983;5:511–25.

Rojanasthien N, Chaichana N, Teekachunhatean S, Kumsorn B, Sangdee C, Chankrachang S. Effect of doses on the bioavailability of phenytoin from a prompt-release and an extended-release preparation: single dose study. J Med Assoc Thai. 2007;90:1883–93.

Ruiz ME, Fagiolino P, Buschiazzo PM, Volonté MG. Is saliva suitable as a biological fluid in relative bioavailability studies? Analysis of its performance in a 4×2 replicate crossover design. Eur J Drug Metab Pharmacokinet. 2011;36:229–36.

Stargel WW, Shand DG. Propranolol: therapeutic use and serum concentration monitoring. In: Taylor WJ, Finn AL, editors. Individualizing drug therapy. Practical applications of drug monitoring, vol. 3. New York: Gross Townsend Frank Inc.; 1981.

Suzuki T, Zhao YL, Nadai M, Naruhashi K, Shimizu A, Takagi K, et al. Gender-related differences in expression and function of hepatic P-glycoprotein and multidrug resistance-associated protein (Mrp2) in rats. Life Sci. 2006;79:455–61.

Uematsu T, Yamaoka M, Matsuura T, Doto R, Hotomi H, Yamada A, et al. P-glycoprotein expression in human major and minor salivary glands. Arch Oral Biol. 2001;46:521–7.

Uematsu T, Yamaoka M, Doto R, Tanaka H, Matsuura T, Furusawa K. Expression of ATP-binding cassette transporter in human salivary ducts. Arch Oral Biol. 2003;48:87–90.

Vázquez M, Fagiolino P, Boronat A, Buroni M, Maldonado C. Therapeutic drug monitoring of vancomycin in severe sepsis and septic shock. Int J Clin Pharmacol Ther. 2008;46:140–5.

Vázquez M, Fagiolino P, Maldonado C, Ibarra M, Boronat A. Impact of severe sepsis or septic shock on drug response. In: Fernández R, editor. Severe sepsis and septic shock. Understanding a serious killer. Rijeka, Croatia: Intech Open Access; 2012.

Wen T, Liu YC, Yang HW, Liu HY, Liu XD, Wang GJ, et al. Effect of 21-day exposure of phenobarbital, carbamazepine and phenytoin on P-glycoprotein expression and activity in the rat brain. J Neurol Sci. 2008;270:99–106.

Chapter 12
Experimental Models to Study Pharmacoresistance in Epilepsy

Cecilia Zavala-Tecuapetla and Luisa Rocha

Abstract At present, there are several experimental models focused on investigating the mechanisms underlying pharmacoresistance in epilepsy. The present chapter aims to briefly describe different experimental models suitable to investigate the mechanisms associated with drug-resistant epilepsy. The in vitro models are useful to evaluate some molecular mechanisms of resistance to antiepileptic drugs, whereas in vivo models allow the identification of animals that are responsive and nonresponsive to pharmacological therapy and detailing of factors associated to these responses. Finally, evaluation of tissue obtained from patients with pharmacoresistant epilepsy submitted to surgery can also be considered as a good strategy to identify the mechanisms related to this neurological disorder and confirm the results obtained from experimental models.

Keywords Drug-resistant epilepsy • Pharmacoresistance • In vitro models • In vivo models • Antiepileptic drugs • Human brain tissue • Drug efflux transporters • P-glycoprotein

12.1 Introduction

Failed response to antiepileptic drugs (AEDs) is a major limitation in the treatment of epilepsy. The reasons for this failure are controversial and multifactorial. Despite advances in AED therapy, seizures remain uncontrolled in a substantial proportion (~30%) of epilepsy patients. In this regard, drug-resistant epilepsy has received important experimental and clinical attention trying to find alternative therapeutic strategies.

C. Zavala-Tecuapetla (✉) • L. Rocha
Department of Pharmacobiology, Center for Research and Advanced Studies,
Calz. Tenorios 235. Col. Granjas Coapa, Mexico City 14330, Mexico
e-mail: cztecua@yahoo.com.mx; lrocha@cinvestav.mx

L. Rocha and E.A. Cavalheiro (eds.), *Pharmacoresistance in Epilepsy: From Genes and Molecules to Promising Therapies*, DOI 10.1007/978-1-4614-6464-8_12,

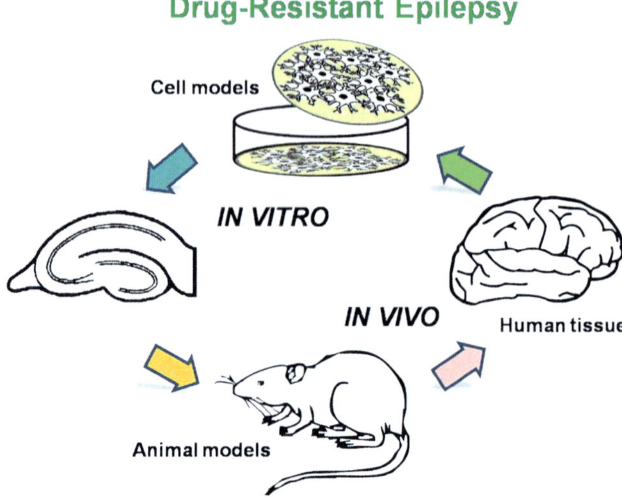

Fig. 12.1 Diagram showing the different experimental approaches to study mechanisms underlying drug resistance in epilepsy

There are three main mechanisms suggested in an attempt to explain the phenomenon of pharmacoresistance: (a) the drug fails to reach the neuronal target; (b) the drug fails to act at the appropriate target and (c) seizure phenotype and history of seizures determine the "level of refractoriness" (Boison et al. 2011).

Currently, a number of experimental models are available and each has some utility and limitations to investigate the mechanisms underlying drug resistance in epilepsy (Fig. 12.1). The in vitro models allow studying molecular mechanisms of resistance to AEDs, while using in vivo models permits the identification and selection of responsive and nonresponsive animals and the evaluation of differences between them. However, since animal models differ from humans, it is necessary to confirm findings in patients with drug-resistant epilepsy and vice versa. Thus, experiments using brain tissue obtained from patients with drug-resistant epilepsy represents an additional strategy to elucidate the mechanisms associated with this disorder. This chapter aims to briefly review the different experimental models employed to investigate the molecular and cellular basis associated with drug-resistant epilepsy (Fig. 12.1).

12.2 In Vitro Cell Models

Since AEDs must cross the blood–brain barrier (BBB) to act on specific targets and exert the desired effects, the over-expression of drug efflux pumps in the endothelial cells of the BBB may contribute to pharmacoresistance in epilepsy (Löscher and

Potschka 2005a). The in vitro cell models allow to study BBB function and transport and to identify which AEDs are substrates of drug efflux transporters (Luna-Tortós et al. 2008; Zhang et al. 2012). Many studies report over-expression of the efflux transporter called P-glycoprotein (P-gp, a product of ABCB1 gene also named MDR1) in capillary endothelial cells of drug-resistant patients (Tishler et al. 1995; Dombrowski et al. 2001; Löscher and Potschka 2005a). Thus, P-gp is one of the most intensively studied transporters evaluated in vitro (Weiss et al. 2003; Yang and Liu 2008; Yang et al. 2008).

The in vitro cell models include the use of isolated brain capillaries, primary brain capillary endothelial cell cultures, immortalized brain endothelial cell lines, and cell lines of non-cerebral origin (e.g., the epithelial cell lines from the intestine and kidney) (Cecchelli et al. 2007). Cells expressing drug transporters can be cultured in a variety of forms (as a monoculture; as a coculture, including endothelial cells and glia; or triple coculture, including brain endothelial cells, pericytes, and astrocytes) (Dehouck et al. 1990; Abbott et al. 2006; Nakagawa et al. 2009; Zhang et al. 2012).

Although the in vitro cell models are useful to evaluate transporters-induced AEDs efflux, a number of drawbacks still limit their application in basic research as well as in drug-screening processes. Use of in vitro cell models is limited because they are time consuming and highly expensive, situations that may hamper their routine use in nonexpert laboratories. Another limitation is that brain endothelial cells rapidly dedifferentiate in vitro, losing their characteristics after a few passages in culture, which limits their long-term use for biochemical or pharmacological studies (Roux and Couraud 2005; Abbott et al. 2006; Cecchelli et al. 2007).

12.3 In Vitro Models Using Slices

Brain slices can be obtained from any area of the brain and they partially preserve inter-area connectivity (e.g., between the entorhinal cortex and the hippocampus) (Dreier and Heinemann 1990), and maintain some of the intrinsic properties of the tissue (Heinemann et al. 2006). In general, in vitro preparations are useful to induce epileptic-like activity and evaluate the effects of AEDs. Interestingly, pharmacoresistant epileptic-like activity can be produced in slices by different procedures.

Different patterns of epileptiform activities in entorhinal cortico-hippocampal slices as well as in organotypic hippocampal slice cultures can be induced when they are incubated in buffer containing low magnesium (Walther et al. 1986; Mody et al. 1987; Albus et al. 2008). Epileptiform activity results from the removal of voltage-dependent blockage of magnesium on the *N*-methyl-D-aspartate (NMDA) receptor-operated ion channels, thereby increasing excitatory neurotransmitter release and augmenting neuronal excitability (Hamon et al. 1987). Epileptiform activity is characterized by the presence of *recurrent short discharges* (RSDs, bursts of population spikes superimposed on positive going field potentials with a frequency of 10–60 discharges/min); seizure-like events (SLEs, characterized by slow negative potential shifts) and late recurrent discharges (LRDs, characterized by 0.8–10-s long negative field potentials shifts recurring with a frequency of 10–50 discharges/min, which appear 20–80 min after the onset of the SLEs) (Dreier and Heinemann 1990; Armand et al. 2000). RSDs and SLEs have been found to be pharmacosensitive, whereas LRDs have demonstrated to be insensitive to clinically employed AEDs (Zhang et al. 1995; Albus et al. 2008; Dreier et al. 1998). The transition from pharmacosensitive to pharmacoresistant events may depend on reduced efficacy of gamma-aminobutyric acid (GABA)-ergic synaptic transmission (Pfeiffer et al. 1996).

The immature cortico-hippocampal slice preparation bathed with low magnesium also develops epileptiform activity that is pharmacoresistant to AEDs (Quilichini et al. 2002, 2003). This situation might relate to incomplete myelination, open BBB, incomplete development of astrocytic properties, delayed expression of ion channels and receptors for neurotransmitters and neuromodulators, as well as immaturity of Cl^- homeostasis (Wahab et al. 2010). It is suggested that this preparation may correspond to a model of generalized convulsive seizures and could be helpful to identify new AEDs for refractory infantile epilepsies (Quilichini et al. 2003).

In the entorhinal cortical-hippocampal slices of rats, LRDs induced by 4-aminopyridine (4-AP 100 μM, which is well known to interfere with different types of K^+ channels) are nonresponsive to AEDs (phenytoin, carbamazepine, valproic acid, and phenobarbital) when GABAergic transmission is blocked by bicuculline (a GABA receptor antagonist; 10–30 μM) (Brückner et al. 1999; Brückner and Heinemann 2000).

These in vitro preparations offer a variety of options for studying the mechanisms leading to generation, spread, and termination of pharmacoresistant seizures and the effects of new drugs on drug-resistant epilepsy that are difficult to evaluate in in vivo conditions (Heinemann et al. 1994; Pfeiffer et al. 1996; Dreier et al. 1998; Armand et al. 2000). However, these models lack the behavioral and motor components of clinical seizures.

12.4 In Vivo Animal Models

In vivo animal models have played a key role in discovering and characterizing AEDs. In contrast to human studies, animal models have the advantage that invasive procedures may be used allowing measurement of both, pharmacokinetic and pharmacodynamic aspects of AEDs in specific brain areas. In drug-resistant epilepsy, these models are useful to identify responsive or nonresponsive animals to specific AEDs and to investigate the mechanisms involved in pharmacoresistance.

12.4.1 6-Hz Psychomotor Seizure Model

This model was initially designated as a "psychomotor" seizure test and employed in screening of AEDs for complex partial seizures (Toman 1951; Toman et al. 1952). In 2001, Barton et al. suggested that the 6-Hz stimulation might provide a useful model of therapy-resistant limbic seizures since phenytoin is ineffective in avoiding convulsive seizures.

This model consists in the corneal application of low frequency (6 Hz), long-duration (3 s) electrical stimulation in mice which produces "psychomotor" seizures characterized by immobility, forelimb clonus, twitching of the vibrissae and Straub-tail. These seizures are not modified by AED administration when the electrical stimulation is applied at high intensity (Barton et al. 2001). The principal advantage of this model is its simplicity compared with other animal models such as the kindling model, allowing screening of several compounds over a relatively short time (Löscher 2006). However, it is important to notice that this is a model of acute seizures, but not epilepsy.

12.4.2 Pharmacoresistant Convulsions Induce by 3-Mercaptopropionic Acid

3-Mercaptopropionic acid (3-MPA) inhibits GABA synthesis as a consequence of competitive inhibition of glutamate decarboxylase (GAD) (de Lores Arnaiz et al. 1973; Tunnicliff 1990; Timmerman et al. 1992). This situation results in myoclonic twitches as well as clonic and tonic-clonic seizures when administered to laboratory animals (Netopilova et al. 1997; DeSarro et al. 2003; Girardi et al. 2004). The repetitive administration of 3-MPA (45 mg/kg i.p.) produces a progressive refractoriness to AEDs that is evident after seven injections (Girardi et al. 2005; Höcht et al. 2007, 2009), a situation associated with over-expression of P-gp (Lazarowski et al. 2006). This model has the advantage of inducing pharmacoresistant seizures in a few days. However, at present this model has not been characterized to determine if it produces long-term changes.

12.4.3 Kindling Model

The kindling process consists in a progressive development of seizure activity in response to repetitive application of initially subthreshold chemical or electrical stimulation that culminates in permanently enhanced seizure susceptibility (Goddard et al. 1969). At present, it has been recognized that kindled animals with a low response to specific AEDs represent a model for drug-resistant epilepsy (Löscher and Rundfeldt 1991).

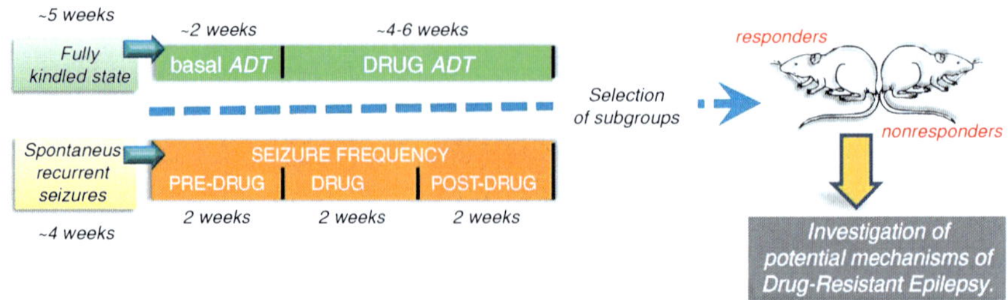

Fig. 12.2 Schematic representation of the selection procedure of responders and nonresponders rats after they achieved the fully kindled state (after about 5 weeks of repetitive kindling stimulation) or when spontaneous recurrent seizures (SRS) appear following a latent period (about 4 weeks) after status epilepticus (SE). Seizure susceptibility of animals with epileptic seizures is evaluated under basal conditions, during and after administration of antiepileptic drugs (AEDs). In kindled rats, the afterdischarge threshold (ADT, the lowest current intensity necessary to produce an afterdischarge) is used to determine the seizure susceptibility. In animals with SRS the parameter evaluated is the frequency of ictal events. Animals showing high ADT or low frequency of SRS during the AED administration are considered responders, whereas rats without changes on ADT or frequency of SRS under AED treatment are classified as nonresponders

12.4.3.1 Electrical Kindling

Once rats achieve the fully kindled stage (five consecutive stage V seizure according to the Racine scale, 1972) as a consequence of repetitive electrical kindling stimulation in brain areas such as the hippocampus or amygdala, animals may differ in their individual anticonvulsant response to AEDs (Löscher and Rundfeldt 1991; Töllner et al. 2011). This situation allows selecting responsive and resistant rats to use them differently in the research for mechanisms underlying pharmacoresistance (Fig. 12.2).

Several nonresponsive animals present higher seizure susceptibility under pre-kindling conditions, faster developing of the kindling process and enhanced interictal glutamate release in the hippocampus when the kindled state is reached (Luna-Munguia et al. 2011), an effect that is similar to that observed in patients with refractory temporal lobe epilepsy (TLE) (Cavus et al. 2005; During and Spencer 1993).

Recently, it was also found that kindled rats responsive and resistant to valproate show different sensitivity in neurons from the substantia nigra pars reticulate (SNr) to this AED (Töllner et al. 2011). SNr is thought to be crucially involved in the propagation and modulation of different types of experimental seizures (i.e., complex-partial seizures as observed in TLE) (Iadarola and Gale 1982; McNamara et al. 1984; Gale et al. 2008). Thus, the low sensitivity of SNr neurons to valproate of nonresponsive animals suggests that the basal ganglia network is involved in pharmacoresistant epilepsy (Töllner et al. 2011).

12.4.3.2 Chemical Kindling

Chemical kindling results from repetitive systemic administration of initially subconvulsant doses of excitatory compounds. Pentylenetetrazol (PTZ), a selective blocker of the chloride channel coupled to the $GABA_A$ receptor, is commonly used to induce chemical kindling when applied at 25–45 mg/kg i.p. or s.c. Liu and coworkers (2007) demonstrated that PTZ-kindling might increase expression and function of efflux transporters in the rat brain, resulting in decreased levels of AEDs in brain tissue.

It has been demonstrated that pretreatment with lamotrigine (5 mg/kg i.p.) before every PTZ administration during kindling acquisition is ineffective in preventing the development of kindling, but leads to subsequent development of pharmacoresistance to this AED and carbamazepine. These findings suggest that PTZ-induced kindling associated with AEDs is able to induce pharmacoresistant epilepsy (Srivastava et al. 2003).

Chemical kindling can also be induced by repetitive administration of coriaria lactone (CL, at 1.75, 1.50 and 1.25 mg/kg i.p. or i.m.) (Wang et al. 2003) that increases the release of glutamate, activates NMDA receptors on the postsynaptic membrane and decreases GABA-mediated inhibition (Yu et al. 1996). CL elicits partial seizures that culminate in secondarily generalized tonic-clonic seizures (Gilbert 2001). Once the rats are fully kindled, AEDs such as carbamazepine, phenytoin and valproate lack a satisfactory control on seizure activity, a situation associated with cerebral over-expression of drug transporters (Wang et al. 2003).

Electrical or chemical kindling represents a good strategy to obtain animals with drug-resistant epilepsy. However, the experimental procedure to obtain them is time consuming and the number of drug-resistant rats is low (about 20%).

12.4.4 Pharmacoresistant Epilepsy as a Consequence of Status Epilepticus

Some animals presenting long-term spontaneous recurrent seizures (SRS) after status epilepticus (SE) induced by prolonged electrical (of the basolateral amygdala) or chemical stimulation (pilocarpine treatment) have been shown to be pharmacoresistant to several AEDs (such as phenobarbital or levetiracetam) (Fig. 12.2). The identification of responsive and nonresponsive animals is based on the frequency of SRS determined during the administration of AEDs (Nissinen et al. 2000; Glien et al. 2002; Brandt et al. 2004, 2006). SE-induced pharmacoresistant rats exhibit a marked brain over-expression of drug efflux transporters (e.g., P-gp) (Volk and Löscher 2005; Guo and Jiang 2010).

Similar to patients with pharmacoresistant epilepsy, animals with SE-induced pharmacoresistant SRS allow the evaluation of such variables as frequency and severity of seizures as indicators of drug resistance (Stables et al. 2003). However, it is technically difficult, time consuming and expensive due to the necessity of continuously monitoring SRS over a period of at least 6 weeks. In addition, AED administration protocols should be based on the pharmacokinetics characteristics of the experimental subjects (rats).

12.4.5 Genetically Deficient Animals

As mentioned above, in addition to the physical barrier, numerous efflux transport proteins are present at the BBB, acting as pumps to actively exclude a wide variety of chemically diverse compounds from the central nervous system. Studies in genetically deficient animals, with a nonfunctional kind of efflux transporters have contributed to our current knowledge about their physiological and pharmacological function (Löscher and Potschka 2005b). In this regard, genetically deficient mice have been generated by gene technology (mdr1a knockout mice; mdr1a/1b double knockout mice; Mrp1 knockout mice; mdr1a/mdr1b/mrp1 triple knockout mice; mrp4 knockout mice; BCRP knockout mice) as well as rats (mdr1a-knockout rats) (Schinkel et al. 1995, 1996; Schinkel 1997; Wijnholds et al. 2000; Assem et al. 2004; Lee et al. 2005; Geurts et al. 2009; Chu et al. 2012). Furthermore, subpopulations of animals with spontaneous mutations in multidrug transporter genes have been identified in different species and breeds (mdr1a deficient mice; subpopulation of Collies and other dog breeds with natural mutations; the GY/TR− rat; the Eisai hyperbilirubinemic rat (EHBR)) (Paul et al. 1987; Buchler et al. 1996; Paulusma et al. 1996; Lankas et al. 1997; Umbenhauer et al. 1997; Neff et al. 2004). In these transporter-deficient animal models, it is possible to investigate how the expression of specific transporter proteins may contribute to seizure refractoriness. An important disadvantage of genetically deficient animals is that they may develop compensatory changes including up-regulation of other transporters (Löscher and Potschka 2005b).

12.5 Human Brain Tissue as a Tool to Investigate Pharmacoresistant Epilepsy

One of the major problems in developing treatments for human brain disorders has been the poor translation of therapeutics in animal models back to patients. The evaluation of brain tissue obtained from patients with pharmacoresistant epilepsy submitted to surgery constitutes an excellent opportunity to identify neuropathological and molecular alterations involved in this disorder. This tissue can be used for different approaches, such as in vitro slice preparations that provide a research environment to study electrical properties of local synaptic networks, or in vitro evaluation of receptor binding, protein or gene expression that allows the identification of changes occurring at the molecular level.

In contrast with post-mortem brain tissue collected from patients with neurological disorders such as Alzheimer's or Parkinson's disease, human tissue samples from patients with medically refractory epilepsy can be obtained fresh and immediately after surgical resection. This situation represents a unique feature of human epilepsy that makes it particularly attractive for molecular profiling. The surgical approach may yield abundant, fresh tissue samples from both epileptic and surrounding structures, such as neocortical and hippocampal regions in patients with TLE, a situation allowing the evaluation of different aspects of neurotransmitters involved in pharmacoresistant epilepsy. Indeed, the freshness of the tissue significantly reduces RNA degradation that is common in post-mortem tissue samples (Stan et al. 2006).

The protocols involving evaluation of human brain tissue have to consider the degree of tissue complexity, relationship of epileptic tissue to structural lesions, availability and appropriateness of "control tissues," relationship of the molecular profiling to the underlying electrical activities as well as clinical aspects (duration of epilepsy, age and gender of the patient, pharmacological treatment, etc.). It is emphasized that the correlation of changes with clinical data is essential to reveal factors associated to the pharmacoresistant process.

At present, functional genomics has been the most widely used biological method to study epilepsy. Proteomics not only measure the amount of a given protein, but also whether there are any modifications of a protein such as phosphorylation. Since the main goal of functional genomics is to foster in-depth understanding of the evaluated processes, results obtained in pharmacoresistant epilepsy will lead to new biomedical and pharmacological applications as well as biosynthetic and biotechnical developments. The continuously increasing knowledge and data bases in the proteomic field offer new prospects for the development of disease biomarkers. Molecular diagnostics using such biomarkers will provide the opportunity for early recognition of diseases. However, the development of consistent diagnostic and prognostic markers and their validation is still in its infancy.

12.6 Conclusion

The use of appropriate experimental models and brain tissue obtained from patients with pharmacoresistant epilepsy represents an excellent opportunity to disclose specific changes associated to this disorder and subsequently develop new therapeutic strategies.

Acknowledgments This work was supported by CONACYT (Proyect 98386). We thank Leticia Neri Bazán and Héctor Vázquez Espinosa for their technical assistance and Dr. Erika Brust-Mascher for English improvement.

References

Abbott NJ, Ronnback L, Hannson E. Astrocyte-endothelial interactions at the blood–brain barrier. Nat Rev Neurosci. 2006;7:41–53.

Albus K, Wahab A, Heinemann U. Standard antiepileptic drugs fail to block epileptiform activity in rat organotypic hippocampal slice cultures. Br J Pharmacol. 2008;154:709–24.

Armand V, Rundfeldt C, Heinemann U. Effects of retigabine (D-23 129) on different patterns of epileptiform activity induced by low magnesium in rat entorhinal cortex hippocampal slices. Epilepsia. 2000;41(1):28–33.

Assem M, Schuetz EG, Leggas M, Sun D, Yasuda K, Reid G, et al. Interactions between hepatic Mrp4 and Sult2a as revealed by the constitutive androstane receptor and Mrp4 knockout mice. J Biol Chem. 2004;279:22250–7.

Barton ME, Klein BD, Wolf HH, White HS. Pharmacological characterization of the 6 Hz psychomotor seizure model of partial epilepsy. Epilepsy Res. 2001;47:217–28.

Boison D, Masino SA, Geiger JD. Homeostatic bioenergetic network regulation: a novel concept to avoid pharmacoresistance in epilepsy. Expert Opin Drug Discov. 2011;6(7):713–24.

Brandt C, Volk HA, Löscher W. Striking differences in individual anticonvulsant response to phenobarbital in rats with spontaneous seizures after status epilepticus. Epilepsia. 2004;45:1488–97.

Brandt C, Bethmann K, Gastens AM, Loscher W. The multidrug transporter hypothesis of drug resistance in epilepsy: proof-of-principle in a rat model of temporal lobe epilepsy. Neurobiol Dis. 2006;24:202–11.

Brückner C, Stenkamp K, Meierkord H, Heinemann U. Epileptiform discharges induced by combined application of bicuculline and 4-aminopyridine are resistant to standard anticonvulsants in slices of rats. Neurosci Lett. 1999;268:163–5.

Brückner C, Heinemann U. Effects of standard anticonvulsant drugs on different patterns of epileptiform discharges induced by 4-aminopyridine in combined entorhinal cortex-hippocampal slices. Brain Res. 2000;859:15–20.

Buchler M, Konig J, Brom M, Kartenbeck J, Spring H, Horie T, et al. cDNA cloning of the hepatocyte canalicular isoform of the multidrug resistance protein, cMrp, reveals a novel conjugate export pump deficient in hyperbilirubinemic mutant rats. J Biol Chem. 1996;271:15091–8.

Cavus I, Kassof WS, Cassaday MP, Jacob R, Gueorguieva R, Sherwin RS, et al. Extracellular metabolites in the cortex and hippocampus of epileptic patients. Ann Neurol. 2005;57: 226–35.

Cecchelli R, Berezowski V, Lundquist S, Culot M, Renftel M, Dehouck MP, et al. Modelling of the blood–brain barrier in drug discovery and development. Nat Rev Drug Discov. 2007;6:650–61.

Chu X, Zhang Z, Yabut J, Horwitz S, Levorse J, Li XQ, et al. Characterization of mdr1a/P-glycoprotein knockout rats generated by zinc finger nucleases. Mol Pharmacol. 2012;81(2):220–7.

Dehouck MP, Méresse S, Delorme P, Fruchart JC, Cecchelli R. An easier, reproducible, and mass-production method to study the blood-brain barrier in vitro. J Neurochem. 1990;54(5): 1798–801.

De Lores Arnaiz GR, de Canal MA, Robiolo B, de Pacheco MM. The effect of the convulsant 3-mercaptopropionic acid on enzymes of the γ-aminobutyrate system in the rat cerebral cortex. J Neurochem. 1973;21:615–23.

DeSarro G, Ferreri G, Gareri P, Russo E, DeSarro A, Gitto R, et al. Comparative anticonvulsant activity of some 2,3-benzodiazepine derivates in rodents. Pharmacol Biochem Behav. 2003;74:595–602.

Dreier JP, Heinemann U. Late low magnesium-induced epileptiform activity in rat entorhinal cortex slices becomes insensitive to the anticonvulsant valproic acid. Neurosci Lett. 1990;119:68–70.

Dreier JP, Zhang CL, Heinemann U. Phenytoin, phenobarbital, and midazolam fail to stop status epilepticus-like activity induced by low magnesium in rat entorhinal slices, but can prevent its development. Acta Neurol Scand. 1998;98:154–60.

Dombrowski SM, Desai SY, Marroni M, Cucullo L, Goodrich K, Bingaman W, et al. Overexpression of multiple drug resistance genes in endothelial cells from patients with refractory epilepsy. Epilepsia. 2001;42:1501–6.

During MJ, Spencer DD. Extracellular hippocampal glutamate and spontaneous seizure in the conscious human brain. Lancet. 1993;341:1607–10.

Gale K, Proctor M, Velískova J, Nehlig A. Basal ganglia and brainstem anatomy and physiology. In: Engel JJ, Pedley TA, editors. Epilepsy: a comprehensive textbook. 2nd ed. Philadelphia, PA: Lippincott Williams and Wilkins; 2008.

Geurts AM, Cost GJ, Freyvert Y, Zeitler B, Miller JC, Choi VM, et al. Knockout rats via embryo microinjection of zinc-finger nucleases. Science. 2009;325:433.

Gilbert ME. Does the kindling model of epilepsy contribute to our understanding of multiple chemical sensitivity? Ann N Y Acad Sci. 2001;933:68–91.

Girardi E, Ramos AJ, Vanore G, Brusco A. Astrocytic response in hippocampus and cerebral cortex in an experimental epilepsy model. Neurochem Res. 2004;29(2):371–7.

Girardi E, González NN, Lazarowski A. Refractory phenotype reversion by nimodipine administration in a model of epilepsy resistant to phenytoin treatment. Epilepsia. 2005;46(S6):212.

Glien M, Brandt C, Potschka H, Löscher W. Effects of the novel antiepileptic drug levetiracetam on spontaneous recurrent seizures in the rat pilocarpine model of temporal lobe epilepsy. Epilepsia. 2002;43:350–7.

Goddard GV, McIntyre DC, Leech CK. A permanent change in brain function resulting from daily electrical stimulation. Exp Neurol. 1969;32:295–330.

Guo Y, Jiang L. Drug transporters are altered in brain, liver and kidney of rats with chronic epilepsy induced by lithium-pilocarpine. Neurol Res. 2010;32(1):106–12.

Hamon B, Stanton PK, Heinemann U. An N-methyl-D-aspartate receptor-independent excitatory action of partial reduction of extracellular [Mg^{2+}] in CA1-region of rat hippocampal slices. Neurosci Lett. 1987;75:240–5.

Heinemann U, Dreier J, Leschinger A, Stabel J, Draguhn A, Zhang C. Effects of anticonvulsant drugs on hippocampal neurons. Hippocampus. 1994;4:291–6.

Heinemann U, Kann O, Schuchmann S. An overview of in vitro seizure models in acute and organotypic slices. In: Pitkanen A, Schwartzkroin PA, Moshe SL, editors. Models of seizures and epilepsy. 1st ed. Boston, MA: Academic; 2006.

Höcht C, Lazarowski A, Gonzalez NN, Auzmendi J, Opezzo JA, Bramuglia GF, et al. Nimodipine restores the altered hippocampal phenytoin pharmacokinetics in a refractory epileptic model. Neurosci Lett. 2007;413(2):168–72.

Höcht C, Lazarowski A, Gonzalez NN, Mayer MA, Opezzo JA, Taira CA, et al. Differential hippocampal pharmacokinetics of phenobarbital and carbamazepine in repetitive seizures induced by 3-mercaptopropionic acid. Neurosci Lett. 2009;453(1):54–7.

Iadarola MJ, Gale K. Substantia nigra: site of anticonvulsant activity mediated by gamma-aminobutyric acid. Science. 1982;218:1237–40.

Lankas GR, Cartwright ME, Umbenhauer D. P-glycoprotein deficiency in a subpopulation of CF-1 mice enhances avermectin induced neurotoxicity. Toxicol Appl Pharmacol. 1997;143:357–65.

Lazarowski A, Czornyj L, Lubieniecki F, Vazquez S, D'Giano C, Sevlever G, et al. Multidrug-resistance (MDR) proteins develops refractory epilepsy phenotype: clinical and experimental evidences. Curr Drug Ther. 2006;1:291–309.

Lee YJ, Kusuhara H, Jonker JW, Schinkel AH, Sugiyama Y. Investigation of efflux transport of dehydroepiandrosterone sulfate and mitoxantrone at the mouse blood–brain barrier: a minor role of breast cancer resistance protein. J Pharmacol Exp Ther. 2005;312:44–52.

Liu X, Yang Z, Yang J, Yang H. Increased P-glycoprotein expression and decreased phenobarbital distribution in the brain of pentylenetetrazole-kindled rats. Neuropharmacology. 2007;53(5): 657–63.

Löscher W. Animal models of drug-refractory epilepsy. In: Pitkanen A, Schwartzkroin PA, Moshe SL, editors. Models of seizures and epilepsy. 1st ed. Boston, MA: Academic; 2006.

Löscher W, Potschka H. Drug resistance in brain diseases and the role of drug efflux transporters. Nat Rev Neurosci. 2005a;6:591–602.

Löscher W, Potschka H. Role of drug efflux transporters in the brain for drug disposition and treatment of brain diseases. Prog Neurobiol. 2005b;76:22–76.

Löscher W, Rundfeldt C. Kindling as a model of drug-resistant partial epilepsy: selection of phenytoin-resistant and nonresistant rats. J Pharmacol Exp Ther. 1991;258(2):483–9.

Luna-Munguia H, Orozco-Suarez S, Rocha L. Effects of high frequency electrical stimulation and R-verapamil on seizure susceptibility and glutamate and GABA release in a model of phenytoin-resistant seizures. Neuropharmacology. 2011;61(4):807–14.

Luna-Tortós C, Fedrowitz M, Löscher W. Several major antiepileptic drugs are substrates for human P-glycoprotein. Neuropharmacology. 2008;55(8):1364–75.

McNamara JO, Galloway MT, Rigsbee LC, Shin C. Evidence implicating substantia nigra in regulation of kindled seizure threshold. J Neurosci. 1984;4:2410–7.

Mody I, Lambert JD, Heinemann U. Low extracellular magnesium induces epileptiform activity and spreading depression in rat hippocampal slices. J Neurophysiol. 1987;57:869–88.

Nakagawa S, Deli MA, Kawaguchi H, Shimizudani T, Shimono T, Kittel A, et al. A new blood–brain barrier model using primary rat brain endothelial cells, pericytes and astrocytes. Neurochem Int. 2009;54(3–4):253–63.

Neff MW, Robertson KR, Wong AK, Safra N, Broman KW, Slatkin M, et al. Breed distribution and history of canine mdr1-1Delta, a pharmacogenetic mutation that marks the emergence of breeds from the collie lineage. Proc Natl Acad Sci USA. 2004;101:11725–30.

Netopilova M, Drsata J, Haugvicova R, Kubova H, Mares P. Inhibition of glutamate decarboxylase activity by 3-mercaptopropionic acid has different time course in the immature and adult rat brains. Neurosci Lett. 1997;226:68–70.

Nissinen J, Halonen T, Koivisto E, Pitkänen A. A new model of chronic temporal lobe epilepsy induced by electrical stimulation of the amygdala in rat. Epilepsy Res. 2000;38:177–205.

Paul AJ, Tranquilli WJ, Seward RL, Todd KSJ, DiPietro JA. Clinical observations in collies given ivermectin orally. Am J Vet Res. 1987;48:684–5.

Paulusma CC, Bosma PJ, Zaman GJ, Bakker CT, Otter M, Scheffer GL, et al. Congenital jaundice in rats with a mutation in a multidrug resistance-associated protein gene. Science. 1996;271:1126–8.

Pfeiffer M, Draguhn A, Meierkord H, Heinemann U. Effects of γ-aminobutyric acid (GABA) agonists and GABA uptake inhibitors on pharmacosensitive and pharmacoresistant epileptiform activity in vitro. Br J Pharmacol. 1996;119:569–77.

Quilichini PP, Diabira D, Chiron C, Ben-Ari Y, Gozlan H. Persistent epileptiform activity induced by low Mg^{2+} in intact immature brain structures. Eur J Neurosci. 2002;16(5):850–60.

Quilichini PP, Diabira D, Chiron C, Milh M, Ben-Ari Y, Gozlan H. Effects of antiepileptic drugs on refractory seizures in the intact immature corticohippocampal formation in vitro. Epilepsia. 2003;44:1365–74.

Racine RJ. Modification of seizure activity by electrical stimulation II. Motor seizure. Electroencephalogr Clin Neurophysiol. 1972;32:281–94.

Roux F, Couraud PO. Rat brain endothelial cell lines for the study of blood–brain barrier permeability and transport functions. Cell Mol Neurobiol. 2005;25(1):41–58.

Schinkel AH. The physiological function of drug-transporting P-glycoproteins. Semin Cancer Biol. 1997;8:161–70.

Schinkel AH, Wagenaar E, van Deemter L, Mol CAAM, Borst P. Absence of the mdr1a P-glycoprotein in mice affects tissue distribution and pharmacokinetics of dexamethasone, digoxin, and cyclosporine A. J Clin Invest. 1995;96:1698–705.

Schinkel AH, Wagenaar E, Mol CA, van Deemter L. P-glycoprotein in the blood–brain barrier of mice influences the brain penetration and pharmacological activity of many drugs. J Clin Invest. 1996;97:2517–24.

Srivastava AK, Woodhead JH, White HS. Effect of lamotrigine, carbamazepine and sodium valproate on lamotrigine-resistant kindled rats. Epilepsia. 2003;44 Suppl 9:42.

Stables JP, Bertram E, Dudek FE, Holmes G, Mathern G, Pitkänen A, et al. Therapy discovery for pharmacoresistent epilepsy and for disease-modifying therapeutics: summary of the NIH/NINDS/AES models II workshop. Epilepsia. 2003;44:1472–8.

Stan AD, Ghose S, Gao XM, Roberts RC, Lewis-Amezcua K, Hatanpaa KJ, et al. Human postmortem tissue: what quality markers matter? Brain Res. 2006;1123:1–11.

Timmerman W, Zwaveling J, Westerink BHC. Characterization of extracellular GABA in the substantia nigra reticulata by means of brain microdialysis. Naunyn Schmiedebergs Arch Pharmacol. 1992;345:661–5.

Tishler DM, Weinberg KI, Hinton DR, Barbaro N, Annett GM, Raffel C. MDR1 gene expression in brain of patients with medically intractable epilepsy. Epilepsia. 1995;36:1–6.

Töllner K, Wolf S, Löscher W, Gernert M. The anticonvulsant response to valproate in kindled rats is correlated with its effect on neuronal firing in the substantia nigra pars reticulata: a new mechanism of pharmacoresistance. J Neurosci. 2011;31(45):16423–34.

Toman JEP. Neuropharmacologic considerations in psychic seizures. Neurology. 1951;1:444–60.

Toman JEP, Everett GM, Richards RK. The search for new drugs against epilepsy. Tex Rep Biol Med. 1952;10:96–104.

Tunnicliff G. Action of inhibitors on brain glutamate decarboxylase. Int J Biochem. 1990;22: 1235–41.

Umbenhauer DR, Lankas GR, Pippert TR, Wise LD, Cartwright ME, Hall SJ, et al. Identification of a P-glycoproteindeficient subpopulation in the CF-1 mouse strain using a restriction fragment length polymorphism. Toxicol Appl Pharmacol. 1997;146:88–94.

Volk HA, Löscher W. Multidrug resistance in epilepsy: rats with drug-resistant seizures exhibit enhanced brain expression of P-glycoprotein compared with rats with drug-responsive seizures. Brain. 2005;128:1358–68.

Wahab A, Albus K, Gabriel S, Heinemann U. In search of models of pharmacoresistant epilepsy. Epilepsia. 2010;51 Suppl 3:154–9.

Walther H, Lambert JDC, Jones RSG, Heinemann U, Hamon B. Epileptiform activity in combined slices of the hippocampus, subiculum and entorhinal cortex during perfusion with low magnesium medium. Neurosci Lett. 1986;69:156–61.

Wang Y, Zhou D, Wang B, Li H, Chai H, Zhou Q, et al. A kindling model of pharmacoresistant temporal lobe epilepsy in Sprague-Dawley rats induced by Coriaria lactone and its possible mechanism. Epilepsia. 2003;44(4):475–88.

Weiss J, Kerpen CJ, Lindenmaier H, Dormann SM, Haefeli WE. Interaction of antiepileptic drugs with human P-glycoprotein in vitro. J Pharmacol Exp Ther. 2003;307(1):262–7.

Wijnholds J, deLange EC, Scheffer GL, van den Berg DJ, Mol CA, van der Valk M, et al. Multidrug resistance protein 1 protects the choroid plexus epithelium and contributes to the blood–cerebrospinal fluid barrier. J Clin Invest. 2000;105:279–85.

Yang ZH, Liu XD. P-glycoprotein-mediated efflux of phenobarbital at the blood–brain barrier evidence from transport experiments in vitro. Epilepsy Res. 2008;78(1):40–9.

Yang HW, Liu HY, Liu X, Zhang DM, Liu YC, Liu XD, et al. Increased P-glycoprotein function and level after long-term exposure of four antiepileptic drugs to rat brain microvascular endothelial cells in vitro. Neurosci Lett. 2008;434(3):299–303.

Yu DJ, Liu YH, Zhou JP. The influence of coriaria lactone on the GABA and glutamate from the cultured hippocampal neuron. J Chin Histochem Cytochem. 1996;5:193–7.

Zhang CL, Dreier JP, Heinemann U. Paroxysmal epileptiform discharges in temporal lobe slices after prolonged exposure to low magnesium are resistant to clinically used anticonvulsants. Epilepsy Res. 1995;20:105–11.

Zhang C, Kwan P, Zuo Z, Baum L. The transport of antiepileptic drugs by P-glycoprotein. Adv Drug Deliv Rev. 2012;64(10):930–42.

Chapter 13
Resistance to Epileptogenesis in the Neotropical Rodent *Proechimys*

Carla A. Scorza and Esper A. Cavalheiro

Abstract About 10 % of people will experience at least one seizure during lifespan, and one third of them will develop epilepsy. Antiepileptic drugs (AEDs) have hugely ameliorated the lives of people with epilepsy; however, 30–40 % of those individuals have seizures that cannot be totally controlled by medication. Ideally, one would like to prevent epilepsy in those with known risk but such therapies do not exist. Currently, treatment is exclusively based on the suppression of seizures by AEDs after epilepsy has already developed. Thus, understanding the basic mechanisms of epileptogenesis and epileptogenicity represents a priority for epilepsy research. In this respect, studies in human beings have a very limited capacity to explain such basic mechanisms. Consequently, animal models are invaluable tools of investigation. In this context, the wild Neotropical rodents *Proechimys* have been investigated in different experimental epilepsy paradigms. Interestingly, findings pointed to natural endogenous antiepileptogenic mechanisms in these rodents. Accordingly, *Proechimys* have been proposed as an animal model of resistance to epilepsy. This chapter sheds light to the potential use of these Neotropical animals in neuroscience research.

Keywords *Proechimys* • Epilepsy • Antiepileptogenesis • Pilocarpine

C.A. Scorza (✉)
Department of Neurology and Neurosurgery, Universidade Federal de São Paulo,
Rua Pedro de Toledo 862, Edificio Leal Prado, São Paulo 04023-900, Brazil
e-mail: carlascorza.nexp@epm.br

E.A. Cavalheiro
Disciplina de Neurologia Experimental, UNIFESP/EPM, São Paulo, Brazil
e-mail: esper.nexp@epm.br

L. Rocha and E.A. Cavalheiro (eds.), *Pharmacoresistance in Epilepsy: From Genes and Molecules to Promising Therapies*, DOI 10.1007/978-1-4614-6464-8_13,

13.1 Introduction

Antiepileptic drugs (AEDs) do not cure epilepsy but they unquestionably have ameliorated the lives of people with epilepsy (Löscher 2002). However, only two-thirds of those diagnosed with epilepsy can control their seizures with proper AEDs (Engel 2011). The current AEDs are suited to combat ictogenesis after epilepsy has already developed (Pitkänen 2010). But, a wide range of brain alterations continue to progress in an epileptic condition, especially in those individuals with drug-resistant epilepsy (Löscher and Brandt 2010). Thus, epileptogenesis refers not only to the gradual processes whereby a normal brain is altered becoming predisposed to generate enduring spontaneous seizures but it also refers to the disease-modifying processes after epilepsy diagnosis (Mani et al. 2011; Pitkänen 2010). Seizures are simply the symptom of epilepsy. In this context, the molecular and biochemical processes of seizure generation (ictogenesis) and those involved in the development of epilepsy and/or seizure modification (epileptogenesis) have particular differences (Klitgaard and Pitkänen 2003). In this scenario, we still do not know the events that need to be targeted. Studies in human beings have a very limited capacity to explain basic mechanisms hence animal models of epilepsy are an invaluable prerequisite. In this context, there are animal models with spontaneously recurrent seizures and, on the other hand, animal models naturally resistant to the development of epilepsy (i.e., the Neotropical *Proechimys*) (Löscher 2011; Arida et al. 2005). *Proechimys* rodents have shown atypical resistance in developing a chronic epileptic condition in the most widely used models of mesial temporal lobe epilepsy (MTLE). Accordingly, *Proechimys* rodents have been suggested as an animal model of resistance to epilepsy (Arida et al. 2005). MTLE is the most frequent form of partial epilepsy in young adult humans and a major medical and social problem since people with MTLE have some of the highest rates of medical intractability to conventional AEDs (Dlugos 2001). In this reasoning, *Proechimys* animals may constitute a fruitful tool for research on antiepileptogenic investigation.

13.2 Neotropical Rodent *Proechimys*

Proechimys sp. are the most abundant and widespread terrestrial lowland small mammals in the rainforests; however, they are one of the less well-known and more taxonomically complex genera among the Neotropical rodents (Machado et al. 2005; Patton et al. 2000). These rodents range from the coastal lands of the Guyanas to the Rio Negro basin and the eastern half of the Amazon basin (Bailão Ribeiro et al. 2011). *Proechimys* is about the size of a white laboratory rat, but with a larger head and protuberant eyes, smaller prominent ears and orange-brown spiny pelage on the upper body and white underneath. Adult proportions are reached at 90 days, the heady/body length is about 16–30 cm and tail length 11–32 cm (Nowak 1999). In captivity, the average weight of a male adult *Proechimys* is 300 g (Weir 1973).

In order to escape, these animals can break off their tails, between the fifth and sixth caudal vertebrae (Weir 1973). One of the main characteristic of these rodents is the high degree of maturity shown by the newborn animal. The animals are born fully haired and with their eyes open. Furthermore, newly born *Proechimys* are active within a few hours; they can walk supporting their full weight. The species breeds throughout the year, the length of gestation period ranges from 55 to about 63 days and litter sizes ranged from 2 to 3. The mean weight at birth is about 20.9 g (Weir 1973). Up to now, *Proechimys*' brain has been little studied and even neglected. However, recent investigations shed light to the potential use of *Proechimys* in the field of neuroscience.

13.3 *Proechimys*: Animal Model of Resistance to Epilepsy

In the framework of comparative studies on animal models of experimental epilepsy, the susceptibility of *Proechimys* to epileptogenic treatments was tested using three different models: the post-*status epilepticus* (SE) (i.e., pilocarpine and Kainate) and amygdala kindling (Fig. 13.1). The findings suggested that the wild Neotropical rodents *Proechimys* may have natural endogenous antiepileptogenic mechanisms (Carvalho 1999; Arida et al. 2005).

13.3.1 Pilocarpine Model

In this model, injection of pilocarpine induces acute SE followed by a seizure-free latent period, referred to as epileptogenesis, which leads to the chronic phase of the model, in which the animal exhibit spontaneous and recurrent seizures (Turski et al. 1983; Cavalheiro et al. 1991). Carvalho (1999) showed that lower doses of pilocarpine (300–320 mg/kg) than those required in Wistar rats (350–380 mg/kg) were effective at triggering acute seizures and SE in *Proechimys*. Additional investigations reported that between 15 and 30 min after pilocarpine administration, *Proechimys* presented behavioral changes characteristic of kindling stage 2, but then remained with the four limbs on the floor, extended fingers and tonic extension of the tail, with sporadic clonic movements of the head or limbs, and then spontaneously recovered to normal behavior (Fabene et al. 2001a; Arida et al. 2005). Interestingly, *Proechimys* had a shorter SE duration, rarely exceeding 2 h, strongly contrasting to the 8–12 h SE observed in the Wistar rats. According to Arida et al. (2005), of 61 *Proechimys* rodents injected with pilocarpine, 48 presented SE and only two of them presented some sporadic spontaneous seizures after silent periods of 60 and 66 days. Histopathological changes were absent in the *Proechimys* hippocampus at 30 days after SE (Fabene et al. 2001a). However, long-term hippocampal and thalamic variations in protein expression were found in those rodents (Fabene et al. 2001a, b). Furthermore, *Proechimys* showed stronger and persistent hippocampal Fos induction

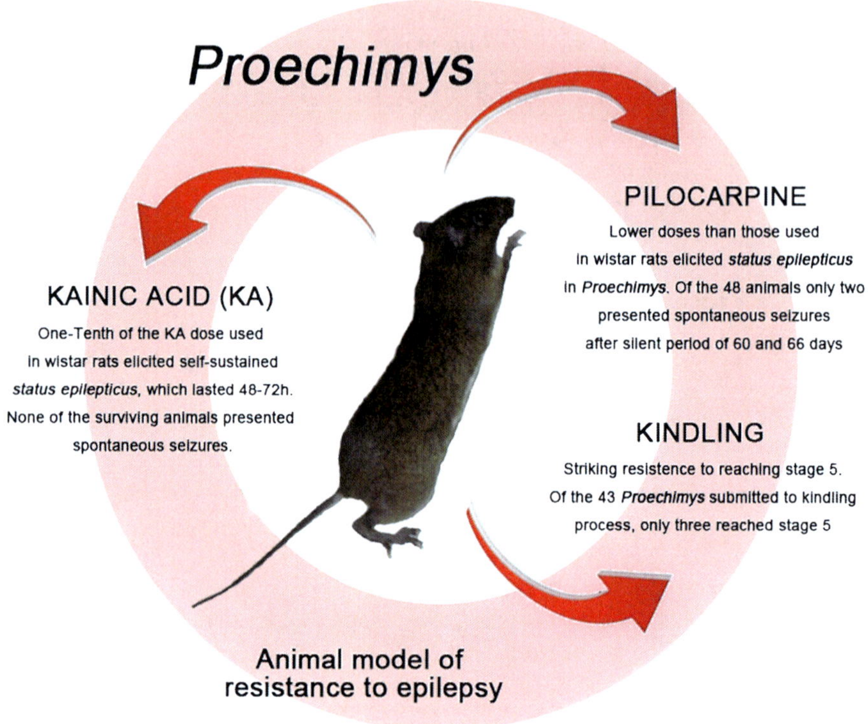

Fig. 13.1 *Proechimys*: animal model of resistance to epilepsy

than Wistar rats (Fabene et al. 2004). Fos-immunoreactivity was observed in almost all the parvalbumin-immunostained cells up to 24 h after SE in the *Proechimys* rodents, contrasting to the lower proportion of the double stained cells found in the white laboratory rats. In addition, Andrioli et al. (2009) described different patterns of thalamic and cortical activation and neuronal death in *Proechimys* versus Wistar rats after pilocarpine-induced seizures.

13.3.2 Kainate Model

Kainic acid (KA) injections were reported to efficiently induce SE and brain damage leading to the development of spontaneous seizures (Dudek et al. 2006). Arida et al. (2005) showed that *Proechimys* were very sensitive to the acute effects of the KA administration. Interestingly, only one-tenth of the KA dose usually used in Wistar rats provoked self-sustained SE lasting between 48 and 72 h, characterized by cataleptic behavior, in the first couple of hours, eventually interrupted by partial complex seizures with generalization and EEG patterns similar to those typically observed in the Wistar rats. Remarkably, the authors showed as well that despite the longer SE and severe neuropathological alterations, none of the *Proechimys* developed spontaneous seizures during the 120 days of observation (Arida et al. 2005).

13.3.3 Kindling Model

Kindling is a progressive enhancement of the neural response to low intensity constant brain stimulation. Some regions of the brain respond to repeated low-level electrical or chemical stimulation by progressively boosting electrical discharges, thereby lowering seizure thresholds. Curiously, adult *Proechimys* rodents submitted to amygdala kindling showed resistance to develop fully generalized seizures (Carvalho et al. 2003). From the 43 animals submitted to the amygdala kindling, only three of them reached stage 5. Of the 40 animals that did not reach stage 5, 16 of them did not get beyond stage 1, 14 stayed at stage 2, 7 on stage 3, and 3 animals did not get beyond stage 4. It is noteworthy that during stages 1–3, *Proechimys*' behavioral changes were similar to those observed in rats and other animal species. However, stages 4 and 5 ($n=3$) of kindling were characterized by an initial behavior similar to catalepsy, suggesting the participation of the opiate system, which lasted 20–30 s, and was then followed by rearing and falling (Carvalho et al. 2003; Arida et al. 2005). Furthermore, in comparison to Wistar rats, afterdischarge duration in *Proechimys* was striking higher in stage 1 and much longer in stages 2–4. One working hypothesis is that kindling process involves three phases: local afterdischarge expression, the recruitment of forebrain regions and, finally, the recruitment of the brainstem. Given this framework, *Proechimys* electrical kindling seems to show a local kindling effect unsuccessful to fully recruit other brain regions.

13.4 *Proechimys*' Brain

Fabene et al. (2001a) described peculiar findings in *Proechimys*' brain, such as the following: large limbic structures and deep rhinal fissure; ventral and dorsal hippocampal commissures constituted by thick bundles at the midline hippocampus; ventral hippocampal commissure similar in size as the corpus callosum; continuous right and left sides of the ventral granular layers of the dentate gyrus at rostral levels and; close contiguity of the two sides of the subicular regions. In addition, a remarkably different *Proechimy*'s cytoarchitecture organization of the hippocampal cornu Ammonis 2 (CA2) subfield has been identified (Scorza et al. 2010). *Proechimys* exhibited a very distinctive CA2 sector with disorganized cell presentation of the pyramidal layer and atypical dispersion of the pyramidal-like cells to the *stratum oriens*, strongly contrasting to the densely packed CA2 cells found in the Wistar rats. In addition, in comparison to the white laboratory rat, higher levels of calcium binding proteins were found in *Proechimys*' CA2 subfield (Scorza et al. 2010). Higher hippocampal expression and different distribution of endocannabinoid receptors CB1 were also encountered in the *Proechimys* rodents (Araujo et al. 2010). The endocannabinoid system, particularly CB1 receptors play a role in both seizure activity and epileptogenesis (Goffin et al. 2011). Another striking finding in *Proechimys* rodents was the presence of large pyramidal-like cells throughout the *stratum oriens* layer from hippocampal CA2 to CA1 sectors (Scorza et al. 2011). Furthermore, this newly identified population of pyramidal-shaped neurons exhibited distinct electrophysiological and morphological properties.

13.5 Conclusions

A great deal of the knowledge that has improved our comprehension of the brain mechanisms has been derived from useful animal models. In this context, the basic science research challenge is to make use of a comparative approach to benefit the most from what each animal model can tell us. Thus, *Proechimys* may represent a relevant tool to investigate the mechanisms underlying epileptogenesis.

Acknowledgments FAPESP/CNPq/MCT-Instituto Nacional de Neurociência Translacional, CAPES and CInAPCe (Brazil).

References

Andrioli A, Fabene PF, Spreafico R, Cavalheiro EA, Bentivoglio M. Different patterns of neuronal activation and neurodegeneration in the thalamus and cortex of epilepsy-resistant *Proechimys* rats versus Wistar rats after pilocarpine-induced protracted seizures. Epilepsia. 2009;50:832–48.

Araujo BH, Torres LB, Cossa AC, Naffah-Mazzacoratti Mda G, Cavalheiro EA. Hippocampal expression and distribution of CB1 receptors in the Amazonian rodent *Proechimys*: an animal model of resistance to epilepsy. Brain Res. 2010;1335:35–40.

Arida RM, Scorza FA, Carvalho RA, Cavalheiro EA. *Proechimys guayannensis*: an animal model of resistance to epilepsy. Epilepsia. 2005;46 Suppl 5:1–9.

Bailão Ribeiro NA, Pieczarka JC, Pereira Soares MC, Nagamachi CY. Identification of a long-standing colony of *Proechimys* at the Instituto Evandro Chagas, Pará, Brazil, based on cytogenetic information. Rev Pan-Amaz Saude. 2011;2:59–66.

Carvalho RA. Caracterização de modelos de epilepsia do lobo temporal em *Proechimys guyannensis*. PhD Thesis, Universidade Federal de São Paulo, SP, Brazil; 1999.

Carvalho RA, Arida RA, Cavalheiro EA. Amygdala kindling in *Proechimys guyannensis* rat: an animal model of resistance to epilepsy. Epilepsia. 2003;44:165–70.

Cavalheiro EA, Leite JP, Bortolotto ZA, Turski WA, Ikonomidou C, Turski L. Long-term effects of pilocarpine in rats: structural damage of the brain triggers kindling and spontaneous recurrent seizures. Epilepsia. 1991;32:778–82.

Dlugos DJ. The early identification of candidates for epilepsy surgery. Arch Neurol. 2001;58:1543.

Dudek FE, Clark S, Williams PA, Grabenstatter HL. Kainate-induced *status epilepticus*: A chronic model of acquired epilepsy. In: Pitkanen A, Schwartzkroin PA, Moshe SL, editors. Models of seizures and epilepsy. Boston: Elsevier Academic; 2006. p. 415–32.

Engel Jr J. Biomarkers in epilepsy: foreword. Biomark Med. 2011;5:529–30.

Fabene PF, Correia L, Carvalho RA, Cavalheiro EA, Bentivoglio M. The spiny rat *Proechimys guyannensis* as model of resistance to epilepsy: chemical characterization of hippocampal cell populations and pilocarpine-induced changes. Neuroscience. 2001a;104:979–1002.

Fabene PF, Bertini G, Correia L, Cavalheiro EA, Bentivoglio M. The thalamus of the Amazon spiny rat *Proechimys guyannensis*, an animal model of resistance to epilepsy, and pilocarpine-induced longterm changes of protein expression. Thal Relat Syst. 2001b;1:117–33.

Fabene PF, Andrioli A, Priel MR, Cavalheiro EA, Bentivoglio M. Fos induction and persistence, neurodegeneration, and interneuron activation in the hippocampus of epilepsy-resistant versus epilepsyprone rats after pilocarpine-induced seizures. Hippocampus. 2004;14:895–907.

Goffin K, Van Paesschen W, Van LaereIn K. In vivo activation of endocannabinoid system in temporal lobe epilepsy with hippocampal sclerosis. Brain. 2011;134:1033–40.

Klitgaard H, Pitkänen A. Antiepileptogenesis, neuroprotection, and disease modification in the treatment of epilepsy: focus on levetiracetam. Epileptic Disord. 2003;5:9–16.

Löscher W. Animal models of epilepsy for the development of antiepileptogenic and disease-modifying drugs. A comparison of the pharmacology of kindling and post-status epilepticus models of temporal lobe epilepsy. Epilepsy Res. 2002;50:105–23.

Löscher W. Critical review of current animal models of seizures and epilepsy used in the discovery and development of new antiepileptic drugs. Seizure. 2011;20:359–68.

Löscher W, Brandt C. Prevention or modification of epileptogenesis after brain insults: experimental approaches and translational research. Pharmacol Rev. 2010;62:668–700.

Machado T, Da Silva MNF, Leal-Mesquita ER, Carmignotto AP, Yonenaga-Yassuda Y. Nine karyomorphs for spiny rats of the genus *Proechimys* (Echimyidae, Rodentia) from North and Central Brazil. Genet Mol Biol. 2005;28:682–92.

Mani R, Pillard J, Dichter MA. Human clinical trials in antiepileptogenesis. Neurosci Lett. 2011;497(3):251–6.

Nowak RM. Walker's mammals of the world, vol II. 6th ed. Baltimore: The Johns Hopkins University; 1999. p. 1688–9.

Patton JL, Da Silva MNF, Malcolm JR. Mammals of the Rio Juruá and the evolutionary and ecological diversification of Amazonia. Bull Am Mus Nat Hist. 2000;244:1–306.

Pitkänen A. Therapeutic approaches to epileptogenesis-hope on the horizon. Epilepsia. 2010;51 Suppl 3:2–17.

Scorza CA, Araujo BH, Arida RM, Scorza FA, Torres LB, Amorim HA, et al. Distinctive hippocampal CA2 subfield of the Amazon rodent *Proechimys*. Neuroscience. 2010;169:965 73.

Scorza CA, Araujo BH, Leite LA, Torres LB, Otalora LF, Oliveira MS, et al. Morphological and electrophysiological properties of pyramidal-like neurons in the stratum oriens of Cornu ammonis 1 and Cornu ammonis 2 area of *Proechimys*. Neuroscience. 2011;177:252–68.

Turski WA, Cavalheiro EA, Schwarz M, Czuczwar SJ, Kleinrok Z, Turski L. Limbic seizures produced by pilocarpine in rats: behavioural, electroencephalographic and neuropathological study. Behav Brain Res. 1983;9:315–35.

Weir BJ. Another hystricomorph rodent: keeping casiragua (*Preochimys guairae*) in captivity. Lab Animal. 1973;7:125–34.

Chapter 14
On the Development of New Antiepileptic Drugs for the Treatment of Pharmacoresistant Epilepsy: Different Approaches to Different Hypothesis

Alan Talevi and Luis E. Bruno-Blanch

Abstract Despite the introduction of 15 new antiepileptic drugs to the market since 1990, around a third of the epileptic patients do not achieve seizure remission with current known medications. The chapter overviews current hypothesis on the causes of drug resistant epilepsy, with an emphasis on the most documented explanations. On the basis of those hypotheses, current approaches to the development of novel antiepileptic medications are overviewed, including adjuvant Pgp-inhibitors, development of Pgp-non substrates, use of nanocarriers to circumvent active transport, design of multi-target directed ligands and adjuvant therapies with antioxidant and anti-inflammatory medications. In line with current discussions on the matter, it is proposed that different hypothesis may serve as explanation for different subgroups of drug-resistant patients, and that—in the light of recent basic research—at least some of the hypotheses may be interrelated.

Keywords Refractory epilepsy • Drug resistant epilepsy • Antiepileptic drugs • Drug design • Transporter hypothesis • Target hypothesis • Intrinsic severity hypothesis • ABC transporters • Multi-target directed drugs • Nanocarriers

14.1 Refractory Epilepsy: Current Explanations

According to the current definition from the International League Against Epilepsy (ILAE) the term refractory (or intractable, or drug resistant) epilepsy refers to the failure of adequate trials of two tolerated, appropriately chosen antiepileptic drug schedules (either as monotherapies or in combination) to achieve sustained seizure

A. Talevi (✉) • L.E. Bruno-Blanch
Department of Biological Sciences, Faculty of Exact Sciences,
National University of La Plata, 47 and 115, La Plata, B1900AJI, Argentina
e-mail: alantalevi@gmail.com; atalevi@biol.unlp.edu.ar; brunoblanch.luis@gmail.com; lbb@biol.unlp.edu.ar;

L. Rocha and E.A. Cavalheiro (eds.), *Pharmacoresistance in Epilepsy: From Genes and Molecules to Promising Therapies*, DOI 10.1007/978-1-4614-6464-8_14,

freedom (Kwan et al. 2010). In the previous definition "appropriate" indicates an intervention that has previously been shown to be effective (preferably in randomized controlled studies) for the patient's epilepsy and seizure type, while "adequate" indicates that the drug has been administered at adequate dosage for a sufficient length of time. Regarding what constitutes and adequate period without seizures for a patient to be regarded as "seizure-free," a minimum of three times the longest pre-intervention inter-seizure period or 12 months (whichever is longer) has been proposed. Application of a standardized definition of refractoriness is not trivial, since depending on the definition chosen the frequency of drug resistant epilepsy varies considerably (between 10 and nearly 40 %) (Beleza 2009). What is more, as discussed later, general applicability of a given hypothesis of drug resistant epilepsy may critically depend on what we actually call "drug resistant epilepsy."

Despite the fact that there are currently more than 20 available antiepileptic drugs (AEDs) and that 15 third generation agents have been introduced to the market since 1990, the clinical need of refractory epilepsy remains unmet (Bialer 2012; Löscher and Schmidt 2011): there are still no solid evidence indicating improved efficacy. There are currently four hypotheses explaining the nature of refractory epilepsy: on the one hand, the traditional transporter and target hypothesis (Löscher and Potschka 2005; Schmidt and Löscher 2005; Kwan and Brodie 2005; Remy and Beck 2006); more recently, the inherent severity hypothesis and the neural network hypothesis have also been proposed (Rogawski and Johnson 2008; Fang et al. 2011). Among them, the transporter hypothesis is so far, without a shadow of doubt, the most extensively studied.

The transporter hypothesis suggests that intractable epilepsy may have a pharmacokinetic basis. It states that drug resistance may emerge, as in other disorders, from intrinsic or acquired activation or over-expression of drug transporters involved in drug distribution, metabolism and elimination. Research supporting this hypothesis has focused in efflux transporters from the ATP-binding cassette (ABC) superfamily. Evidence abounds indicating high expression levels of members of this family such as P-glycoprotein (Pgp), breast cancer resistance protein (BCRP), and multidrug resistance proteins (MRPs) at the neurovascular unit of nonresponsive patients (either at the blood–brain barrier or glial cells or neurons) (Tishler et al. 1995; Dombrowski et al 2001; Sisodiya et al. 2002, 2006; Aronica et al. 2003, 2005; Lazarowski et al. 2004; Calatozzollo et al. 2005; Kubota et al. 2006; Ak et al. 2007). Lack of efficacy of those AEDs which are substrates of any of the up-regulated efflux transporter would be a consequence of limited bioavailability of the therapeutic agent in the brain or specifically at the epileptic focus. In fact, some studies showed reduced AEDs concentrations in the brain extracellular fluid and epileptic tissue of refractory patients (Marchi et al. 2005; Rambeck et al. 2006). A general pharmacokinetic mechanism underlying refractory epilepsy is consistent with the fact that available AEDs act through a wide range of molecular mechanisms. The transporter hypothesis has been fully verified in animal models of epilepsy. Several animal models of epilepsy (chronic models) have provided evidence of Pgp over-expression in brain tissue from animals with refractory epilepsy (Zhang et al. 2012), and drug resistance has been reverted by co-administration of Pgp inhibitors together with the AED (van Vliet et al. 2006; Brandt et al. 2006). Nevertheless, conclusive evidence of the validity of the transporter hypothesis in humans remains elusive. There are some (anecdotical) cases of patients who have showed improvement when AED were co-administered with Verapamil, a known Pgp-inhibitor (Summers et al. 2004; Ianetti et al. 2005; Schmitt et al. 2010; Pirker and Baumgartner 2011). It is still not clear, however, if the observed results are due to the intrinsic antiepileptic activity of verapamil, to Pgp inhibition or another effect on AEDs pharmacokinetics, and randomized control trials with more selective inhibitors are needed to obtain definitive proof of concept. The main argument against the transporter hypothesis is the fact that numerous but not all AEDs are substrates of human Pgp (Zhang et al. 2012). At this point one should bear in mind that current definition of drug resistant epilepsy requires only two adequate, appropriate, well-tolerated AED interventions to consider that a patient presents refractory epilepsy. It is then conceivable that (if the transporter hypothesis were valid) a patient would be diagnosed as drug resistant if at least one of those two AEDs interventions does not include a Pgp-non-substrate (e.g., Carbamazepine). It has been suggested that the transporter hypothesis may be valid for a subgroup of the epileptic patients (Löscher and Delanty 2009).

The target hypothesis states that structural (transcriptional or posttranscriptional) alterations in AEDs molecular targets might explain pharmacoresistance. This hypothesis is based, essentially, in reported loss of sensitivity to voltage-gated sodium channel blockers such as carbamazepine and phenytoin in patients and animal models of epilepsy (Schmidt and Löscher 2009). It has been observed that the inactivation effect of Phenytoin on sodium channels is transiently reduced in kindling models (Vreugdenhil and Wadman 1999), while the use-dependent effect of Carbamazepine and Phenytoin is permanently lost or reduced in the pilocarpine model and in temporal lobe epilepsy patients (Remy et al. 2003a, b; Jandová et al. 2006). Numerous changes in the expression of sodium channels subunits have been described in animal models of seizure and epilepsy, and in epileptic patients (Bartolomei et al. 1997; Gastaldi et al. 1998; Aronica et al. 2001; Whitaker et al. 2001; Ellerkmann et al. 2003), suggesting seizures or epileptogenesis may alter AEDs targets. Mutations at accessory subunit β1 have been linked to a dramatic loss in the use-dependent effect of phenytoin (Lucas et al. 2005). On the other hand, associations between alterations at $GABA_A$ receptor subunits and resistance to phenobarbital in animal models of temporal lobe epilepsy have been reported (Volk et al. 2006; Bethmann et al. 2008). The main objection to the target hypothesis is that, as has been already mentioned, there exist clinical AEDs associated to different mechanisms of action. Even those AEDs that share a common mechanism (e.g., $GABA_A$ receptor allosteric modulators) frequently bind to different sites of the same receptor. Thus, the target hypothesis by itself would only satisfactorily explain the phenomenon of multidrug resistance involving drugs that share their mechanism of action.

A third hypothesis, the hypothesis of the intrinsic severity, proposes the inherent severity of the disorder as determinant of the treatment outcome (Rogawski and Johnson 2008). It relies on epidemiologic data which indicates that the single most important factor linked to the prognosis of epilepsy is the number of episodes at the early phase of the disorder (MacDonald et al. 2000; Williamson et al. 2006; Sillampää and Schmidt 2006; Mohanraj and Brodie 2006; Kim et al. 2006; Hitiris et al. 2007; Sillampää and Schmidt 2009). Some limitations of the intrinsic severity hypothesis have been highlighted (Schmidt and Löscher 2009): the lack of studies on the biological basis of disease severity; the lack of genetic studies comparing patients with low seizure frequency versus patients with high seizure frequency at the disorder onset and; the fact that there are reports of nonresponsive patients with low frequency of episodes at the early phase of epilepsy (Spooner et al. 2006).

Very recently, a fourth hypothesis has arisen. The neural network hypothesis states that the adaptive remodeling of neural circuits that follows seizures may contribute to the development of refractory epilepsy. However, one should remember that remodeling of neural circuits also occurs in responsive patients. Therefore, differences between the degree of neural reorganization in responsive and nonresponsive patients should be studied to support this latest explanation to drug resistance.

This short overview suggests that either different hypothesis may explain the drug resistance phenomenon in different subgroups of patients (understanding that refractory epilepsy is a complex, multi-factor phenomenon and conceiving that in some patients more than one factor may be present simultaneously) or that the previous hypothesis may be integrated (Schmidt and Löscher 2009), with the two first hypothesis (partially) providing a biological basis for the others. Most importantly to the scope of this chapter, different hypothesis claim for different strategies to develop novel therapeutic answers. In the next sections we discuss potential implications of the first three hypothesis in the field of AEDs development.

14.2 Possible Therapeutic Answers to the Transporter Hypothesis

The obvious answer to overcome efflux transporter-mediated drug resistance is to develop therapeutic systems to circumvent this barrier to achieving adequate concentrations of the drug in its site of action. An excellent review on this matter has recently been published (Potschka 2012). The general strategies studied in the last 15 years to overcome ABC transporters can be synthesized as (Talevi and Bruno-Blanch 2012): (a) modulation of ABC transporters (i.e., reversal of multidrug resistance and down-regulation of transporters); (b) design of novel drugs which are not efflux transporter-substrates; (c) bypassing drug transport (or the Trojan horse strategy). Most of the research on these strategies has focused on the best known representative of the ABC superfamily, Pgp (note that Pgp was purified back in 1979 and it was not until 1990s that MRPs were identified). However, it is now established that there exist numerous transporters involved in transport of endogenous and exogenous compounds and that the levels of expression of different ABC transporters are interrelated (in some cases, a co-expression pattern has been observed; in others, an inverse relationship has been established) (Miller et al. 2008; Cisternino et al. 2004; Bark et al. 2008; Choi et al. 1999; Bordow et al. 1994). Taking into consideration that the spectra of substrates of different ABC transporters overlap to a certain degree, it might be hypothesized that up-regulation of a given transporter might have a compensatory role in the transient or permanent disturbance of other, which might explain the observed development of tolerance to some interventions aimed at regulating Pgp function (van Vliet et al. 2006). One must consider that development of tolerance is not acceptable when dealing with long-term drug treatments such as AEDs.

Regarding transporters modulation, the most advanced research relates to add-on therapies of specific inhibitors of ABC transporters, a strategy that was originally conceived for cancer treatment. Although preclinical and initial clinical results in the field of cancer treatment were encouraging at first, trials of first, second and even third generation agents had to be stopped at clinical stage due to serious adverse effects (Deeken and Löscher 2007; Lhommé et al. 2008; Tiwari et al. 2011; Fox and Bates 2007). These results have called into question the general validity of this approach of overcoming cellular drug resistance by the use of transporters inhibitors, even though trials continue in order to find more effective and safe inhibitors for Pgp and other transporters (Deeken and Löscher 2007; Akhtar et al. 2011). At this point it is important to remember that ABC transporters comprise a concerted, complex efflux and influx dynamic system whose substrates are not only drugs but also endogenous compounds (e.g., waste products) and toxins. They are implicated in the inflammatory response to several stress and harmful stimuli, and, apparently, they have a role in neurodegenerative diseases such as Alzheimer's and Parkinson's disease (Hartz and Bauer 2010). Thus, their permanent impairment or disruption is likely to result in severe side effects (again, one should bear in mind the chronic nature of epilepsy, which demands long-term treatment). A similar outcome to RNA interference technologies to down-regulate a given gene codifying a member of the ABC superfmailiy may be expected (Potschka 2012). Recent research has then focused on elucidating intracellular signaling pathways that control ABC transporters (their expression, intracellular trafficking, activation and inactivation). It is proposed that finding the molecular switches of these transporters will allow selective modulation of transporters function and or expression for therapeutic purposes in different clinical scenarios (Hartz and Bauer 2010), which includes turning the efflux mechanisms off for short, controlled periods of time.

Another strategy which should provide delivery of a drug to the brain without the toxic issues associated to the impairment of the efflux transport is virtual screening or computer-aided design of novel AEDs which are not recognized by ABC transporters (Demel et al. 2008, 2009). A review on in silico models for early detection of Pgp substrates has been recently published (Chen et al. 2012). A 2D QSAR model to detect anti-maximal electroshock seizures (MES) drug candidates (Talevi et al. 2007a, b, 2012), an ensemble of 2D models to identify Pgp-susbtrates (Di Ianni et al. 2011) and a structure-based approach based on homology modeling of human Pgp were jointly applied in a virtual screening campaign to ZINC and DrugBank databases (Irwin and Shoichet 2005; Knox et al. 2011). From 360 compounds predicted as Pgp-non-substrates anticonvulsants, ten diverse candidates

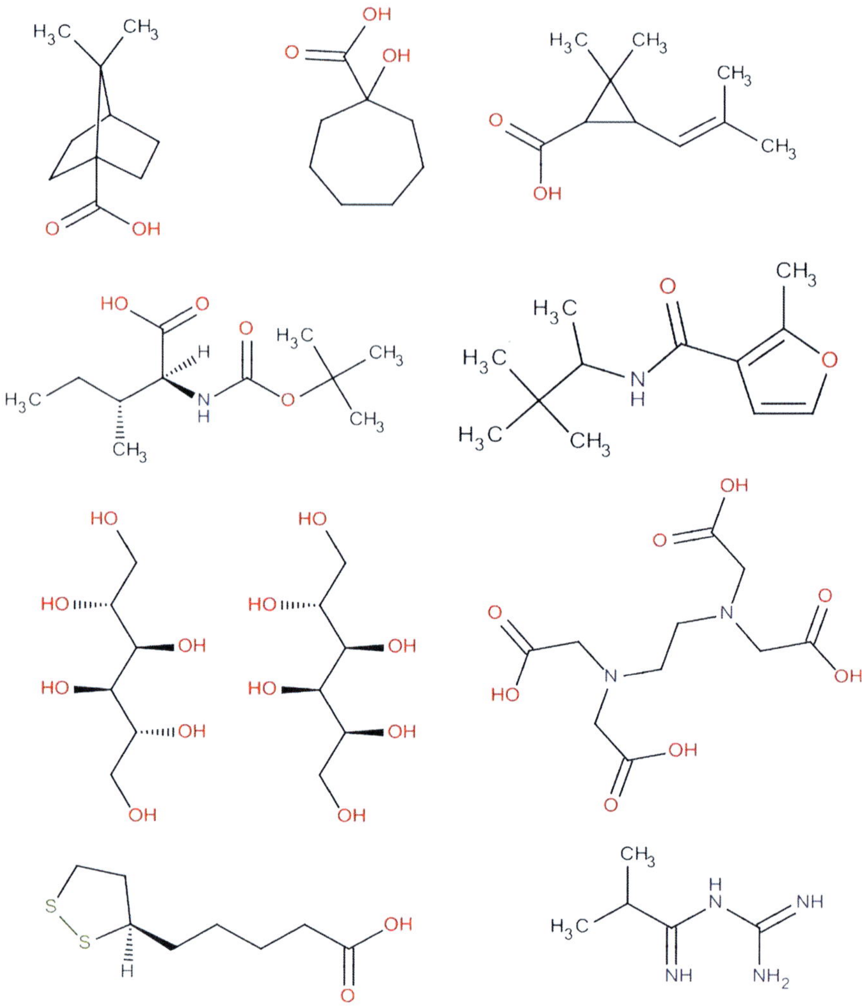

Fig. 14.1 A series of novel anticonvulsants emerging from a multistep virtual screening campaign aiming at novel treatments for refractory epilepsy

(Fig. 14.1) were acquired and tested in the MES test, with good results (Di Ianni et al. 2012, submitted).

The last strategy implies the application of a carrier system to "hide" the drug from the efflux pump. Different carrier systems have been tested to increase the bioavailability of drugs to the brain, among them nanosystems (polymer nanoparticles, nanogels, lipid nanocapsules, liposomes) (Bansal et al. 2009; Patel et al. 2009; Bennewitz and Saltzman 2009; Alam et al. 2010,). An exhaustive review of all the carriers that have been tested in brain drug targeting to avoid recognition by transporters will deserve an entire chapter or even a book, so we are including some

Table 14.1 Increment of brain bioavailability of VPA when administered intranasally with nanostructured lipid carriers [adapted from Eskandari et al. (2011)]

Formulation	Route	Dose (mg/kg)	Plasma concentration 60 min after administration (μg/ml), mean ± SD	Brain concentration 60 min after administration (μg/g) mean ± SD	Brain:plasma ratio
NLC of VPA	Intranasal	4	7.96 ± 2.9	64.35 ± 5.7	8.4
NLC of VPA	IP	20	11.35 ± 5.8	19.85 ± 8.5	1.65
Sodium VPA solution	Intranasal	30	3.87 ± 1.9	23.36 ± 8.3	6.77
Sodium VPA solution	IP	150	275.85 ± 39.5	112 ± 16	0.42

NLC nanostructured lipid carriers, *VPA* valproic acid

examples for illustrative purposes. A 60-fold increase in the brain localization of doxorubicin (a known Pgp-substrate) in rats, when administered i.v. as polysorbate 80-coated nanoparticles (compared to: i.v. administration in saline solution; in polysorbate 80 solution and; bound to nanoparticles without polysorbate 80 coating) (Gulyaey et al. 1999). Much more recently, a 2.6-fold increase in coumarin-6 localization in the brain through encapsulation of the drug in poly(ε-caprolactone)-block-poly(ethyl ethylene phosphate) nanomicelles was achieved (Zhang et al. 2010). Regarding specific application of this strategy to antiepileptic agents, different nanosystems have been studied for the delivery of Clonazepam, Diazepam, Phenytoin, Ethosuximide, 5-5-diphenyl hydantoin, carbamazepine, and valproic acid (VPA) and NMDA receptor antagonists (Fresta et al. 1996; Kim et al. 1997; Jeong et al. 1998; Nah et al. 1998; Ryu et al. 2000; Darius et al. 2000; Friese et al. 2000; Thakur and Gupta 2006; Abdelbary and Fahmy 2009; Varshosaz et al. 2010; Eskandari et al. 2011). A valid question would be whether this galenic artifices do improve availability of the drug in the central nervous system (CNS) and, if so, the molecular basis of such improvement. Unfortunately, most of this reports limit to physical characterization and in vitro behavior of the proposed systems. However, some of them explore the in vivo behavior of the nanosystems, with variable results. Darius et al. (2000) found that the brain tissue levels of VPA were not altered by administration with nanoparticles, though the nanosystem inhibits metabolism of VPA via mitochondrial beta-oxidation. Friese et al. (2000) reported that poly(butylcyanoacrylate) nanoparticles coated with polysorbate 80 prolong the duration of the anticonvulsive activity of NMDA receptor antagonist MRZ 2/576, presumably by prevention of active transport processes at the choroid plexus. More recently, Eskandari et al. (2011) have found an increased protective effect of VPA in the MES test when the drug was administered in nanostructured lipid carriers to rats. Intranasal administration of a dose of 4 mg/kg of nanostructured lipid carriers of VPA lead to almost three times higher brain concentrations than an intranasally administered solution of 30 mg/kg of the drug; brain–plasma ratio was also increased with the nanosystem (Table 14.1).

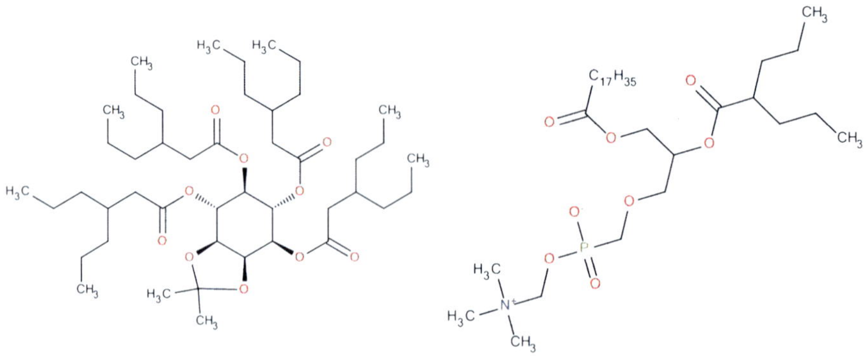

Fig. 14.2 Two prodrugs of VPA designed for improvement of VPA bioavailability at the epileptic focus: a prodrug of myo-inositol (*left*) and DP-VPA (*right*)

Prodrugs are another option to circumvent the blood–brain barrier, sometimes making use of influx transporters (e.g., dopamine is administered as its precursor L-dopa, which is transported into the brain by the L-type amino acid transporter and bio-transformed to dopamine in situ) (Mandaya et al. 2010). Numerous prodrugs of different anticonvulsant agents such as phenytoin, gabapentin, VPA and eslicarbazepine have been developed in order to improve bioavailability by regulation of drug absorption, distribution and elimination (Bennewitz and Saltzman 2009; Trojnar et al. 2004; Bialer and Soares-da-Silva 2012). DP-VPA (Fig. 13.2) was designed to be specifically activated at the epileptic focus. It is a prodrug of VPA in which the VPA moiety is covalently bound to a phospholipid, lecithin, leading to a 50-fold increase in efficacy in the pentylenetetrazol-induced seizures test (Trojnar et al. 2004). Similarly, our group has developed prodrugs of VPA with myo-inositol (Fig. 14.2) aiming at capitalizing the active influx of inositol enantiomers into the brain; the activity of these prodrugs in animal models of seizure is also increased compared to VPA, seemingly by improving CNS bioavailability (Bodor et al. 2000; Moon et al. 2007; Bruno-Blanch and Moon 2010). Whether these prodrugs interact with efflux transporters and bypass up-regulated transporter molecules at the neurovascular unit has yet to be studied.

It is noteworthy that in the last few years it has been proven that, besides helping bypassing Pgp, many pharmaceutical excipients which are usually incorporated into carrier-systems can inhibit or modulate Pgp function by different mechanisms (Bansal et al. 2009). For example, it has been proposed that PEG and surfactans such as sorbitans and polysorbates can disrupt the lipid arrangement of the cellular membrane and that these perturbations have been shown to modulate Pgp activity (Lo 2003). This kind of modulation is interesting since it may increase drug bioavailability in a transient manner, without the undesired effects of direct inhibition. Besides its possible role modulating transporters, cumulative evidence indicates that nanoparticle's coating leads to adsorption of elements from the blood such as apolipoproteins, which in turn allows distribution to the brain by receptor-mediated transcytosis (Wohlfart et al. 2012 and references therein).

14.3 Possible Therapeutic Answers to the Target Hypothesis

Several CNS disorders (either neurological or affective) present a complex etiology which includes a combination of polygenic, environmental, and neuro-developmental factors. Empiric evidence with effective treatments for some of such diseases (e.g., antidepressants) shows that searching for polyspecific, selective non-selective drugs (multi-target directed-ligands or "magic shotguns" or polyvalent drugs) may prove more safe and effective than the development of highly selective, single-target drugs (Roth et al. 2004). There are plenty examples of recent developments in the field of CNS medications based on this new paradigm, including developing drugs for Alzheimer and Parkinson's diseases (Cavalli et al. 2008; Youdim and Buccadfasco 2005), schizophrenia, depression and other mood disorders (Decker and Lehmann 2007; Wong et al. 2010).

There are many reasons why multi-target therapies are attractive in the field of epilepsy. First, evidence indicate that—if total drug load is carefully watched—some refractory patients may achieve seizure remission on poly-pharmacy, especially if the pharmacologic properties of the specific AEDs being combined is taken into account (Canevini et al. 2010; Kwan and Brodie 2006). A recent study on 131 patients who underwent successful epilepsy surgery seems to indicate that, at least in the early postoperative stage, dual-therapy may be more effective than monotherapy to achieve seizure remission (Zeng et al. 2012). Second, the normal function of neural networks may be more likely preserved by multiple small adjustments than by a single, strong perturbation, reducing not only the likelihood of central side-effects but also the induction of counter-regulatory processes which may relate with drug resistance (Löscher and Schmidt 2011; Bianchi et al. 2009). What is more: many currently used AEDs are in fact unintended multi-target agents (Bianchi et al. 2009).

In the light of the evidence that refractoriness may be in some cases related to modifications in drug targets, the design of novel multi-target AEDs seems as a natural answer to the second hypothesis of drug resistance, considering that it seems to be less likely that two distinct drug targets are altered simultaneously. Therefore, even if one target of a multi-target drug has lost sensitivity, one can speculate that the other/s will remain sensitive.

From the drug design perspective, in silico, rational approaches to develop multifunctional agents can be classified in two strategies (Ma et al. 2010). On the one hand, the combinatorial approach, in which parallel Virtual Screening searches against each target of interest are conducted, retaining those hits that simultaneously gather all the structural requisites needed to interact with each individual target. In other words, the common hits from parallel Virtual Screening searches (one for every model associated to a particular target) are retained. In the background of multi-target drug discovery, the Virtual Screening for ligands for each individual target must be highly sensitive (i.e., a reduced number of false negatives should be observed) since the collective retrieval rate for multiple targets will tend to be relatively low than when aiming to individual targets (one might speculate that, naturally, it is more difficult to find compounds that selectively interact with different targets without being excessively promiscuous). In contrast, when drugs that selectively interact with a single target are being searched, in certain contexts one might sacrifice sensitivity in order to gain specificity. The second strategy is the fragment-based approach. Here, multiple elements or scaffolds that bind to each of the targeted targets are combined (usually through a linker) into a single, often larger molecule. The main drawback of this later approach relates to the poorer pharmacokinetic and toxicological profile of the final drug. Unless small, highly specific blocks/fragments are combined, it is unlikely that a given compound will gather the features for a CNS drug-like drug.

14.4 Possible Therapeutic Answers to the Intrinsic Severity Hypothesis

If the intrinsic severity hypothesis was valid, AEDs research would face to elemental questions. Firstly, what are the determinants of epilepsy severity? And, if the answer to that initial question was answered, how could one control, through a therapeutic intervention, such determinants? During the last 10 years, basic research has begun to provide us some knowledge to attempt some very draft answers to these issues.

Acquired epilepsy is typically initiated by a brain insult followed by a latent, silent period whereby molecular, biochemical and cellular alterations occur in the brain and eventually lead to chronic epilepsy (Waldbaum and Patel 2010a). In the last 10–15 years a link between epileptogenesis and oxidative stress, mitochondrial impairment and inflammation has been established by a large body of studies (Waldbaum and Patel 2010b; Waldbaum et al. 2010; Devi et al 2008; Liang and Patel 2006; Shin et al. 2008; Patel 2004; Sudha et al 2001; Vezzani and Granata 2005; Vezzani et al. 2011; Choi and Koh 2008). These phenomena seem to be both cause and consequence of seizures, constituting a vicious circle which results in a chronic disorder, e.g., inflammatory mediators are released during seizures, and inflammatory mediators take part in seizure generation and exacerbation. It is also interesting to note that chronic inflammation and oxidative unbalance take part in the physiopathology of a diversity of neurological disorders. The brain combines a peculiar set of factors which makes it particularly vulnerable to reactive species: high rate of oxidative metabolism, low antioxidant defenses and abundant polyunsaturated lipids (Devi et al 2008).

In line with the integrative approach towards explaining refractory epilepsy, a series of studies developed in the last decade agree that pro-inflammatory signals and Reactive Oxygen Species play a role in the regulation of ABC transporters' expression and activity. For example, exposing isolated rat brain capillaries to nanomolar concentrations of ET-1 and TNF-α for long periods of time (above 4 h) increased Pgp-mediated transport compared to control levels, and after a 6-h exposure Pgp transport was roughly doubled (Bauer et al. 2007). Von Wedel-Parlow et al. (2009) reported that Pgp levels were increased by TNF-α within 6 h but decreased later (Von Wedel-Parlow et al. 2009). Poller et al. reported similar results working with a human cell line of immortalized brain microvessels endothelial cells; they also noted that IL-6 treatment produced a slight decrease in Pgp mRNA expression (Poller et al. 2010). Regarding the influence of Reactive Oxygen Species on efflux transporters expression levels, the first evidence of up-regulation of Pgp came from in vitro experiments on primary culture of rat brain endothelial cells (Felix and Barrand 2002). Four hours after exposure to 100 μM H_2O_2, up-regulation of Pgp was observed at both mRNA and protein levels, which continue to increase up to a maximum at 48 h. A biphasic up-regulation was also observed after a 6-h hypoxia and subsequent reoxigenation (H/R) treatment; in this case, return to basal levels was observed following reoxigenation by 48 h. More recently, Robertson et al. (2009) reproduced the previous experiments comparing the effects of H_2O_2 H/R treatments in primary rat brain endothelial cells and immortalized rat brain endothelial cells. Although the production of Reactive Oxygen Species after H_2O_2 was more pronounced in immortalized cells lines, similar up-regulation of Pgp, at the protein level, was observed after the oxidative stress treatments in both types of cells. Similar results were obtained with other models, such as exposure to diesel exhaust particles or glutathione depletion (Hartz et al. 2008; Hong et al. 2006; Wu et al. 2009).

The discovery of the role of pro-inflammatory mediators and oxidative stress in epilepsy explains current interest in immune, antiinflammatory and neuroprotective therapies as potential strategies to improve disease prognosis. For example, it was observed that ascorbic and lipoic acids ameliorate oxidative stress in experimental seizures (Santos et al. 2009; Militão et al. 2010). ACTH—a peptide that releases endogenous steroids in the patient—is used as a treatment for infantile spasms, a childhood refractory epilepsy; its efficacy has been confirmed in controlled trials (Pellock et al. 2010), while the use of other anti-inflammatory therapies such as steroids remains controversial due to current lack of controlled clinical studies (Vezzani et al. 2011).

14.5 Conclusions

There are currently four different hypotheses for drug resistant epilepsy. None of them seems to completely explain all cases of refractory epilepsy, but subgroups of unresponsive patients instead. At first sight, each of them claims for a different therapeutic approach. Among the strategies proposed to overcome transporter-mediated refractory epilepsy, computer-aided research on new AEDs which are not recognized by ABC transporters, and circumventing transport by either prodrug design or nanoscale drug carriers seem as the best alternatives. Considering the efflux transporters' role in the disposal of potentially toxic endogenous and exogenous compounds, we do not believe adjuvant inhibitory therapies as a feasible option in the case of long-term treatments (e.g., AEDs). Still, one should consider that inhibition of a given transporter is often compensated by up-regulation of another member of the ABC superfamiliy. Regarding the target hypothesis, design of multi-target agents that introduce mild perturbations to several AED targets seems to be a good alternative for the treatment of those patients with certain altered, unsensitive target. Finally, considering the intrinsic severity hypothesis, and since inflammation and oxidative stress seem to have a role in generation and exacerbation of seizures, controlled trials on the possible effects of antioxidants, immune and anti-inflammatory medication on epilepsy may have an impact on disease prognosis and severity, and consequently improve the chance of seizure remission.

Recent findings on the effect of oxidative stress and inflammation on ABC transporters expression confirm the idea that some (if not all) of the hypothesis of drug resistant epilepsy can be integrated. More research on the relationship between oxidative stress and alterations to AED targets should be explored. Revealing the fine mechanisms that govern biochemical pathways and cellular events involved in epileptogenesis (e.g., angiogenesis, inflammation) would create new opportunities for the development of innovative antiepileptic medications.

Acknowledgments A. Talevi is a member of the Scientific Research Career at CONICET. L.E. Bruno-Blanch is a researcher of Facultad de Ciencias Exactas, Universidad Nacional de La Plata. The authors would like to thank UNLP (Incentivos X-597), CONICET (PIP 11220090100603), and ANPCyT (PICTs 2010-2531 and 2010-1774) for providing funds to develop our research.

References

Abdelbary G, Fahmy RH. Diazepam-loaded solid lipid nanoparticles: design and characterization. AAPS Pharm Sci Tech. 2009;10:211–9.

Ak H, Ay B, Tanrivedi T, Sanus GZ, Is M, Sar M, et al. Expression and cellular distribution of multidrug resistance-related proteins in patients with focal cortical dysplasia. Seizure. 2007;16:493–503.

Akhtar N, Ahad A, Khar RK, Jaggi M, Ágil M, Igbal Z, Ahmad FJ, Talegaonkar S. The emerging role of P-glycoprotein inhibitors in drug delivery: a patent review. Expert Opin Ther Pat. 2011;21:561–76. doi: 10.1517/13543776.2011.561784.

Alam MI, Beg S, Samad A, Baboota S, Kohli K, Ali J, et al. Strategy for effective brain drug delivery. Eur J Pharm Sci. 2010;40:385–403.

Aronica E, Yankaza B, Troost D, van Vliet FA, Lopes da Silva FH, Gorter JA. Induction of neonatal sodium channel II and III alpha-isoform mRNAs in neurons and microglia after status epilepticus in the rat hippocampus. Eur J Neurosci. 2001;13:1261–6.

Aronica E, Gorter JA, Jansen GH, van Veelen CW, van Rijen PC, Leenstra S, et al. Expression and cellular distribution of multidrug transporter proteins in two major causes of medically intractable epilepsy: focal cortical dysplasia and glioneuronal tumors. Neuroscience. 2003;118:417–29.

Aronica E, Gorter JA, Redeker S, van Vliet EA, Ramkema M, Scheffer GL, et al. Localization of breast cancer resistance protein (BCRP) in microvessel endothelium of human control and epileptic brain. Epilepsia. 2005;46:849–57.

Bansal T, Akhtar N, Jaggi M, Khar RK, Talegaonkar S. Novel formulation approaches for optimizing delivery of anticancer drugs based on P-glycoprotein modulation. Drug Discov Today. 2009;14:1067–74.

Bark H, Xu HD, Kim SH, Yun J, Choi CH. P-glycoprotein down-regulates expression of breast cancer resistance protein in a drug-free state. FEBS Lett. 2008;582:2595–600.

Bartolomei F, Gastaldi M, Massacrier A, Planells R, Nicolas S, Cau P. Changes in the mRNAs encoding subtypes I, II and III sodium cannel alpha subunits following kainate-induced seizures in rat brain. J Neurocytol. 1997;26:667–78.

Bauer B, Hartz AM, Miller DS. Tumor necrosis factor alpha and endothelin-1 increase P-glycoprotein expression and transport activity at the blood–brain barrier. Mol Pharmacol. 2007;71:667–75.

Beleza P. Refractory epilepsy: a clinically oriented review. Eur Neurol. 2009;62:65–71.

Bennewitz MF, Saltzman, WM. Nanotechnology for delivery of drugs to the brain for epilepsy. Neurotherapeutics. 2009;6:323–36. doi: 10.1016/j.nurt.2009.01.018.

Bethmann K, Fritschy JM, Brandt C, Löscher W. Antiepileptic drug resistant rats differ from drug responsive rats in $GABA_A$ receptor subunit expression in a model of temporal lobe epilepsy. Neurobiol Dis. 2008;31:169–87.

Bialer M. Chemical properties of antiepileptic drugs (AEDs). Adv Drug Deliv Rev. 2012;64:887–95.

Bialer M, Soares-da-Silva P. Pharmacokinetics and drug interactions of eslicarbazepine acetate. Epilepsia. 2012;53:935–46.

Bianchi MT, Pathmanathan J, Cash SS. From ion channels to complex networks: magic bullet versus magic shotgun approaches to anticonvulsant pharmacotherapy. Med Hypotheses. 2009;72:297–305.

Bodor N, Moon SC, Bruno-Blanch LE. Synthesis and pharmacological evaluation of prodrugs of valproic acid. Pharmazie. 2000;55:184–6.

Bordow SB, Haber M, Madafigli J, Cheung B, Marshall GM, Norris MD. Expression of the multidrug resistance-associated protein (MRP) gene correlates with amplification and overexpression of the N-myc oncogene in childhood neuroblastoma. Cancer Res. 1994;54:5036–40.

Brandt C, Nethmann K, Gastens AM, Löscher W. The multidrug transporter hypothesis of drug resistance in epilepsy: proof-of-principle in a rat model of temporal lobe epilepsy. Neurobiol Dis. 2006;24:202–11.

Bruno-Blanch L, Moon SC. US Patent 7,763,650; 2010.

Calatozzollo C, Gelati M, Ciusani E, Sciacca FL, Pollo B, Cajola L, et al. Expression of drug resistance proteins Pgp, MRP1, MRP3, MRP5 and GST.pi in human glioma. J Neurooncol. 2005;74:113–21.

Canevini MP, De Sarro G, Galimberti CA, Gatti G, Licchetta L, Malerba A, et al. Relationship between adverse effects of antiepileptic drugs, number of coprescribed drugs, and drug load in a large cohort of consecutive patients with drug-refractory epilepsy. Epilepsia. 2010;51:797–804.

Cavalli A, Bolognesi ML, Minarini A, Rosini M, Tumiatti V, Recanatini M, et al. Multi-target-directed ligands to combat neurodegenerative diseases. J Med Chem. 2008;51:347–72.

Chen L, Li Y, Yu H, Zhang L, Hou T. Computational models for predicting substrates or inhibitors of P-glycoprotein. Drug Discov Today. 2012;17:343–51.

Choi J, Koh S. Role of brain infalmmation in epileptogenesis. Yonsei Med J. 2008;49:1–18.

Choi CH, Kim SH, Rha HS, Jeong JH, Park YH, Min YD, et al. Drug concentration-dependent expression of multidrug resistance-associated protein and P-glycoprotein in the doxorubicin-resistant acute myelogenous leukemia sublines. Mol Cell. 1999;9:314–9.

Cisternino S, Mercier C, Bourasset F, Roux F, Scherrmann JM. Expression, upregulation, and transport activity of the multidrug-resistance protein abcg2 at the mouse blood–brain barrier. Cancer Res. 2004;64:3296–301.

Darius J, Meyer FP, Sabel BA, Schroeder U. Influence of nanoparticles on the brain-to-serum distribution and the metabolism of valproic acid in mice. J Pharm Pharmacol. 2000;52:1043–7.

Decker M, Lehmann J. Agonistic and antagonistic bivalent ligands for serotonin and dopamine receptors including their transporters. Curr Top Med Chem. 2007;7:347–53.

Deeken JF, Löscher W. The blood–brain barrier and cancer: transporters, treatment and Trojan horses. Clin Cancer Res. 2007;13:1663–74.
Demel MA, Schwha R, Krämer O, Ettmayer P, Haaksma EE, Ecker GF. In silico prediction of substrate properties for ABC-mulridrug transporters. Expert Opin Drug Metab Toxicol. 2008;4:1167–80.
Demel MA, Krämer O, Ettmayer P, Haaksma EE, Ecker GF. Predicting ligand interactions with ABC transporters in ADME. Chem Biodivers. 2009;6:1960–9.
Devi PU, Manocha A, Vohora D. Seizures, antiepileptics, antioxidants and oxidative stress: an insight for researchers. Expert Opin Pharmacother. 2008;9:3169–77.
Di Ianni M, Talevi A, Castro EA, Bruno-Blanch LE. Development of a highly specific ensemble of topological models for early identification of P-glycoprotein substrates. J Chemometr. 2011;25:313–22.
Di Ianni M, Enrique A, Palestro P, Gavernet L, Talevi A, Bruno-Blanch L. Several new diverse anticonvulsant agents discovered in a virtual screening campaign aime at novel antiepileptic drugs to treat refractory epilepsy. J Chem Inf Model. 2012;52:3325–30. doi: 10.1021/ci300423q.
Dombrowski SM, Desai SY, Marroni M, Cucullo L, Goodrich K, Bingaman W, et al. Overexpression of multiple drug resistance genes in endothelial cells from patients with refractory epilepsy. Epilepsia. 2001;42:1501–6.
Ellerkmann RK, Remy S, Chen J, Sochiyko D, Elger CE, Urban BW, et al. Molecular and functional changes in voltage-dependent Na(+) channels following pilocarpine-induced status epilepticus in rat dentrate granule cells. Neuroscience. 2003;119:323–33.
Eskandari S, Varshosaz J, Minaiyan M, Tabbakhian M. Brain delivery of valproic acid via intranasal administration of nanostructured lipid carriers: in vivo pharmacodynamic studies using rat electroshock model. Int J Nanomedicine. 2011;6:363–71.
Fang M, Xi ZQ, Wu Y, Wang XF. A new hypothesis of drug refractory epilepsy: neural network hypothesis. Med Hypotheses. 2011;76:871–6.
Felix RA, Barrand MA. P-glycoprotein expression in rat brain endothelial cells: evidence for regulation by transient oxidative stress. J Neurochem. 2002;80:64–72.
Fox E, Bates SE. Tariquidar (XR9576): a P-glycoprotein drug efflux pump inhibitor. Expert Rev Anticancer Ther. 2007;7:447–59.
Fresta M, Cavallaro G, Giammona G, Wehrli E, Puglisi G. Preparation and characterization of polyethyl-2-cyanoacrylate nanocapsules containing antiepileptic drugs. Biomaterials. 1996;17:751–8.
Friese A, Seiller E, Quack G, Lorenz B, Kreuter J. Increase of the duration of the anticonvulsive activity of a novel NMDA receptor antagonist using poly(butylcyanoacrylate) nanoparticles as a parenteral controlled release system. Eur J Pharm Biopharm. 2000;49:103–9.
Gastaldi M, Robaglia-Schlupp A, Massacrier A, Planells R, Cau P. mRNA coding for voltage-gated sodium channel beta2 subunit in rat central nervous system: cellular distribution and changes following kainate induced seizures. Neurosci Lett. 1998;249:53–6.
Gulyaey AE, Gelperina SE, Skidan IN, Antropoy AS, Kivman GY, Kreuter J. Significant transport of doxorubicin into the brain with polysorbate 80-coated nanoparticles. Pharm Res. 1999;16:1564–9.
Hartz AM, Bauer B. Regulation of ABC transporters at the blood–brain barrier: new targets for CNS therapy. Mol Interv. 2010;10:293–304.
Hartz AM, Bauer B, Block ML, Hong JS, Miller DS. Diesel exhaust particles induce oxidative stress proinflammatory signaling and P-glycoprotein up-regulation at the blood–brain barrier. FASEB J. 2008;22:2723–33.
Hitiris N, Mohanraj R, Norrie J, Sills GJ, Brodie MJ. Predictors of pharmacoresistant epilepsy. Epilepsy Res. 2007;75:192–6.
Hong H, Lu Y, Ji ZN. Up-regulation of P-glycoprotein expression by glutathione depletion-induced oxidative stress in rat brain microvessel endotelial cells. J Neurochem. 2006;98:1465–73.
Ianetti P, Spalice A, Parisi P. Calcium-channel blocker verapamil administration in prolonged and refractory status epilepticus. Epilepsia. 2005;46:967–9.

Irwin JJ, Shoichet BK. ZINC – a free database of commercially available compounds for virtual screening. J Chem Inf Model. 2005;45:177–82.

Jandová K, Päsler D, Leite Antonio L, Raue C, Ji S, Njunting M, et al. Carbamazepine-resistance in the epileptic dentate gyrus of human hippocampal slices. Brain. 2006;129:3290–306.

Jeong YI, Cheon JB, Kim SH, Nah JW, Lee YM, Sung YK, et al. Clonazepam release from core-shell type nanoparticles *in vitro*. J Control Release. 1998;51:169–78.

Kim HJ, Jeong YI, Kim SH, Lee YM, Cho CS. Clonazepam release from core-shell type nanoparticles *in vitro*. Arch Pharm Res. 1997;20:324–9.

Kim LG, Johnson TL, Marson AG, Chadwick DW, Medical Research Council MESS Study Group. Predicting risk of seizure recurrence after a single seizure and early epilepsy: further results from the MESS trial. Lancet Neurol. 2006;5:317–22.

Knox C, Law V, Jewison T, Liu P, Ly S, Frlokis A, et al. DrugBank: a comprehensive resource for "omics" research on drugs. Nucleic Acid Res. 2011;39(Database Issue):D1035–41.

Kubota H, Ishihara H, Langmann T, Schmitz G, Stieger B, Wieser HG, et al. Distribution and functional activity of P-glycoprotein and multidrug resistance-associated proteins in human brain microvascular endothelial cells in hippocampal sclerosis. Epilepsy Res. 2006;68: 213–28.

Kwan P, Brodie MJ. Potential role of drug transporters in the pathogenesis of medically intractable epilepsy. Epilepsia. 2005;46:224–35.

Kwan P, Brodie MJ. Combination therapy in epilepsy: when and what to use. Drugs. 2006;66:1817–29.

Kwan P, Arzimanoglou A, Berg AT, Brodie MJ, Allen Hauser W, Mathern G, et al. Definition of drug resistant epilepsy: consensus proposal by the *ad hoc* task force of the ILAE Comission on therapeutic strategies. Epilepsia. 2010;51:1069–77.

Lazarowski A, Massaro M, Schteinschnaider A, Intruvini S, Sevlever G, Rabinowicz A. Neuronal MDR-1 gene expression and persistent low levels of anticonvulsants in a child with refractory epilepsy. Ther Drug Monit. 2004;26:44–6.

Lhommé C, Joly F, Walker JL, Lissoni AA, Nicoletto MO, Manikhas GM, et al. Phase III study of valspodar (PSC 833) combined with paclitaxel and carboplatin compared with paclitaxel and carboplatin alone in patients with stage IV or suboptimally debulked stage III epithelial ovarian cancer or primary peritoneal cancer. J Clin Oncol. 2008;26:2674–82.

Liang LP, Patel M. Seizure-induced changes in mitochondrial redox status. Free Radic Biol Med. 2006;40:16–22.

Lo YL. Relationships between the hydrophilic–lipophilic balance values of pharmaceutical excipients and their multidrug resistance modulating effect in Caco-2 cells and rat intestines. J Control Release. 2003;90:37–48.

Löscher W, Delanty N. MDR1/ABCB1 polymorphisms and multidrug resistance in epilepsy: in and out of fashion. Pharmacogenomics. 2009;10:711–3.

Löscher W, Potschka H. Role of drug efflux transporters in the brain disposition and treatment of brain diseases. Prog Neurobiol. 2005;76:22–76.

Löscher W, Schmidt D. Modern antiepileptic drug development has failed to deliver: ways out of the current dilemma. Epilepsia. 2011;52:667–78.

Lucas PT, Meadows LS, Nicholls J, Ragsdale DS. An epilepsy mutation in the beta1 subunit of the voltage-gated sodium channel results in reduced channel sensitivity to Phenytoin. Epilepsy Res. 2005;64:77–84.

Ma X, Shi Z, Tan C, Jiang Y, Go ML, Low BC. *In silico* approaches to multi-target drug discovery. Computer aided multi-target drug design, multi-target virtual screening. Pharm Res. 2010;27:739–49.

MacDonald NK, Johnson AL, Goodridge DM, Cockerell OC, Sander JW, Shorvon SD. Factors predicting prognosis of epilepsy after presentation with seizures. Ann Neurol. 2000;48:833–41.

Mandaya N, Oberoi RK, Minocha M, Mitra AK. Transporter targeted drug delivery. J Drug Deliv Sci Technol. 2010;20:89–99.

Marchi N, Guiso G, Rizzi M, Pirker S, Novak K, Czech T, Baumgastner C, Janigro D, Caccia S, Vezzani A. Pilot study on brain-to-plasma partition of 10,11-Dyhydro-10-hydroxy-5H-dibenzo(b,f)azepine-5-carboxamide and MDR1 brain expression in epilepsy patients not responding to oxcarbazepine. Epilepsia. 2005;46:1613–9. doi: 10.1111/j.1528-1167.2005.00265.x.

Militão GC, Ferreira PM, de Freitas RM. Effects of lipoic acid on oxidative stress in rat striatum after pilocarpine-induced seizures. Neurochem Int. 2010;56:16–20.

Miller DS, Bauer B, Hartz AMS. Modulation of P-glycoprotein at the blood–brain barrier: opportunities to improve CNS pharmacotherapy. Pharmacol Rev. 2008;60:196–209.

Mohanraj R, Brodie MJ. Diagnosing refractory epilepsy: response to sequential treatment schedules. Eur J Neurol. 2006;13:277–82.

Moon SC, Echeverria GA, Punte G, Ellena J, Bruno-Blanch LE. Crystal structure and anticonvulsant activity of (+/–)-1,2:4,5-di-O-isopropylidene-3,6-di-O-(2-propylpentanoyl)-myoinositol. Carbohydr Res. 2007;342:1456–61.

Nah JW, Paek YW, Jeong YI, Kim DW, Cho CS, Kim SH, et al. Clonazepam release from poly(DL-lactide-co-glycolide) nanoparticles prepared by dialysis method. Arch Pharm Res. 1998;21:418–22.

Patel M. Mitochondrial dysfunction and oxidative stress: cause and consequence of epileptic seizures. Free Radic Biol Med. 2004;37:1951–62.

Patel MM, Goval BR, Bhadada SV, Bhatt JS, Amin AF. Getting into the brain: approaches to enhance brain drug delivery. CNS Drugs. 2009;23:35–58.

Pellock JM, Hrachovy R, Shinnar S, Baram TZ, Bettis D, Dlugos DJ, et al. Infantile spasms: A U.S. consensus report. Epilepsia. 2010;51:2175–89.

Pirker S, Baumgartner C. Termination of refractory focal status epilepticus by the P-glycoprotein inhibitor verapamil. Eur J Neurol. 2011;18:e151.

Poller B, Drewe J, Krähenbühl S, Huwyer J, Gutmann H. Regulation of BCRP (ABCG2) and P-glycoprotein (ABCB1) by cytokines in a model of the human blood–brain barrier. Cell Mol Neurobiol. 2010;30:63–70.

Potschka H. Role of CNS efflux drug transporters in the antiepileptic drug delivery: overcoming CNS efflux drug transport. Adv Drug Deliv Rev. 2012;64:896–910.

Rambeck B, Jürgens UH, May TW, Pannek HW, Behne F, Ebner A, Gorij A, Straub H, Speckmann EJ, Pohlmann-Eden B, Löscher W. Comparison of brain extracellular fluid, brain tissue, cerebrospinal fluid, and serum concentrations of antiepileptic drugs measured intraoperatively in patients with intractable epilepsy. Epilepsia. 2006;47:681–94. doi: 10.1111/j.1528-1167.2006.00504.x.

Remy S, Beck H. Molecular and cellular mechanisms of pharmacoresistance in epilepsy. Brain. 2006;129:18–35.

Remy S, Gabriel S, Urban BW, Dietrich D, Lehmann TN, Elger CE, et al. A novel mechanism underlying drug resistance in chronic epilepsy. Ann Neurol. 2003a;53:469–79.

Remy S, Urban BW, Elger CE, Beck H. Anticonvulsant pharmacology of voltage-gated Na+ channels in hippocampal neurons of control and chronically epileptic rats. Eur J Neurosci. 2003b;17:2648–58.

Robertson SJ, Kania KD, Hladky SB, Barrand MA. P-glycoprotein expression in immortalized rat brain endothelial cells: comparisons following exogenously applied hydrogen peroxide and after hypoxia-reoxygenation. J Neurochem. 2009;111:132–41.

Rogawski MA, Johnson MR. Intrinsic severity as a determinant of antiepileptic drug refractoriness. Epilepsy Curr. 2008;8:127–30.

Roth BL, Sheffler DJ, Kroeze WK. Magic shotguns versus magic bullets: selectively non-selective drugs for mood disorders and schizophrenia. Nat Rev Drug Discov. 2004;3:353–9.

Ryu J, Jeong YI, Kim IS, Lee JH, Nah JW, Kim SH. Clonazepam release from core-shell type nanoparticles of poly(epsilon-caprolactone)/poly(ethyleneglycol)/poly(epsilon-caprolactone) triblock copolymers. Int J Pharm. 2000;200:231–42.

Santos IM, Tomé Ada R, Saldanha GB, Ferreira PM, Militão GC, Freitas RM. Oxidative stress in the hippocampus during experimental seizures can be ameliorated with the antioxidant ascorbic acid. Oxid Med Cell Longev. 2009;2:214–21.

Schmidt D, Löscher W. Drug resistance in epilepsy: putative neurobiologic and clinical mechanisms. Epilepsia. 2005;46:858–77. doi:10.1111/j.1528-1167.2005.54904.x.
Schmidt D, Löscher W. New developments in antiepileptic drug resistance: and integrative view. Epilepsy Curr. 2009;9:47–52.
Schmitt FC, Dehnicke C, Merschhemke M, Meencke HJ. Verapamil attenuates the malignant treatment course in recurrent status epilepticus. Epilepsy Behav. 2010;17:565–8.
Shin EJ, Ko KH, Kim WK, Chae JS, Yen TP, Kim HJ, et al. Role of glutathione peroxidase in the ontogeny of hippocampal oxidative stress and kainate seizure sensitivity in the genetically epilepsy-prone rats. Neurochem Int. 2008;52:1134–47.
Sillampää M, Schmidt D. Natural history of treated childhood onset epilepsy: prospective long-term population based study. Brain. 2006;129:617–24.
Sillampää M, Schmidt D. Early seizure frequency and aetiology predict long-term medical outcome in childhood-onset epilepsy. Brain. 2009;132:989–98.
Sisodiya SM, Lin WR, Harding BN, Squier MV, Thorn M. Drug resistance in epilepsy: expression of drug resistance proteins in common causes of refractory epilepsy. Brain. 2002;125:22–31.
Sisodiya SM, Martinian L, Scheffer GL, van der Valk P, Scheper RJ, Harding BN, et al. Vascular colocalization of P-glycoprotein, multidrug resistance associated protein 1, breast cancer resistance protein and major vault protein in human epileptogenic pathologies. Neuropathol Appl Neurobiol. 2006;32:51–63.
Spooner CG, Berkovik SF, Mitchell LA, Wrennall JA, Harvey AS. New-onset temporal lobe epilepsy in children: lesion on MRI predicts poor seizure outcome. Neurology. 2006;67:2117–8.
Sudha K, Rap AV, Rao A. Oxidative stress and antioxidants in epilepsy. Clin Chim Acta. 2001;303:19–24.
Summers MA, Moore JL, McAuley JW. Use of verapamil as a potential P-glycoprotein inhibitor in a patient with refractory epilepsy. Ann Pharmacother. 2004;38:1631–4.
Talevi A, Bruno-Blanch LE. Efflux transporters at the blood–brain barrier: Therapeutic opportunities. In: Montenegro PA, Juárez SM, editors. Blood–brain barrier: new research. 1st ed. New York: Nova Science; 2012.
Talevi A, Sella-Cravero M, Castro EA, Bruno-Blanch LE. Discovery of anticonvulsant activity of abietic acid through application of linear discriminant analysis. Bioorg Med Chem Lett. 2007a;17:1684–90.
Talevi A, Bellera CL, Castro EA, Bruno-Blanch LE. A successful virtual screening application: prediction of anticonvulsant activity en MES test of widely-used pharmaceutical and food preservatives methylparaben and propylparaben. J Comput Aided Mol Des. 2007b;21:527–38.
Talevi A, Enrique AV, Bruno-Blanch LE. Anticonvulsant activity of artificial sweeteners: a structural link between sweet-taste receptor T1R3 and brain glutamate receptors. Bioorg Med Chem Lett. 2012;22:4072–4.
Thakur R, Gupta RB. Formation of phenytoin nanoparticles using rapid expansion of supercritical solution with solid cosolvent (RESS-SC) process. Int J Pharm. 2006;308:190–9. doi: 10.1016/j.ijpharm.2005.11.005.
Tishler DM, Weinberg KI, Hinton DR, Barbaro N, Annett GM, Raffel C. MDR1 gene expression in brain of patients with medically intractable epilepsy. Epilepsia. 1995;36:1–6.
Tiwari A, Sodani K, Dai CL, Ashby CR, Chen ZS. Revisiting the ABCs of multidrug resistance in cancer chemotherapy. Curr Pharm Biotechnol. 2011;12:570–94.
Trojnar MK, Wierzchowska-Cioch E, Krzyżanowski M, Jargiełło M, Czuczwar SJ. New generation of valproic acid. Pol J Pharmacol. 2004;56:283–8.
van Vliet EA, van Schaik R, Edelbroek PM, Redeker S, Aronica E, Wadman WJ, et al. Inhibition of the multidrug transporter P-glycoprotein improves seizure control in pehnytoin-treated chronic epileptic rats. Epilepsia. 2006;47:672–80.
Varshosaz J, Eskandari S, Tabakhian M. Production and optimization of valproic acid nanostructured lipid carriers by the Taguchi design. Pharm Dev Technol. 2010;15:89–96.
Vezzani A, Granata T. Brain inflammation in epilepsy: experimental and clinical evidence. Epilepsia. 2005;46:1724–43.

Vezzani A, Fench J, Bartfai T, Baram TZ. The role of inflammation in epilepsy. Nat Rev Neurol. 2011;7:31–40.

Volk HA, Arabadzisz D, Fritschy JM, Brandt C, Bethmann K, Löscher W. Antiepileptic drug resistant rats differ from drug responsive rats in hippocampal neurodegeneration and $GABA_A$ receptor ligand-binding in a model of temporal lobe epilepsy. Neurobiol Dis. 2006;21: 633–46.

Von Wedel-Parlow M, Wölte P, Galla HJ. Regulation of major efflux transporters under inflammatory conditions at the blood–brain barrier *in vitro*. J Neurochem. 2009;111:111–8.

Vreugdenhil M, Wadman WJ. Modulation of sodium currents in rat CA1 neurons by carbamazepine and valproate after kindling epileptogenesis. Epilepsia. 1999;40:1512–22.

Waldbaum S, Patel M. Mitochondrial dysfunction and oxidative stress: a contributing link to acquired epilepsy? J Bioenerg Biomembr. 2010a;42:449–55.

Waldbaum S, Patel M. Mitochondria, oxidative stress, and temporal lobe epilepsy. Epilepsy Res. 2010b;88:23–45.

Waldbaum S, Liang LP, Patel M. Persistent impairment of mitochondrial and tissue redox stratus during lithium–pilocarpine-induced apileptogenesis. J Neurochem. 2010;115:1172–82.

Whitaker WR, Faull RL, Dragunow M, Mee EW, Emson PC, Clare JJ. Changes in the mRNAs encoding voltage-gated sodium channel types II and III in human epileptic hippocampus. Neuroscience. 2001;106:275–85.

Williamson PR, Marson AG, Coffey AJ, Middleditch C, Rogers J, Bentley DR, et al. Clinical factors and ABCB1 polymorphisms in prediction of antiepileptic drug response: a prospective cohort study. Lancet Neurol. 2006;5:668–76.

Wohlfart S, Gelperina S, Kreuter J. Transport of drugs across the blood–brain barrier by nanoparticles. J Control Release. 2012;161:264–73.

Wong EH, Tarazi FI, Shahid M. The effectiveness of multitarget agents in schizophrenia and mood disorders: relevance of receptor signature to clinical action. Pharmacol Therapeut. 2010; 126:173–85.

Wu J, Ji H, Wang Y, Li YQ, Li WG, Long Y, et al. Glutathione depletion upregulates P-glycoprotein expression at the blood–brain barrier in rats. J Pharm Pharmacol. 2009;61:819–24.

Youdim MBH, Buccadfasco JJ. Multi-functional drugs for various CNS targets in the treatment of neurodegenerative disorders. Trends Pharmacol Sci. 2005;26:27–35.

Zeng TF, An DM, Li JM, Li YH, Chen L, Hong Z, et al. Evaluation of different antiepileptic drug strategies in medically refractory epilepsy patients following epilepsy surgery. Epilepsy Res. 2012;101:14–21.

Zhang P, Hu L, Wang Y, Wang J, Feng L, Li Y. Poly(ε-caprolactone)-blockpoly(ethyl ethylene phosphate) micelles for brain-targeting drug delivery: *in vitro* and *in vivo* valuation. Pharm Res. 2010;27:2657–69.

Zhang C, Kwan P, Zuo Z, Baum L. The transport of antiepileptic drugs by P-glycoprotein. Adv Drug Deliv Rev. 2012;64:930–42.

Chapter 15
Modulating P-glycoprotein Regulation as a Therapeutic Strategy for Pharmacoresistant Epilepsy

Heidrun Potschka

Abstract Experimental data suggest a role of blood–brain barrier P-glycoprotein over-expression as a factor contributing to drug-resistant epilepsy. Therefore, efforts are made developing and validating therapeutic approaches which aim to overcome transporter-mediated drug resistance.

Considering the physiological function of efflux transporters it will be advantageous to preserve the basal transport function. Thus, recent studies focused on the elucidation of key signaling factors driving P-glycoprotein up-regulation in response to epileptic seizure activity. Based on these investigations novel concepts have been developed blocking the signaling pathway and controlling P-glycoprotein expression despite recurrent seizure activity. Further development of respective approaches is based on ongoing studies which explore the relevance of the signaling mechanisms in human capillaries.

In general, the success of respective strategies will depend on the question whether patients exist in which P-glycoprotein over-expression constitutes a predominant factor contributing to therapeutic failure.

Keywords P-glycoprotein • Efflux transporters • Glutamate • Cyclooxygenase-2 • Drug resistance • Epilepsy

H. Potschka (✉)
Institute of Pharmacology, Toxicology, and Pharmacy, Ludwig-Maximilians-University, Koeniginstr. 16, Munich 80539, Germany
e-mail: potschka@pharmtox.vetmed.uni-muenchen.de

L. Rocha and E.A. Cavalheiro (eds.), *Pharmacoresistance in Epilepsy: From Genes and Molecules to Promising Therapies*, DOI 10.1007/978-1-4614-6464-8_15,

15.1 Introduction

Efflux transport mediated by blood–brain barrier P-glycoprotein is considered as a limiting factor in brain penetration of different antiepileptic drugs (Potschka 2010a). Up-regulation in the epileptic brain might therefore contribute to therapeutic failure.

Rodent studies supported a respective functional contribution to drug resistance in several studies (Potschka 2010a). However, although high expression rates have repeatedly been reported in tissue from patients with drug-resistant epilepsy (Tishler et al. 1995; Sisodiya et al. 1999, 2006; Aronica et al. 2003), data confirming a functional relevance in patients is still limited. Thus, further studies will be necessary to explore the role of P-glycoprotein over-expression in clinical drug resistance. Respective investigations will be of utmost importance considering that drug resistance reflects a multifactorial problem with several contributing factors also including target alterations and network alterations. In addition, epidemiology, intrinsic severity and genetics are known to affect pharmacosensitivity (Loscher and Sills 2007). Considering the multifactorial nature of drug resistance success of any strategy targeting P-glycoprotein as one of the efflux transporters will depend on the question whether patients exist with predominance of P-glycoprotein over-expression among different resistance factors. Moreover, it will be necessary to identify respective patients based on biomarkers such as positron emission tomography with P-glycoprotein substrate radiotracers.

15.2 Strategies to Overcome P-glycoprotein Mediated Efflux Transport

Various options have been discussed as putative strategies overcoming P-glycoprotein mediated efflux transport of antiepileptic drugs (Potschka 2010a).

One obvious strategy is based on pharmacological inhibition and modulation of P-glycoprotein function. Whereas first and second generation inhibitors of P-glycoprotein (e.g., verapamil, cyclosporin A, valspodar) were characterized by additional pharmacodynamic and pharmacokinetic effects which might hamper their use, more selective and potent third generation inhibitors (e.g., tariquidar, elacridar, zosuquidar) have been developed (Thomas and Coley 2003). These efforts in particular aimed to develop compounds for combination with cytostatic drugs in cancer patients in which transporter over-expression contributes to therapeutic failure. However, clinical studies have failed related to a relevant increase of the toxic effects of the cytostatic drugs likely to be due to enhanced distribution in various sensitive tissues and cells, which are known to be protected by P-glycoprotein from exposure to harmful xenobiotics (Fox and Bates 2007).

Considering a long-term add-on therapy with potent P-glycoprotein modulators in patients with drug-resistant epilepsy also needs to take into account that this will limit the protective function of P-glycoprotein throughout the body. Therefore one should only consider an interval therapy with a transient add-on of P-glycoprotein modulators until P-glycoprotein expression returns to control levels and antiepileptic drugs are efficacious again when administered alone. However, this hypothetical regime has not been validated so far, neither experimentally or clinically. So far experimental evidence has been obtained that tariquidar add-on treatment can help to overcome drug resistance in chronic models of drug-resistant temporal lobe epilepsy in rats (Brandt et al. 2006). Clinical experience with P-glycoprotein modulation is only limited to case reports, which can not be interpreted clearly as verapamil, which possesses additional pharmacodynamic and pharmacokinetic effects, has been used for P-glycoprotein modulation (Summers et al. 2004; Iannetti et al. 2005, 2009). Moreover, testing add-on therapy in a pilot translational study in canine patients with drug-resistant epilepsy indicated that verapamil might also aggravate seizure control (Jambroszyk et al. 2011).

As an alternate approach bypassing efflux transporters or bypassing the blood–brain barrier might be considered (Potschka 2010c). Nanoparticle encapsulation of antiepileptic drugs has been suggested as one approach. However, brain penetration and distribution rates are still not satisfying, so that further efforts seem to be necessary to optimize respective delivery tools. Local administration approaches are characterized by the invasiveness of the approach.

Considering the disadvantages or limitations of the different strategies efforts have been made to develop further alternatives. In particular it has been tried to identify targets in signaling pathways contributing to P-glycoprotein up-regulation in the epileptic brain. These targets might help to further develop add-on strategies preventing over-expression of P-glycoprotein in epilepsy patients (Potschka 2010b).

15.3 Regulation of P-glycoprotein Expression

In order to develop respective strategies it was crucial to identify key signaling factors which contribute to P-glycoprotein regulation in response to epileptic seizure activity. Glutamate was among the obvious candidate factors as it is released in high concentrations during an epileptic seizure and as first evidence has been described that glutamate might affect P-glycoprotein expression in brain capillaries. Glutamate incubation in ex vivo preparations of rodent brain capillaries confirmed that this neurotransmitter causes transcriptional activation of the P-glycoprotein encoding gene resulting in enhanced functional surface expression of the efflux transporter (Bauer et al. 2008). The in vivo role was substantiated by injecting glutamate in the right hippocampus of rats in concentrations that did not induce electrographic or behavioral seizure activity (Bauer et al. 2008). In this study glutamate obviously induced a local up-regulation of brain capillary P-glycoprotein expression. The effect of the neurotransmitter proved to be mediated by NMDA receptor signaling as an antagonist of this receptor prevented the impact of glutamate on P-glycoprotein (Bauer et al. 2008).

NMDA receptor activation seems to mediate its effects on transcriptional activation of the P-glycoprotein encoding gene via arachidonic acid signaling (Potschka 2010b). In this context, the role of the inflammatory enzyme cyclooxygenase-2 has been confirmed based on pharmacological inhibition as well genetic deficiency studies in isolated rodent brain capillaries (Bauer et al. 2008). In contrast, pharmacological modulation of cyclooxygenase-1 had no impact on glutamate-mediated increases in P-glycoprotein.

Among the prostanoid products of arachidonic acid signaling PGE_2 effects via its EP1 receptor were identified as another key element in the P-glycoprotein regulatory signaling pathway (Pekcec et al. 2009).

15.4 Targeting Signaling Pathways of P-glycoprotein

The elucidation of the key signaling factors, which drive P-glycoprotein expression in the epileptic brain raised the main question whether targeting of these factors might help to control P-glycoprotein expression at control levels and might help to overcome drug resistance (Fig. 15.1).

The cyclooxygenase-2 inhibitor celecoxib proved to be efficacious in a rat electrical status epilepticus model with prevention of seizure-associated P-glycoprotein

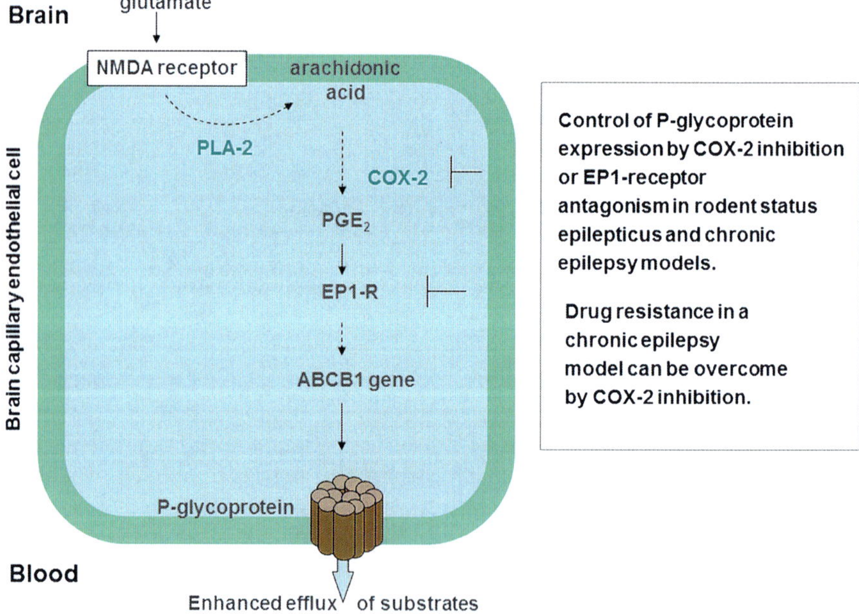

Fig. 15.1 Signaling pathway that up-regulates P-glycoprotein in response to seizure activity. Targets are indicated and main findings from animal experiments evaluating respective targeting strategies are summarized. *COX-2*-cyclooxygenase-2. Figure is modified from Potschka (2010b). Data are from Bauer et al. (2008), Zibell et al. (2009), Pekcec et al. (2009), Van Vliet et al. (2010), and Schlichtiger et al. (2010)

up-regulation in different areas of the hippocampus and cortex (Zibell et al. 2009). Even more importantly, cyclooxygenase-2 inhibition helped to bring brain P-glycoprotein expression rates back to control levels in a chronic rat epilepsy model with recurrent spontaneous seizures (van Vliet et al. 2010). In the same experimental setup pharmacological targeting of cyclooygenase-2 increased the brain penetration rate of the antiepileptic drug phenytoin (van Vliet et al. 2010).

As a next experimental step phenobarbital non-responders were selected in a chronic model with recurrent spontaneous seizures. Following the selection procedure rats were treated for 6 days with the cyclooxygenase-2 inhibitor celecoxib and then following withdrawal of celecoxib the efficacy of phenobarbital was tested again in the same group of animals (Schlichtiger et al. 2010). In this second drug treatment phase seizure control was significantly improved as a consequence of celecoxib pretreatment. In addition to the impact on P-glycoprotein further effects of the anti-inflammatory treatment might have contributed to the therapeutic success in this experimental setup. In particular, it is known that inflammatory processes can contribute to ictogenesis, might enhance signaling via glutamate receptors and decrease GABAergic signaling due to an impact on receptor subunit expression or due to a modulation of the functional state of the receptors (Vezzani et al. 2011).

Targeting of the EP1 receptor was further confirmed as an alternate approach to cyclooxygenase-2 inhibition. EP1 receptor antagonism kept P-glycoprotein expression at control levels in a rat status epilepticus model (Pekcec et al. 2009). Moreover, sub-chronic treatment with an EP1 receptor antagonist during a massive kindling phase with frequent elicitation of seizures improved the efficacy of phenobarbital on kindled seizures evaluated following withdrawal of the EP1 receptor antagonist. However, the efficacy in a model of drug-resistant epilepsy still needs to be evaluated.

In addition to targeting of the arachidonic acid signaling cascade one might also consider targeting of the NMDA receptor (Bankstahl et al. 2008; Bauer et al. 2008). However, earlier experimental and clinical studies have demonstrated that epilepsy causes a significantly enhanced sensitivity to the side effects of competitive and noncompetitive NMDA receptor antagonists (Loscher and Honack 1991a, b; Sveinbjornsdottir et al. 1993). Thus, translational development of respective experimental approaches, which proved that blocking of the NMDA receptor associated ion channel controls P-glycoprotein expression in a status epilepticus, can not be considered based on tolerability issues. Targeting of the co-agonist glycine binding site of the NMDA receptor might render an alternate target, which needs to be further studied.

In addition, it will be necessary to rule out species differences in the signaling pathways. Therefore, current investigations study the regulation in brain capillaries prepared from surgical specimen dissected from patients with drug-resistant epilepsy.

Considering that the clinical data supporting a functional relevance of transporter over-expression is still limited, it will be necessary to further assess the impact in patients. Moreover, taking the multifactorial nature of drug-resistance into account it needs to be determined whether a subgroup of patients exists in which a specific resistance mechanism predominates.

15.5 Biomarkers of P-glycoprotein Associated Drug Resistance

As outlined above it is of utmost importance to further assess the relevance of P-glycoprotein up-regulation in patients. In addition a tool will be needed to identify patients with P-glycoprotein over-expression for any application of therapeutic approaches aiming to overcome transporter-mediated resistance.

Considering the complexity of the regulatory events driving P-glycoprotein expression in the epileptic brain it is rather unlikely that genetic analyses will be helpful in this context (Potschka 2010d). Positron emission tomography has been suggested as an imaging tool for the analyses of blood–brain barrier P-glycoprotein function based on a clinical pilot study using [^{11}C] verapamil (Langer et al. 2007). Meanwhile the concept has been developed further with the performance of two subsequent scans using a P-glycoprotein substrate radiotracer with or without administration of a pharmacological P-glycoprotein modulator. In one of these studies [^{18}F] MPPF has been validated as a suitable radiotracer. In control rats tariquidar pretreatment significantly affected the influx and efflux rates of [^{18}F] MPPF confirming that the tracer is subject to blood–brain barrier efflux transport mediated by P-glycoprotein (la Fougere et al. 2010). Based on these findings, the tracer kinetics was compared between phenobarbital responder and non-responder rats in a chronic epilepsy model. The findings revealed that in line with the hypothesis non-responder rats exhibited a more pronounced response to the P-glycoprotein modulator tariquidar in that the influx and the efflux rate of [^{18}F] MPPF was affected more intensely in non-responders as compared to responders (Bartmann et al. 2010).

Based on these data respective positron emission tomography (PET) studies are currently performed in patients. However, it needs to be considered that the variance will be much higher in patients including differences in the pathology and differences in the treatment regime which might affect tracer brain penetration as well as its modulation by tariquidar. In particular, it will be difficult to predict the interaction between the tracer, the modulator and those antiepileptic drugs which are P-glycoprotein substrates. The large binding pocket of the transporter molecule allows different scenarios in the interaction between compounds that bind to P-glycoprotein in parallel. Some might competitively inhibit each others binding and transport, whereas others might be co-transported.

15.6 Future Perspectives

Whereas experimental data obviously confirm a contribution of the efflux transporter P-glycoprotein to drug resistance, respective clinical data are still limited. Thus, further studies are urgently needed to finally conclude about the functional relevance in the clinical setting. Moreover, translational development of any strategy overcoming efflux transport is based on the assumption that a subgroup of patients exists in which this mechanism of resistance predominates among others such as network and target alterations. Provided that clinical proof-of-principle is obtained in the future, it will be necessary to select patients with transporter overexpression for respective clinical studies.

References

Aronica E, Gorter JA, Jansen GH, van Veelen CW, van Rijen PC, Leenstra S, et al. Expression and cellular distribution of multidrug transporter proteins in two major causes of medically intractable epilepsy: focal cortical dysplasia and glioneuronal tumors. Neuroscience. 2003;118:417–29.

Bankstahl JP, Hoffmann K, Bethmann K, Loscher W. Glutamate is critically involved in seizure-induced overexpression of P-glycoprotein in the brain. Neuropharmacology. 2008;54: 1006–16.

Bartmann H, Fuest C, la Fougere C, Xiong G, Just T, Schlichtiger J, et al. Imaging of P-glycoprotein-mediated pharmacoresistance in the hippocampus: proof-of-concept in a chronic rat model of temporal lobe epilepsy. Epilepsia. 2010;51:1780–90.

Bauer B, Hartz AM, Pekcec A, Toellner K, Miller DS, Potschka H. Seizure-induced up-regulation of P-glycoprotein at the blood–brain barrier through glutamate and cyclooxygenase-2 signaling. Mol Pharmacol. 2008;73:1444–53.

Brandt C, Bethmann K, Gastens AM, Loscher W. The multidrug transporter hypothesis of drug resistance in epilepsy: proof-of-principle in a rat model of temporal lobe epilepsy. Neurobiol Dis. 2006;24:202–11.

Fox E, Bates SE. Tariquidar (XR9576): a P-glycoprotein drug efflux pump inhibitor. Expert Rev Anticancer Ther. 2007;7:447–59.

Iannetti P, Spalice A, Parisi P. Calcium-channel blocker verapamil administration in prolonged and refractory status epilepticus. Epilepsia. 2005;46:967–9.

Iannetti P, Parisi P, Spalice A, Ruggieri M, Zara F. Addition of verapamil in the treatment of severe myoclonic epilepsy in infancy. Epilepsy Res. 2009;85:89–95.

Jambroszyk M, Tipold A, Potschka H. Add-on treatment with verapamil in pharmacoresistant canine epilepsy. Epilepsia. 2011;52:284–91.

la Fougere C, Boning G, Bartmann H, Wangler B, Nowak S, Just T, et al. Uptake and binding of the serotonin 5-HT1A antagonist [18 F]-MPPF in brain of rats: effects of the novel P-glycoprotein inhibitor tariquidar. Neuroimage. 2010;49:1406–15.

Langer O, Bauer M, Hammers A, Karch R, Pataraia E, Koepp MJ, et al. Pharmacoresistance in epilepsy: a pilot PET study with the P-glycoprotein substrate R-[(11)C]verapamil. Epilepsia. 2007;48:1774–84.

Loscher W, Sills GJ. Drug resistance in epilepsy: why is a simple explanation not enough? Epilepsia. 2007;48:2370–2.

Loscher W, Honack D. Anticonvulsant and behavioral effects of two novel competitive N-methyl-D-aspartic acid receptor antagonists, CGP 37849 and CGP 39551, in the kindling model of epilepsy. Comparison with MK-801 and carbamazepine. J Pharmacol Exp Ther. 1991a; 256:432–40.

Loscher W, Honack D. The novel competitive N-methyl-D-aspartate (NMDA) antagonist CGP 37849 preferentially induces phencyclidine-like behavioral effects in kindled rats: attenuation by manipulation of dopamine, alpha-1 and serotonin1A receptors. J Pharmacol Exp Ther. 1991b;257:1146–53.

Pekcec A, Unkruer B, Schlichtiger J, Soerensen J, Hartz AM, Bauer B, et al. Targeting prostaglandin E2 EP1 receptors prevents seizure-associated P-glycoprotein up-regulation. J Pharmacol Exp Ther. 2009;330:939–47.

Potschka H. Modulating P-glycoprotein regulation: Future perspectives for pharmacoresistant epilepsies? Epilepsia. 2010a;51(8):1333–47.
Potschka H. Targeting regulation of ABC efflux transporters in brain diseases: a novel therapeutic approach. Pharmacol Ther. 2010b;125:118–27.
Potschka H. Targeting the brain – surmounting or bypassing the blood–brain barrier. Handb Exp Pharmacol. 2010c;197:411–31.
Potschka H. Transporter hypothesis of drug-resistant epilepsy: challenges for pharmacogenetic approaches. Pharmacogenomics. 2010d;11:1427–38.
Schlichtiger J, Pekcec A, Bartmann H, Winter P, Fuest C, Soerensen J, et al. Celecoxib treatment restores pharmacosensitivity in a rat model of pharmacoresistant epilepsy. Br J Pharmacol. 2010;160:1062–71.
Sisodiya SM, Heffernan J, Squier MV. Over-expression of P-glycoprotein in malformations of cortical development. Neuroreport. 1999;10:3437–41.
Sisodiya SM, Martinian L, Scheffer GL, van der Valk P, Scheper RJ, Harding BN, et al. Vascular colocalization of P-glycoprotein, multidrug-resistance associated protein 1, breast cancer resistance protein and major vault protein in human epileptogenic pathologies. Neuropathol Appl Neurobiol. 2006;32:51–63.
Summers MA, Moore JL, McAuley JW. Use of verapamil as a potential P-glycoprotein inhibitor in a patient with refractory epilepsy. Ann Pharmacother. 2004;38:1631–4.
Sveinbjornsdottir S, Sander JW, Upton D, Thompson PJ, Patsalos PN, Hirt D, et al. The excitatory amino acid antagonist D-CPP-ene (SDZ EAA-494) in patients with epilepsy. Epilepsy Res. 1993;16:165–74.
Thomas H, Coley HM. Overcoming multidrug resistance in cancer: an update on the clinical strategy of inhibiting p-glycoprotein. Cancer Control. 2003;10:159–65.
Tishler DM, Weinberg KI, Hinton DR, Barbaro N, Annett GM, Raffel C. MDR1 gene expression in brain of patients with medically intractable epilepsy. Epilepsia. 1995;36:1–6.
van Vliet EA, Zibell G, Pekcec A, Schlichtiger J, Edelbroek PM, Holtman L, et al. COX-2 inhibition controls P-glycoprotein expression and promotes brain delivery of phenytoin in chronic epileptic rats. Neuropharmacology. 2010;58:404–12.
Vezzani A, Aronica E, Mazarati A, Pittman QJ. Epilepsy and brain inflammation. Exp Neurol. 2011;232:143–8. (in press).
Zibell G, Unkruer B, Pekcec A, Hartz AM, Bauer B, Miller DS, et al. Prevention of seizure-induced up-regulation of endothelial P-glycoprotein by COX-2 inhibition. Neuropharmacology. 2009;56:849–55.

Chapter 16
Vagus Nerve Stimulation for Intractable Seizures

Mario A. Alonso-Vanegas

Abstract Vagus nerve stimulation (VNS) is the most widely used non-pharmacological treatment for pharmacoresistant epilepsy since 1988 based on experimental and clinical observations over several decades. In 1997, the FDA approved VNS "as an adjunctive treatment for partial refractory epilepsy in adults and adolescents over 12 years of age". Considering that polytherapy seldom contributes to seizure control after monotherapy has failed, the need for options—even if only palliative—to address the devastating health, psychosocial, and economic consequences of refractory epilepsy in selected groups and the increasing concern about adverse effects of medications on neurological development, VNS usage has been extended to younger age groups and patients with generalized seizures, who are not candidates for resective surgery. VNS therapy involves implantation of a battery-operated device in the upper chest with two subcutaneously placed wires with electrodes attached to the left vagus nerve in the carotid sheath. The generator is programmed by a telemetry wand attached to a laptop computer. Stimulation is usually initiated 15 days alter implantation and adjusted over time on the basis of patient tolerance and response. The safety, tolerability, and efficacy of the procedure and therapy have been repeatedly demonstrated in prospective randomized clinical trials, uncontrolled retrospective series and long-term follow-up series. Complications of surgery are rare with infection being the most often reported, while stimulation related side effects are usually mild and in most cases decrease over time or can be resolved by changing stimulation parameters. Series have shown a remarkably consistent average reduction in seizure frequency of 40–50% responder rate (i.e., the proportion of patients whose seizure frequency is reduced by at least 50%) with no obvious indication of tolerance and generally a long-term increase

M.A. Alonso-Vanegas, M.D. (✉)
ABC Hospital, Santa Fé, Neurology Center, and National Institute of Neurology and Neurosurgery "Manuel Velasco Suárez", Mexico city, Mexico
e-mail: alonsovanegasm@gmail.com

L. Rocha and E.A. Cavalheiro (eds.), *Pharmacoresistance in Epilepsy: From Genes and Molecules to Promising Therapies*, DOI 10.1007/978-1-4614-6464-8_16,

of efficacy. The number of patients who become seizure free is relatively small. The use of on-demand stimulation triggered by a handheld magnet that may help to prevent or abort seizures has also been cited as a substantial benefit. Other positive outcome measures include improvement in mood, alertness, memory and postictal recovery period, which have been collectively seen as improvement in quality of life. Cost-benefit of the therapy has also been documented, although in many countries the deterrent to the use of VNS is currently the initial cost of the device. However, despite extensive clinical studies and studies on experimental animal models, three aspects of VNS remain elusive (a) the exact mechanisms of action, (b) the definition of stimulation parameters for optimal seizure control, and (c) the precision of factors that can predict which patients will respond and to what extent. Given these evidences, VNS should be considered within a comprehensive epilepsy surgery center on a patient to patient basis, following a detailed bio-psycho-social workup and review of expenses ands risks weighted against expectations, and potential improvements in seizures and quality of life.

Keywords Vagus nerve stimulation • Intractable seizures • VNS mechanisms of action • Stimulation parameters • Seizure outcome • Other measures of outcome • Predictive factors

16.1 Introduction

During the 15 years since the FDA approved vagus nerve stimulation (VNS) therapy in 1997, and its earlier approval in the European community in 1994, VNS has become a mainstay in the comprehensive treatment of epilepsy. In a book dealing with pharmacoresistant epilepsy, the reason for this trend should be fairly evident, since we are faced with the—also evident and permanently latent—reality that there are—despite new antiepileptic medications (AEDs) and dramatic improvements in resective surgical procedures—still many patients with refractory epilepsy who do not benefit from any of these advances and carry a great burden on quality of life and overall cost of the disease. As other neuromodulation techniques are explored as alternative therapies for these subsets of refractory epilepsy patients, VNS, which consists in the chronic and intermittent stimulation of the vagus nerve (VN) in its intracranial cervical segment, remains the only approved modality. The safety and effectiveness of the procedure have been established in prospective randomized clinical trials and uncontrolled retrospective series (Ben-Menachem 2001; Schachter and Wheless 2002) showing a remarkably consistent average reduction in seizure frequency of 40–50% responder rate (i.e., the proportion of patients whose seizure frequency is reduced by at least 50%) with no obvious indication of tolerance, and, these have been compelling reasons to continue its use in treatment of intractable seizures. However, there are three basic considerations that render the precise role of VNS in the treatment of refractory epilepsy, as yet, uncharacterized and, practically, a palliative approach, (a) the fact that the pathophysiology of stimulation remains elusive, (b) the imprecise definition of stimulation protocols/parameters and (c) the lack o prognostic factors that reliably predict its effectiveness (Elliott et al. 2011a). Hence the most important consideration to keep in mind is that VNS should be considered within a comprehensive epilepsy program as an option based on exclusion criteria: the selection should be assessed on a patient to patient basis, ensuring that potential benefits on seizure reduction and quality of life justify the risks and expense of VNS therapy.

16.2 Mechanisms of Action (MOA)

The mechanisms leading to seizure suppression remain undefined, despite numerous experimental and clinical studies focusing primarily on four areas: neurophysiology, neuroanatomy, neurochemistry and cerebral blood flow (CBF). Since this therapy build on the work of Bailey and Bremmer in the 1930s and Dell, Olsen, and Zanchetti in the 1950s, as Zabara proposed to "desynchronize" cerebral cortical activity, thereby attenuating seizure frequency, by applying intermittent electrical current to the cervical VN, it was assumed VNS would produce changes in the electroencephalogram (EEG) in humans, and many initial studies focused on these changes (Hammond et al. 1992). However, no conclusive changes in basal activity have been demonstrated. Several investigators have reported EEG changes during sleep and awake states, as well as acute and chronic changes in EEG and evoked potentials (Marrosu et al. 2005; Hammond et al. 1992; Koo 2001) documented a progressive EEG change characterized by grouping of epileptic activity followed by increasingly longer periods without seizures. One study that evaluated interictal epileptiform discharges documented an important decrease of such discharges when compared to a basal recording without VNS (Kuba et al. 2002). The differences in animal and human effects of VNS may be largely explained because VNS efficacy in animals has been primarily assessed in acute models (3-mercaptopropionate, pentylenetetrazole, maximal electroshock, penicillin or strychnine application), and only a few studies have used chronic animal models of epilepsy (Lockard et al. 1990; Muñana et al. 2002). In the Genetic Absence Epilepsy Rats of Strasbourg, acute VNS applied shortly after the onset of Spike wave discharges (SWD) prolonged the mean duration of SWD during the first day of VNS, but chronic stimulation hardly affected SWD (Dedeurwaerdere et al. 2005). It has also been shown that VNS exerts a powerful acute anticonvulsant effect on spontaneous seizures occurring in rats, previously submitted to full electrical kindling of the amygdala. In particular, this VNS-treated kindled rat model has been proposed as clinically relevant since it affects limbic seizures, which are most responsive to VNS in epilepsy patients (Rijkers et al. 2010). Another point that has been made to explain differences in animal and human studies is that in animal experiments the effect of VNS is evaluated when stimulation is performed in close relation to time of seizure onset, testing the antiseizure effect of VNS. In human beings, VNS is used in an intermittent mode. Seizures are also suppressed when the stimulator is in the "off" mode, suggesting an antiepileptic rather than an antiseizure effect only. This finding is supported by the animal studies by Takaya et al. (1996) who demonstrated that the efficacy of VNS outlasts duration of the stimulation train. There may be different pathways involved in antiseizure and antiepileptic effects.

The fact that seizures recur after the end of battery life has been reached, is a strong argument against VNS having an antiepileptic effect. However, as development of more relevant animal model progresses, the antiepileptic potential of neuromodulation in general is being explored and some promising results have been reported. VNS significantly delayed amygdaloid kindling (AK) in cats and stage VI was not reached despite 50 AK trials (Fernandez-Guardiola et al. 1999) but this effect was absent when VNS was started after the cats had already reached a more severe seizure stage (Magdaleno-Madrigal et al. 2004). Kindling in rats was slowed as well: 1 h of VNS prior to the kindling pulse increased the mean number of stimuli needed to reach the generalized seizure state (Naritoku and Mikels 1997). These anti-epileptogenic effects of VNS, however, could not be confirmed by another study, where the kindling rate did not differ between animals treated with 2 h of VNS prior to the kindling stimulus and controls (Dedeurwaerdere et al. 2006). The authors suggested that VNS treatment could have rendered the amygdala more excitable because after discharge threshold determination evoked generalized seizures in all VNS treated animals and only in half of the controls. There is one report of long lasting seizure control after explantation of the VNS device (Labar and Ponticello 2003).

The early hypothesis of cortical desynchronization induced by activation of unmyelinated afferent vagal fibers through the reticular activating system was contradicted in human studies, because, effective therapeutic parameters were subthreshold for fibers C. Krahl et al. (2001) found strong evidence that vagal fibers C are neither responsible nor necessary for the seizure-suppressing effect of VNS. According to their experiments in awake and freely moving cats, activation of myelinated A and B fibers is responsible for seizure suppression.

Other studies have focused on activation/deactivation of certain brain areas using regional blood flow mapping, single-photon emission computed tomography (SPECT), positron emission tomography (PET), and functional MRI (fMR). Increased bilateral brain activity in the rostral medulla, thalamus, hypothalamus, insula, and postcentral gyrus, with greater contralateral activation has been documented. Reduced perfusion during stimulation in the ipsilateral brain stem and limbic system has also been evidenced (Barnes et al. 2003). One study carried out with SPECT and EEG during VNS activation/deactivation demonstrated that with short-cycle stimulation (7-s stimulation, 12-s turned off) there was a relative reduction in the medial bilateral thalamus (Ring et al. 2000). Studies carried out using fMR found induced activation by left VNS in the thalamus (bilateral and towards the left side), bilateral insular cortex, postcentral gyrus and ipsilateral basal ganglia, right temporal posterosuperior gyrus and inferomedial occipital gyrus (higher on left side). The highest activity was found in the left thalamus and insular cortex. This suggests that these areas play an important role in modulation of brain cortex activity (Narayanan et al. 2002). It is likely that VNS also causes antiseizure effects at non-thalamic sites, including the locus coeruleus, which produces most of the cerebral norepinephrine (NE), and the raphe nuclei, which produce most brain serotonin. Another structure identified in the anticonvulsant effect of VNS is the nucleus of the solitary tract (NST), which receives 95% of the vagal afferent fibers and is regulated by cholinergic innervation. Moreover, the NST projects the sensory information to different areas of the brain, including the amygdala, cerebellum, hypothalamus, thalamus, parabrachial nucleus, raphe nuclei, and locus coeruleus. Thus, the VN is projecting sensory information via NST to NE and serotonin (5-HT) systems, which are associated with the regulation of mood, anxiety, emotion, and seizure activity. Interestingly, it has been found that changes in γ-aminobutyric acid (GABA)-ergic and glutamatergic transmission in the NST can regulate the susceptibility to seizures (Walker et al. 1999). In particular, an increase in GABA transmission or a decrease in glutamate transmission in the rat NST reduces susceptibility to limbic motor seizures evoked by systemic and focal bicuculline and systemic pentylenetetrazol. However, hippocampal GABA levels were not changed after VNS (Meurs et al. 2008).

Other investigations on MOA focus on metabolites expressed in VNS cases or activation areas. An increase in 5-hydroxyindoleacetic acid, homovanillic acid, aspartate, 5-HT and dopamine metabolites, which are significantly associated with seizure control, has been demonstrated. Also, some studies have documented an increase in GABA and ethanolamine in responders. VNS protects cortical glutamic acid decarboxylase (GAD) positive neurons from death subsequent to brain lesions, and may increase GAD cell count in the hippocampal hilus of the injured brain (Neese et al. 2007). Using a SPECT study in patients with pharmacoresistant epilepsy, it was described that VNS may modulate cortical excitability of brain areas associated with epileptogenesis and that GABA-A receptor plasticity contributes to this effect (Marrosu et al. 2003).

Concerning growth factors known to play a crucial role in neuronal trophism, acute VNS in normal rats increases expression of brain-derived neurotrophic factor (BDNF) and fibroblast growth factor in the hippocampus and cerebral cortex, and decreases the abundance of nerve growth factor mRNA in the hippocampus (Follesa et al. 1994). Furthermore, progenitor cell proliferation in the dentate gyrus increases after 3–48 h of VNS (Revesz et al. 2008) and is still detectable 3 weeks later. Chronic VNS for 4 weeks on the other hand did not affect the number of proliferating cells (Biggio et al. 2009). Survival of progenitor cells is also not enhanced by VNS (Revesz et al. 2008). Since, both NE and 5-HT can influence progenitor cell proliferation (Kulkarni et al. 2002), these VNS-induced plastic changes may be the result of reported neurotransmitter changes.

The VN is also implicated in immunomodulation as efferent vagus nerve fibers systemically inhibit pro-inflammatory cytokine release (Pavlov and Tracey 2005). Although it is still unclear to what extent VNS affects this so-called "cholinergic anti-inflammatory pathway", VNS appears to exert an afferent neuroimmunomodulatory effect since 2 h of continuous VNS induced expression of the pro-inflammatory cytokin interleukin-1beta in the hippocampus and hypothalamus of rats (Hosoi et al. 2000). Furthermore, VNS activates the hypothalamic–pituitary–adrenal axis. This was demonstrated by VNS-induced increased hippocampal expression of corticotrophin releasing factor and increased plasma levels of adrenocorticotropic hormone and corticosterone after VNS (Hosoi et al. 2000).

Given these experimental observations and the variable clinical response in different patient subgroups (according to age/type of seizures/etiology) it seems plausible to propose that the MOA of VNS involve a number of neural pathways and networks, with some synergistic actions, possibly with AED regimens, as well. As described in a recently published review article of animal models for VNS (Aalbers et al. 2011), future studies should be directed at more precise elucidation of the MOA. More knowledge about the pathways and networks involved may eventually lead to a more effective target for antiepileptic neuromodulation. Furthermore, these studies should make an attempt to identify VNS responder characteristics to find (bio)markers that can be used in clinical practice to identify responders.

16.3 Patient Selection and Indications

Physicians often differ in their opinions about when it is appropriate to begin discussing the possibility of VNS therapy. In the 30–40% of patients who are evaluated for pharmacoresistant epilepsy, there is often a controversy whether polytherapy is appropriate after two trials of monotherapy have failed, but most agree that patients with localization-related seizures should be evaluated for epilepsy surgery if the third drug trial fails to control the seizures (Fig. 16.1). It is our practice to follow a

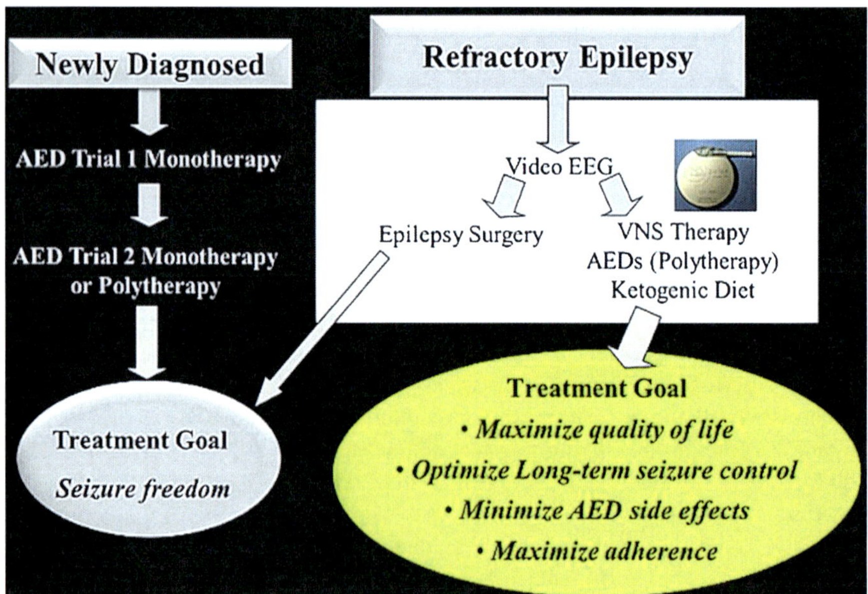

Fig. 16.1 Decision making of treatment stages and goals

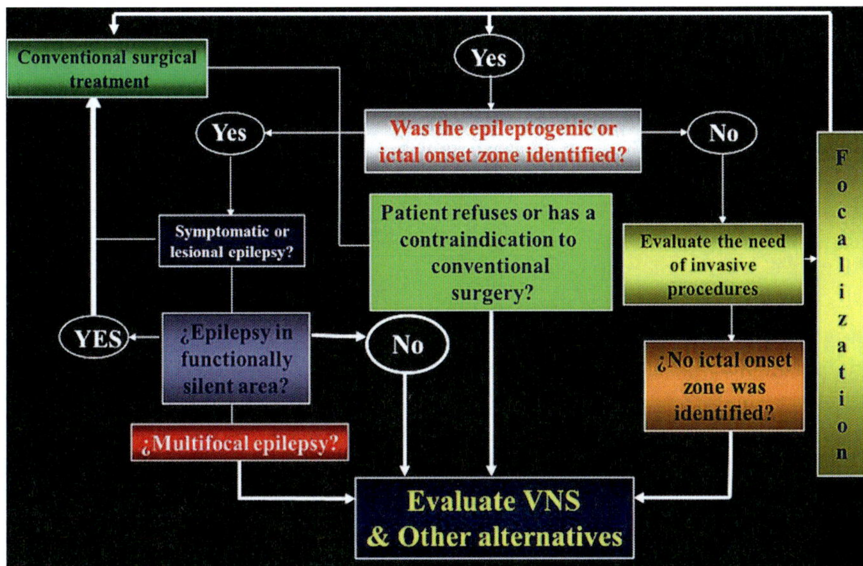

Fig. 16.2 Study algorithm for refractory epilepsy patients

protocolized presurgical evaluation in these patients that includes at least history and physical examination, EEG, MR imaging and in most cases video-EEG and functional imaging studies, and offer or discuss surgical options only once a detailed description or working hypothesis of the seizure type, epileptic syndrome and possible epileptogenic area has been determined (Fig. 16.2). As has been stated, the author considers VNS as a last resort option when other surgical treatments have been discarded.

Initially the FDA approved the use of VNS as an adjunctive therapy in adults and adolescents with partial onset seizures. However, this therapy has been increasingly applied to diverse groups of patients, obtaining benefits in cases with tuberous sclerosis (Parain et al. 2001), Lennox–Gastaut syndrome (Frost et al. 2001), hypothalamic hamartomas (Murphy et al. 2000), ring chromosome 20 syndrome with intractable epilepsy (Chawla et al. 2002), and bitemporal epilepsy (Kuba et al. 2003). Because polytherapy trials seldom contribute to seizure control after monotherapy has failed and because of the increasing concern about adverse effects of medications on neurological development, VNS usage was extended to patients <12 years old. During the initial experience it was observed that 61% of the pediatric population presented a seizure frequency reduction >50% at 12 months (Wheless and Maggio 2002) and even more favorable rates were suggested as typical response for this population (Murphy et al. 2003). The findings by Thompson et al. (2012) in 146 patients followed up for a mean of 41 months, 32% with partial epilepsy and 68% generalized epilepsy, showing reduction in seizure frequency in 91% of patients, seizure duration in 50%, postictal period in 49%, and antiepileptic medication use in 75% clearly suggest limitations on the FDA-approved indications for

VNS therapy, which reflect the design of the original preapproval prospective studies, and do not accurately delineate the patient population able to benefit from this approach.

Another three scenarios have been considered as possible indications, namely cases in which patients, for personal reasons emphatically refuse brain surgery; patients with severe epilepsy in whom surgery carries significant risk of failure and/or functional postoperative deficits and caregivers decide that the expense of VNS is preferable as an initial option, and selected cases with failed surgical results (Amar et al. 2008; Vale et al. 2011).

Once the VNS option is discussed with the patient, there should be an extensive explanation about the cost of the device, the reduced possibility that the patient will be seizure free and all other risks and potential benefits, assuring a well-informed decision. Patients/caregivers should be informed that the antiepileptic effect is generally delayed after the procedure, as well as about the difficulty of removing the vagal electrode and the need to replace the battery after its useful life.

16.4 Surgical Procedure

Surgical implantation usually takes 1–2 h (Fig. 16.3). General anesthesia is preferred although, in principle, local anesthesia is feasible. It is often stated that the procedure can be performed by neurosurgeons, vascular surgeons, or ear, nose, and throat specialists, familiar with the surgical anatomy of the vagus nerve adjacent to the carotid artery. This is evidently correct, but it must always be considered that the implantation procedure must be preceded by a protocolized presurgical evaluation and followed up by the programming of the device in a comprehensive program that specializes in intractable seizures. The patient is positioned supine with a shoulder roll beneath the scapula to provide mild neck extension and the head rotated 30° towards the right. Prior asepsis and antisepsis, sterile drapes are placed and a 3 cm horizontal incision in the lateral neck is made, from the internal border of the sternocleidomastoid muscle to the midline; the platysma muscle is divided vertically and the investing layer of deep cervical fascia is opened along the anterior border of the sternocleidomastoid muscle, allowing it to be mobilized laterally to place a Weitlander retractor. The thyroid, trachea, esophagus and laryngeal recurrent nerve contained in the pretracheal fascia are retracted in bloc medially. The carotid sheath is incised with Metzenbaum scissors and the deep aponeurosis is dissected to identify the jugular vein, the vagus nerve and common carotid artery. An automatic valve retractor is placed to contain the structures of the midline medially and the muscular mass laterally. The dissection of the vagus nerve, at least 3.5 cm in length, is carried out carefully with Metzenbaum scissors and DeBakey tweezers. In case of bleeding, a bipolar coagulator should be used. Next a transversal 5 cm incision along the lateral border of the pectoralis major muscle and a subcutaneous pocket in the subcutaneous-muscle juncture is created to contain the generator. A tunneling tool is then used to create a subcutaneous tract between the two incisions. The field

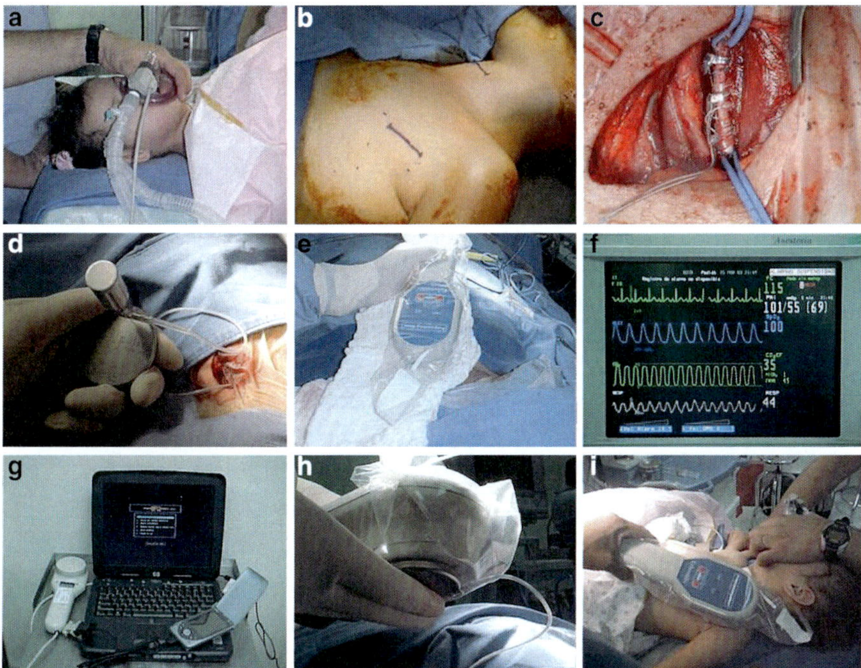

Fig. 16.3 Sequence of the surgical procedure: showing general anesthesia (**a**), positioning of the patient showing markers for cutaneous incisions (**b**), electrodes wrapped around the VN (**c**), with the hair pin resistor inserted into the receptacles for the lead connector pins, the telemetry wand interrogates the device from within a sterile sheath (**d**, **e**), monitoring of electrocardiographic and vital signs during the stimulation test (**f**), external programming equipment (**g**), final impedance test (**h**), and percutaneous tests (**i**)

is irrigated with physiological solution and antibiotic. Depending on the relative size of the exposed nerve, either a small or large helical electrode is selected. The lead connector pins are passed through the tunnel and emerge from the chest incision, while the helical electrodes remain exposed in the cervical region. The surgeon should grasp the suture tail at either end gently and apply each coil by stretching it over the nerve. The central turn of the unfurled coil is applied either obliquely or perpendicularly across or beneath the vagus trunk and wrapped around the nerve. The coil is then redirected parallel to the nerve as the remaining loops are applied proximal and distal to this midpoint. During these maneuvers the generator is tested. With the hair pin resistor inserted into the receptacles for the lead connector pins, the telemetry wand interrogates the device from within a sterile sheath to measure the internal impedance. Once the generator passes the pre-implantation test, it is ready for insertion. The lead connector pins are inserted into the pulse generator and secured to their receptacles with setscrews, using the included hexagonal torque wrench. A 1-min lead test is performed at a frequency of 20 Hz with an output current of 1mA and a pulse width of 500 μs, during which the patient's vital signs and electrocardiographic changes are monitored. After the stimulation test, the generator is restored to its inactive status. The distal lead is secured to the fascia of the carotid sheath. Finally the generator is retracted into the pocket and secured to the pectoralis fascia using nonabsorbable suture, using the suture hole contained within the epoxy resin holder. Wound closure proceeds in the standard multilayer fashion.

In children a subpectoral technique for generator implantation has been described and should be considered given the increased soft tissue coverage, improved cosmesis, lower risk of tampering or trauma and a comparable risk of infection (Bauman et al. 2006).

The device is usually activated 1–2 weeks postoperatively, often at the first outpatient follow-up. Continuous electrical stimulation of the vagus nerve in animal models has been shown to produce fibrosis and ultimately failure of the nerve, so stimulation is provided in an intermittent manner.

16.5 Magnet Use

Patients or caregivers can pass a handheld magnet over the implanted generator to initiate on demand stimulation, typically when a seizure is anticipated or is in progress. Commonly the current delivered by magnet-induced activation is set slightly higher than the regular level. The magnet also provides a means for the patient to deactivate the device. If the magnet is placed over the generator box and it remains there for more than a few seconds it becomes switched off. When the magnet is subsequently removed, it reactivates at the previous settings. Boon et al. (2001) described magnet use by 35 patients followed at a single center for an average of 35 months. Of the 21 patients who used the magnet, 7 reported no effect and 14 (67%) noted positive effects. Morris (2003) analyzed the data on magnet-activated VNS therapy from the double-blind, randomized E03 study (The Vagus Nerve Stimulation Study Group 1995) and the nonrandomized E04 study (Labar et al. 1999). This retrospective analysis of E03 and E04 data found that approximately half of the VNS therapy patients who used the magnet to activate stimulation gained some control over their seizures. About one-fifth of the patients in the treatment arm of the E03 study and the E04 study reported that they could abort seizures with the magnet. The E03 study analysis showed no correlation between the extent of magnet use and change in seizure frequency with programmed VNS therapy as measured during the acute phase of the trial. In a similar finding from the E04 trial, about two-thirds of the patients reporting magnet-activated improvement of more than 90% of their seizures were classified as non-responders to programmed VNS therapy because they experienced seizure frequency reductions of 50% or less. For these patients, magnet-activated, on-demand stimulation appears to have been VNS therapy's most important contribution to gaining a sense of control over their seizures. Achieving the best results from magnet-activated stimulation requires both appropriate VNS device settings and proper instruction in magnet use for patients and caregivers. Additional studies of programming settings for magnet-activated stimulation and analysis of quality-of-life aspects, such as increased sense of control or empowerment may provide a better understanding of this unique mode of delivering antiseizure therapy.

16.6 Stimulation Protocols

Standard parameter settings, as determined from the clinical trials range from 20 to 30 Hz at a pulse width of 250–500 μs and an output current of 0.25–3.5 mA for 30 s on time and 5 min off time. Initial stimulation is set at the low end of these ranges and slowly adjusted over time on the basis of patient tolerance and response. The position of the fascicles and key fascicles needed for effective stimulation may vary among patients and depending on the size of the nerve, the electrode may not fully encircle it. If the fibers of interest are in the uncovered region, they may require more current for activation. Patients should be closely monitored during the dose adjustment phase, typically every 2–4 weeks for the first 2 months following implantation. Optimizing response can be done by increasing output current or modifying ON/OFF times (duty cycles). Managing side effects can be done by decreasing signal frequency (from 30 to 20 Hz), decreasing output current (by 0.25 mA), reducing pulse width (from 500 to 250 μs) or reducing output current by 0.25 mA. Once a patient responds to a tolerated stimulation dose, further parameter adjustments are performed only as clinically required. Currently, the best approach is to guide stimulation parameter titration on an individual basis, but future studies should be directed at identifying noninvasive measures that can guide individual titration. Routine assessment of lead wire integrity and generator function should be performed at regular visits. Battery life, which depends on output and magnet use, is now likely to exceed 6 years even at higher output levels, after which the pulse generator will need to be replaced. The device should be checked regularly and an early replacement indicator or "near end of service" (NEOS) alert warns the clinician of impending battery exhaustion.

16.7 Complications and Adverse Effects

Various complications and adverse effects have been well documented, although their incidence varies greatly in different reports and in most cases adverse effects decrease over time or can be resolved by changing stimulation parameters. Secondary stimulation related effects (viscerosensory symptoms, cough, hoarseness, dyspnea, dysphonia, dysphagia, neck, throat and chin numbness) are usually described as mild. Reported complications from a large (436 patients) single center study are described in Elliott et al. (2011a). Early clinical studies reported that if electrodes were placed below the cardiac branch of the VN, no cardiac effects would be manifested during stimulation. However, some ventricular asystole cases during impedance tests were reported (Ascanope et al. 1999) and according to the manufacturer's database, 98 patients from 60,014 implantations developed asystole or bradycardia during implantation (Cyberonics data on file, May 2008). The main reason for this phenomenon is lack of dissection of the cardiac branch during the procedure or lack of anatomic knowledge.

Surgical infection is the most commonly described complication, although the rates of 2–20 and 0.7–7.7% (Air et al. 2009; Benifla et al. 2006; Elliott et al. 2011a, b) in adults and children, respectively have varied considerably. It is interesting to note that larger series have generally reported lower infection rates, i.e., 0.7% infection rate in the series reported by Elliott et al. (2011a, b), 2.7% in the series by Thompson et al. (2012) and the author's own series of 100 consecutive cases with a 0% infection rate, which suggests that a proper and careful surgical technique, surgical volume, and experience contribute to beneficial outcomes for VNS therapy.

The possibility of tissue damage has been a concern; however, stimulation parameters have not been associated with nerve damage. Diathermy (shortwave, microwave, ultrasound) should not be used on VNS therapy patients. It has been demonstrated that cellular phones, security systems at airports and commercial centers do not affect pulse generator or electrodes. There is, however, some concern regarding limitations of new generation MRI, including patients in whom the device has been removed but the wire remains. The potential risks of performing MRI on patients with an implanted VNS include heating effects, especially of the stimulation electrodes, inadvertent resetting of the device or magnet activation, image distortion and artifacts, magnetic field interactions and device malfunction or damage. If an MRI scan has to be performed, VNS output should be set to zero beforehand and reset afterwards. VNS is approved in MRI scanning using only transmit-and-receive type head coils at both 1.5 and 3 T field strength. Some modern head coils are of the phased-array type, which should not be used. In practice, good diagnostic quality brain scanning can be achieved if appropriate precautions are in place; however, body or extremity imaging (receive only coils) and experimental brain protocols are discouraged, even if the generator has been explanted and only the wire remains. It is advisable to consult the device manufacturer if there is any doubt.

16.8 Device Revisions and Removals

As use of VNS devices increases and patients meet longer follow-up periods, revisions and removals has become more of an issue to be considered. In the retrospective review of a prospectively created database of 436 consecutive patients (Elliott et al. 2011a) who underwent VNS for pharmacoresistant epilepsy, 129 patients (29.6%) underwent a total of 155 VNS revisions after primary implantation. The most common indication for revision was generator power depletion and occurred at a mean of 47.7 ± 18.9 months following implantation or last generator change (range: 23–106 months). Lead fracture occurred in 20 devices and presented with delayed neck pain in synchrony with the duty cycle in 17 cases or by loss of device efficacy in three. Seventy-four patients (17.0%) underwent device removal following primary insertion at a mean of 40.4±30.6 months. Indications for VNS device removal were nonefficacy/worse seizures in 32, MRI for possible or planned IES or other MRI indications in 31, infection in 7, AED success in 3, and vocal cord paralysis in 1 case. There were no complications during device removal.

16.9 Results

16.9.1 Seizure Reduction

The meta-analysis performed by Englot et al. (2011) through a PubMed query for all articles in the English literature published up to November 2010 using the search terms alone and in combination: "seizure," "epilepsy," "vagus," "vagal," "nerve," "stimulation," "stimulator," and "surgery" identified 74 clinical studies of VNS in epilepsy including 3,321 patients. These studies consisted of three blinded, randomized controlled trials (Class I evidence); two nonblinded, randomized controlled trials (Class II evidence); ten studies reporting prospective data (Class III evidence); and numerous retrospective studies. Among prospective studies, seizure reduction rates were 17–55% after 3–64 months of VNS therapy, with 21–50% of patients experiencing ≥50% decrease in seizure frequency. Across all studies, VNS reduced seizure frequency by approximately 45%, although the rate of seizure reduction increased from 36% at the 3- to 12-month follow-up to 51% after >1 year of therapy. In examining outcomes using the Engel outcome scale, the authors found that ≈50% of patients attained a clinically significant reduction in seizure frequency ≥50%, with about 12% experiencing ≥90% decrease in seizures. Overall, VNS predicted ≥50% reduction in seizures with a main effects odds ratio (OR) of 1.83 (95% CI 1.80–1.86). The summary of class of data, number of patients studied, minimum follow-up, and percentage of patients achieving seizure freedom and 50% or greater reduction in seizure frequency in publications investigating outcome in VNS was recently reported by Connor et al. (2012). Approximately 25% of the patients in the published literature did not receive a measurable clinical benefit and complete seizure freedom was rarely (<5%) attained. The authors also stratified outcomes by patient age and seizure type and observed that children experienced a slightly better outcome than adults (55 vs. 50% reduction in seizures, respectively), with patients younger than 6 years old achieving a 62% decrease in seizure frequency. Furthermore, patients with generalized epilepsy received increased benefit compared with those with partial seizures (58 vs. 43% reduction in seizures). Caution must be used in interpreting these results, as data on age and type of seizure is frequently missing in source studies. Therefore, while the data are insufficient to determine if VNS truly conveys increased benefit in children and in patients with generalized epilepsy, available data do suggest that both patient groups may receive benefit from VNS therapy despite initial exclusion during device approval.

16.9.2 Quality of Life and Other Neuropsychological Variables

Preliminary studies reported additional effects of VNS on neuropsychological variables, such as mood, alertness, memory, postictal recovery periods. Although different mood scales were used, several studies have demonstrated mood improvements after treatment with VNS (Elger et al. 2000; Aldenkamp et al. 2001). None of these studies have found an association between seizure reduction and mood improvement. This may indicate specific additional effects of VNS on mood, which may be independent of improved seizure control. This treatment effect became relevant for the treatment of mood disorders in general, and after a randomized controlled trial and several clinical trial data the FDA approved VNS as treatment for therapy resistant depression in 2005 (FDA 2005). The effects of VNS on QoL, which is more difficult to assess quantitatively, remain controversial. Some studies have reported increased health-related QoL (McLachlan et al. 2003), where McGlone et al. (2008) have found no change in QoL. Klinkenberg et al. (2012b) studied 41 patients with refractory epilepsy and found significant improvements for both mood and QoL after 6 months of VNS; based on the results in the profile of mood states (POMS) and QoLIE-89 questionnaires ($P<0.05$). There was no significant change in cognition. Mean percentage change in seizure frequency was −9.0%, while 20% of the patients achieved a seizure frequency reduction of 50% or more. No significant correlation was found between changes in seizure frequency and improvements in mood or QOL. Concerning cognition, both Dodrill and Morris (2001) and Hoppe et al. (2001) report no change in cognition in VNS therapy. Aldenkamp et al. (2002) have demonstrated an improvement in mental age in children independent of seizure control. A possible explanation for this improvement of functioning might be the improved quality of sleep (Hallbook et al. 2005). Although statistically significant, the IQ increase observed in the high level stimulation group in the controlled trial by (Klinkenberg et al. 2012a, 2013) is considered too modest to be clinically relevant and in fact could no longer be demonstrated at the end of the follow-up period. One may conclude that VNS at least does not have any negative effects on cognition, in contrast to some AEDs, especially in case of polytherapy.

Many reports have sustained an—often subjective—improvement in QoL, as a conglomerate of variables including seizure frequency, seizure severity, AED burden, mood and other psychological factors perceived by patients and/or caregivers, and many authors suggest that given the great incapacity of these patients even this improvement, independently of seizure reduction is a well acceptable outcome.

16.9.3 AEDs

The possibility of reducing AEDs in the postsurgical period is a common and often controverted topic in every surgical option for intractable epilepsy, and it has been mentioned as a potential advantage of VNS, which would be particularly beneficial in the pediatric population. However, in the authors experience (Alonso-Vanegas et al. 2010) as well as in reports of long-term studies, it is generally not possible to reduce the number of AEDs, though a reduction in dosage can often be used during some periods. In a study (Majkowska-Zwolińska et al. 2012) in 57 children and adolescents the average number of AEDs taken over time decreased from 2.71 drugs per subject at 6 months to 2.27 drugs per subject at 48 months. This modest decrease is consistent with the results reported in other studies (De Herdt et al. 2007; Vonck et al. 2004) but it is noteworthy that two thirds of children receiving benzodiazepines at baseline are able to withdraw from the drugs completely. This is important from a clinical point of view since chronic use of these drugs is associated with cognitive impairment, sedation, and tolerance. Reduction in the number of AEDs has generally only been found in small series (Hornig et al. 1997; Shahwan et al. 2009). It has proven difficult to evaluate the impact that changes in AED regimens have on seizure frequency in the setting of VNS. In fact, as stated by Elliott et al. (2011a) the increase in VNS efficacy over time may be due to alteration in device parameters, changes in AED regimen, or an undefined, synergistic effect of both.

16.10 Cost-Effectiveness

Several studies have reported clinical and economic benefits of VNS. A study in Sweden reported an annual cost savings of $3,000 when comparing 18 months before and after VNS implantation among 43 patients, stating that the purchase price of a VN stimulator can be absorbed in 2—3 years (Ben-Menachem et al. 2002). Another study reported that the average annual direct medical costs decreased from $4,826 to $2,496 for 25 patients who underwent VNS in Belgium (Boon et al. 2002). The cost estimates in both studies were reported in 1999 US dollars. In 2007, the average quarterly resource utilization for 12 months before implantation was compared with that 48 months after implantation in 138 patients treated in the USA, and the investigators found that use of health care resources, such as emergency room and outpatient visits, decreased after implantation (Bernstein et al. 2007). The first study (Helmers et al. 2011) to evaluate the long-term impact of VNS on resource utilization, epilepsy-related clinical events, and costs, simultaneously in a very large cohort of 1,655 patients found that average quarterly health care resource utilization (overall and seizure-related) decreased in the post-VNS period versus the pre-VNS period, even after adjusting for potential confounding factors. Hospitalizations decreased post-VNS compared with pre-VNS (adjusted IRR=0.59, $P<0.001$). Grand mal status events decreased post-VNS compared with pre-VNS (adjusted IRR=0.79, $P<0.001$). Average total health care costs were lower post-VNS than pre-VNS ($18,550 vs. $19,945 quarterly, $P<0.001$). The average cost in the first quarter after implantation, including the cost of the device and implantation, was high at $42,540 per patient per quarter, but this cost was outweighed at about 1.5 years postimplantation, producing net health care cost savings. Naturally, it must be kept in mind that conclusions from cost-effectiveness studies can often not be generalized to broader populations, and to different health care system; it is very likely that different subsets of patients (including different epileptic syndromes, public or private health care system) derive differential economic benefits from VNS.

16.11 Prognostic Factors

Several studies have tried to identify a profile of responders. The first prospective randomized active controlled trial in children evaluating the effects of VNS frequency, comparing low versus high stimulation parameters (Klinkenberg et al. 2012b) found a trend towards a correlation between age at onset and response to VNS in line with the previous results of Patwardhan et al. (2000). According to Janszky et al. (2005) absence of bilateral interictal epileptic discharges and presence of malformation of cortical development were factors predicting a favorable outcome. In this randomized trial, seven out of nine participants in whom 50% or more seizure frequency reduction was achieved had bilateral interictal epileptic dischargers compared with 18 out of 25 non-responders. However, only one of the eight participants with malformation of cortical development had a 50% or more seizure frequency reduction. Callosotomy before VNS treatment has been reported to be associated with a positive response, but this was not the case in one participant in the randomized trial.

Other factors, presumably associated to a better response, have also proven controversial. For instance, in the meta-anlysis by Englot et al. (2011) the greatest benefit from VNS was seen in patients with posttraumatic epilepsy (79% reduction in seizures) and with tuberous sclerosis (68% decrease in seizures), while individuals with an unknown or idiopathic epilepsy etiology experienced 51% fewer seizures, and patients suffering from Lennox–Gastaut syndrome or other epileptic encephalopathies had a 48% decrease in seizures, but only 517 of 3,321 patients from the literature could be disaggregated by epilepsy etiology.

A recent pilot study (de Vos et al. 2011) explored predictive interictal EEG features for seizure reduction in 19 patients with medically refractory epilepsy submitted to VNS. They found that a quantitative symmetry measure, the pair wise derived brain symmetry index (pdBSI), was on average higher for delta, theta, alpha and beta bands for non-responders (nine patients) than for responders (ten patients). The average pdBSI of the theta and alpha bands could significantly discriminate between responders and non-responders. Additional validation of the proposed pdBSI features and the creation of a prediction model are subjects that should be further explored and might provide answers as to predictive response factors.

16.12 Conclusions

As most articles evaluating the effect of VNS on intractable seizures in the current literature conclude, VNS is a safe, feasible, and well-tolerated option, with minimal side effects and complication, and improvement in seizure frequency and severity that often increase over time in selected groups of children and adults with partial or generalized seizures. Pending the still elusive precision in the understanding of MOA, factors that can predict a good response and stimulation parameters/protocols that can be applied to subsets of patients according to measurable clinical evidences, its use in a comprehensive epilepsy program is still a function of the multidisciplinary team's experience and individual evidence-based judgment. It cannot be stressed enough that a careful presurgical evaluation of refractory epilepsy patients, that excludes resective surgical options with a higher probability of seizure freedom, and proposes VNS with detailed regard to expense and risks weighted against potential improvements in seizures and quality of life is of paramount importance.

References

Aalbers M, Vles J, Klinkenberg S, Hoogland G, Majoie M, Rijkers K. Animal models for vagus nerve stimulation in epilepsy. Exp Neurol. 2011;230(2):167–75.

Air EL, Ghomri YM, Tyagi R, Grande AW, Crone K, Mangano FT. Management of vagal nerve stimulator infections: do they need to be removed? Clinical article. J Neurosurg Pediatr. 2009;3:73–8.

Aldenkamp AP, Van de Veerdonk SH, Majoie HJ, Berfelo MW, Evers SM, Kessels AG, et al. Effects of 6 months of treatment with vagus nerve stimulation on behavior in children with Lennox-Gastaut syndrome in an open clinical and nonrandomized study. Epilepsy Behav. 2001;2(4):343–50.

Aldenkamp AP, Majoie HJ, Berfelo MW, Evers SM, Kessels AG, Renier WO, Wilmink J. Long-term effects of 24-month treatment with vagus nerve stimulation on behaviour in children with Lennox-Gastaut syndrome. Epilepsy Behav. 2002;3(5):475e9.

Alonso-Vanegas MA, Austria-Velásquez J, López Gómez M, Brust-Mascher E. Estimulación crónica intermitente del nervio vago en el tratamiento de epilepsia refractaria: experiencia en México con 35 casos. Cir Cir. 2010;78:15–24.

Amar AP, Apuzzo ML, Liu CY. Vagus nerve stimulation therapy after failed cranial surgery for intractable epilepsy: results from the vagus nerve stimulation therapy patient outcome registry. Neurosurgery. 2008;62 Suppl 2:506–13.

Ascanope JJ, Moore DD, Zipes DP, Hartman LM, Duffel Jr WH. Bradycardia and asystole with the use of vagus nerve stimulation for the treatment of epilepsy: a rare complication of intraoperative device testing. Epilepsia. 1999;40:1452–4.

Barnes A, Duncan R, Chisholm JA, Lindsay K, Patterson J, Wyper D. Investigation into the mechanisms of vagus nerve stimulation for the treatment of intractable epilepsy, using 99mTc-HMPAO SPET brain images. Eur J Nucl Med Mol Imaging. 2003;30:301–5.

Bauman JA, Ridgway EB, Devinsky O, Doyle WK. Subpectoral implantation of the vagus nerve stimulator. Neurosurgery. 2006;58 ONS:322–5.

Benifla M, Rutka JT, Logan W, Donner EJ. Vagal nerve stimulation for refractory epilepsy in children: indications and experience at The Hospital for Sick Children. Childs Nerv Syst. 2006;22:1018–26.

Ben-Menachem E. Vagus nerve stimulation, side effects and long-term safety. J Clin Neurophysiol. 2001;18:415–8.

Ben-Menachem E, Hellström K, Verstappen D. Analysis of direct hospital costs before and 18 months after treatment with vagus nerve stimulation therapy in 43 patients. Neurology. 2002;59 Suppl 4:S44–7.

Bernstein AL, Barkan H, Hess T. Vagus nervestimulation therapy for pharmacoresistant epilepsy: effect on health care utilization. Epilepsy Behav. 2007;10:134–7.

Biggio F, Gorini G, Utzeri C, Olla P, Marrosu F, Mocchetti I, et al. Chronic vagus nerve stimulation induces neuronal plasticity in the rat hippocampus. Int J Neuropsychopharmacol. 2009;12:1209–21.

Boon P, Vonck K, Van Walleghem P, D'Havé M, Goossens L, Vandekerckhove T, et al. Programmed and magnet-induced vagus nerve stimulation for refractory epilepsy. J Clin Neurophysiol. 2001;18:402–7.

Boon P, D'Havé M, Van Walleghem P, Michielsen G, Vonck K, Caemaert J, et al. Direct medical costs of refractory epilepsy incurred by three different treatment modalities: a prospective assessment. Epilepsia. 2002;43:96–102.

Chawla J, Suscholeiki R, Jones C, Silver K. Intractable epilepsy with ring chromosome 20 syndrome treated with vagal nerve stimulation: case report and review of the literature. J Child Neurol. 2002;17:778–80.

Connor Jr DE, Nixon M, Nanda A, Guthikonda B. Vagal nerve stimulation for the treatment of medically refractory epilepsy: a review of the current literature. Neurosurg Focus. 2012;32(3):E12.

De Herdt V, Boon P, Ceulemans B, Hauman H, Lagae L, Legros B, et al. Vagus nerve stimulation for refractory epilepsy: a Belgian multicenter study. Eur J Paediatr Neurol. 2007;11:261–9.

de Vos CC, Melching L, van Schoonhoven J, Ardesch JJ, de Weerd AW, van Lambalgen HC, et al. Predicting success of vagus nerve stimulation (VNS) from interictal EEG. Seizure. 2011;20(7):541–5.

Dedeurwaerdere S, Vonck K, Van Hese P, Wadman W, Boon P. The acute and chronic effect of vagus nerve stimulation in genetic absence epilepsy rats from Strasbourg (GAERS). Epilepsia. 2005;46 Suppl 5:94–7.

Dedeurwaerdere S, Gilby K, Vonck K, Delbeke J, Boon P, McIntyre D. Vagus nerve stimulation does not affect spatial memory in fast rats, but has both anti-convulsive and pro-convulsive effects on amygdala-kindled seizures. Neuroscience. 2006;140:1443–51.

Dodrill CB, Morris GL. Effects of vagal nerve stimulation on cognition and quality of life in epilepsy. Epilepsy Behav. 2001;2(1):46–53.

Elger G, Hoppe C, Falkai P, Rush AJ, Elger CE. Vagus nerve stimulation is associated with mood improvements in epilepsy patients. Epilepsy Res. 2000;42(2–3):203–10.

Elliott RE, Morsi A, Kalhorn SP, Marcus J, Sellin J, Kang M, et al. Vagus nerve stimulation in 436 consecutive patients with treatment-resistant epilepsy: long-term outcomes and predictors of response. Epilepsia. 2011a;20:57–63.

Elliott RE, Rodgers SD, Bassani L, Morsi A, Geller EB, Carlson C, et al. Vagus nerve stimulation for children with treatment-resistant epilepsy: a consecutive series of 141 cases. J Neurosurg Pediatr. 2011b;7:491–500.

Englot DJ, Chang EF, Auguste KI. Vagus nerve stimulation for epilepsy: a meta-analysis of efficacy and predictors of response. J Neurosurg. 2011;115(6):1248–55.

FDA. VNS therapy system for adjunctive long-term treatment of chronic or recurrent depression for patients 18 years of age or older. FDA approvals, 2005. 2005. Available from: http://www.fda.gov/MedicalDevices/ProductsandMedicalProcedures/DeviceApprovalsandClearances/Recently-ApprovedDevices/ucm078532.htm. Accessed on 12 Sept 2011.

Fernandez-Guardiola A, Martinez A, Valdes-Cruz A, Magdaleno-Madrigal VM, Martinez D, Fernandez-Mas R. Vagus nerve prolonged stimulation in cats: effects on epileptogenesis (amygdala electrical kindling): behavioral and electro-graphic changes. Epilepsia. 1999;40:822–9.

Follesa P, Gale K, Mocchetti I. Regional and temporal pattern expression of nerve growth factor and basic fibroblast growth factor mRNA in rat brain following electroconvulsive shock. Exp Neurol. 1994;127:37–44.

Frost M, Gates J, Helmers SL, Wheless JW, Levisohn P, Tardo C, et al. Vagus nerve stimulation in children with refractory seizures associated with Lennox-Gastaut syndrome. Epilepsia. 2001; 42:1148–52.

Hallbook T, Lundgren J, Kohler S, Blennow G, Strömblad LG, Rosén I. Beneficial effects on sleep of vagus nerve stimulation in children with therapy resistant epilepsy. Eur J Paediatr Neurol. 2005;9(6):399–407.

Hammond E, Uthmann B, Reid S, Wilder B. Electrophysiological studies of cervical vagus nerve stimulation in humans. I. EEG effects. Epilepsia. 1992;33:1013–20.

Helmers SL, Duh MS, Guérin A, Sarda SP, Samuelson TM, Bunker MT, et al. Clinical and economic impact of vagus nerve stimulation therapy in patients with drug-resistant epilepsy. Epilepsy Behav. 2011;22(2):370–5.

Hoppe C, Helmstaedter C, Scherrmann J, Elger CE. No evidence for cognitive side effects after 6 months of vagus nerve stimulation in epilepsy patients. Epilepsy Behav. 2001;2(4):351–6.

Hornig GW, Murphy JV, Schallert G, Tilton C. Left vagus nerve stimulation in children with refractory epilepsy: an update. South Med J. 1997;90:484–8.

Hosoi T, Okuma Y, Nomura Y. Electrical stimulation of afferent vagus nerve induces IL-1beta expression in the brain and activates HPA axis. Am J Physiol Regul Integr Comp Physiol. 2000;279:R141–7.

Janszky J, Hoppe M, Behne F, Tuxhorn I, Pannek HW, Ebner A. Vagus nerve stimulation: predictors of seizure freedom. J Neurol Neurosurg Psychiatry. 2005;76:384–9.

Klinkenberg S, Aalbers MW, Vles JS, Cornips EM, Rijkers K, Leenen L, et al. Vagus nerve stimulation in children with intractable epilepsy: a randomized controlled trial. Dev Med Child Neurol. 2012a;54(9):855–61.

Klinkenberg S, Majoie HJM, van der Heijden MMAA, Rijkers K, Leenen L, Aldenkamp AP. Vagus nerve stimulation has a positive effect on mood in patients with refractory epilepsy. Clin Neurol Neurosurg. 2012b;114:336–40.

Klinkenberg S, van den Bosch CN, Majoie HJ, Aalbers MW, Leenen L, Hendriksen J, Cornips EMJ, Rijkers K, Vles JS, Aldenkamp AP. Behavioural and cognitive effects during vagus nerve stimulation in children with intractable epilepsy – A randomized controlled trial. Eur J Paediatr Neurol. 2013;17(1):82–90.

Koo B. EEG changes with vagus nerve stimulation. J Clin Neurophysiol. 2001;18:434–41.

Krahl S, Senanayake S, Handforth A. Destruction of peripheral C-fibers does not alter subsequent vagus nerve stimulation-induced seizure suppression in rats. Epilepsia. 2001;42:586–9.

Kuba R, Guzaninova M, Brazdil M, Novak Z, Chrastina J, Rektor I. Effect of vagal nerve stimulation on interictal epileptiform discharges: a scalp EEG study. Epilepsia. 2002;43(10):1181–8.

Kuba R, Brazdil M, Novak Z, Chrastina J, Rector I. Effect of vagal nerve stimulation on patients with bitemporal epilepsy. Eur J Neurol. 2003;10:91–4.

Kulkarni VA, Jha S, Vaidya VA. Depletion of norepinephrine decreases the proliferation, but does not influence the survival and differentiation, of granule cell progenitors in the adult rat hippocampus. Eur J Neurosci. 2002;16:2008–12.

Labar D, Ponticello L. Persistent antiepileptic effects after vagus nerve stimulation ends? Neurology. 2003;61:1818.

Labar D, Murphy J, Tecoma E. Vagus nerve stimulation for medication-resistant generalized epilepsy. E04 VNS Study Group. Neurology. 1999;52:1510–2.

Lockard JS, Congdon WC, DuCharme LL. Feasibility and safety of vagal nerve stimulation in monkey model. Epilepsia. 1990;31:20–6.

Magdaleno-Madrigal V, Valdes-Cruz A, Martinez-Vargas D, Almazan-Alvarado S, Fernandez-Mas R, Fernandez-Guardiola A. Effect of vagus nerve stimulation on later stages of amygdaloid kindling in freely-moving cats. FENS Abstr. 2004;2:A124.118.

Majkowska-Zwolińska B, Zwoliński P, Roszkowski M, Drabik K. Long-term results of vagus nerve stimulation in children and adolescents with drug-resistant epilepsy. Childs Nerv Syst. 2012;28:621–8.

Marrosu F, Serra A, Maleci A, Puligheddu M, Biggio G, Piga M. Correlation between GABA(A) receptor density and vagus nerve stimulation in individuals with drug-resistant partial epilepsy. Epilepsy Res. 2003;55(1–2):59–70.

Marrosu F, Santoni F, Puligheddu M, Barberini L, Maleci A, Ennas F, et al. Increase in 20–50 Hz (gamma frequencies) power spectrum and synchronization after chronic vagal nerve stimulation. Clin Neurophysiol. 2005;116:2026–36.

McGlone J, Valdivia I, Penner M, Williams J, Sadler RM, Clarke DB. Quality of life and memory after vagus nerve stimulator implantation for epilepsy. Can J Neurol Sci. 2008;35(3):287–96.

McLachlan RS, Sadler M, Pillay N, Guberman A, Jones M, Wiebe S, et al. Quality of life after vagus nerve stimulation for intractable epilepsy: is seizure control the only contributing factor? Eur Neurol. 2003;50(1):16–9.

Meurs A, Clinckers R, Raedt R, El Tahry R, De Herdt V, Vonck K, et al. Vagus nerve stimulation suppressess pilocarpine- induced limbic seizures and increases hippocampal extracellular noradrenalin concentration. Epilepsia. 2008;49:350.
Morris III GL. A retrospective analysis of the effects of magnet-activated stimulation in conjunction with vagus nerve stimulation therapy. Epilepsy Behav. 2003;4:740–5.
Muñana KR, Vitek SM, Tarver WB, Saito M, Skeen TM, Sharp NJ, et al. Use of vagal nerve stimulation as a treatment for refractory epilepsy in dogs. J Am Vet Med Assoc. 2002;221:977–83.
Murphy JV, Wheeles JW, Schmoll CM. Left vagal nerve stimulation in six patients with hypothalamic hamartomas. Pediatr Neurol. 2000;23:167–8.
Murphy JV, Torkelson R, Dowler I, Simon S, Hudson S. Vagal nerve stimulation in refractory epilepsy: the first 100 patients receiving vagal nerve stimulation at a pediatric epilepsy center. Arch Pediatr Adolesc Med. 2003;157:560–4.
Narayanan JT, Watts R, Hadad N, Labar DR, Li PM, Filippi CG. Cerebral activation during vagus nerve stimulation: a functional MR study. Epilepsia. 2002;43:1509–14.
Naritoku D, Mikels JA. Vagus nerve stimulation (VNS) is antiepileptogenic in the electrical kindling model. Epilepsia. 1997;38:220.
Neese SL, Sherill LK, Tan AA, Roosevely RW, Browning RA, Smith DC, et al. Vagus nerve stimulation may protect GABAergic neurons following traumatic brain injury in rats: an immunocytochemical study. Brain Res. 2007;1128(1):157–63.
Parain D, Penniello MJ, Berquen P, Delangre T, Billard C, Murphy JV. Vagal nerve stimulation in tuberous sclerosis complex patients. Pediatr Neurol. 2001;25:213–6.
Patwardhan RV, Stong B, Bebin EM, Mathisen J, Grabb PA. Efficacy of vagal nerve stimulation in children with medically refractory epilepsy. Neurosurgery. 2000;47:1353–7.
Pavlov VA, Tracey KJ. The cholinergic anti-inflammatory pathway. Brain Behav Immun. 2005;19:493–9.
Revesz D, Tjernstrom M, Ben-Menachem E, Thorlin T. Effects of vagus nerve stimulation on rat hippocampal progenitor proliferation. Exp Neurol. 2008;214:259–65.
Rijkers K, Aalbers M, Hoogland G, van Winden L, Vles J, Steinbusch H, et al. Acute seizure-suppressing effect of vagus nerve stimulation in the amygdala kindled rat. Brain Res. 2010;1319:155–63.
Ring HA, White S, Costa DC, Pottinger R, Dick JP, Koeze T, et al. A SPECT study of the effect of vagal nerve stimulation on thalamic activity in patients with epilepsy. Seizure. 2000;9:380–4.
Schachter SC, Wheless JW (eds). Vagus nerve stimulation therapy 5 years after approval: a comprehensive update. Neurology. 2002;59 Suppl 4:S1–61.
Shahwan A, Bailey C, Maxiner W, Harvey AS. Vagus nerve stimulation for refractory epilepsy in children: more to VNS than seizure frequency reduction. Epilepsia. 2009;50:1220–8.
Takaya M, Terry W, Naritoku D. Vagus nerve stimulation induces a sustained anticonvulsant effect. Epilepsia. 1996;37:1111–6.
The Vagus Nerve Stimulation Study Group. A randomized controlled trial of chronic vagus nerve stimulation for treatment of medically intractable seizures. Neurology. 1995;45:224–30.
Thompson EM, Wozniak SE, Roberts CM, Kao A, Anderson VC, Selden NR. Vagus nerve stimulation for partial and generalized epilepsy from infancy to adolescence. J Neurosurg Pediatr. 2012;10(3):200–5.
Vale FL, Ahmadian A, Youssef AS, Tatum WO, Benbadis SR. Long-term outcome of vagus nerve stimulation therapy after failed epilepsy surgery. Seizure. 2011;20(3):244–8.
Vonck K, Thadani V, Gilbert K, Dedeurwaerdere S, De Groote L, De Herdt V, et al. Vagus nerve stimulation for refractory epilepsy: a transatlantic experience. J Clin Neurophysiol. 2004; 21:283–9.
Walker BR, Easton A, Gale K. Regulation of limbic motor seizures by GABA and glutamate transmission in nucleus tractus solitarius. Epilepsia. 1999;40:1051–7.
Wheless JW, Maggio V. Vagus nerve stimulation therapy in patients younger than 18 years. Neurology. 2002;59 Suppl 4:S21–5.

Chapter 17
The Role of Neuromodulation in the Treatment of Refractory Epilepsy

Ana Luisa Velasco and Francisco Velasco

Abstract Neuromodulation or electrical stimulation of the neural tissue instead of performing lesions is a current trend in neurosurgery. Regarding epilepsy, neuromodulation is currently under intensive research. The field is growing at a fast pace every day. This work has the purpose of reviewing the various targets that have been stimulated in the search of the possibility to control refractory seizures. A consideration is made of how the different targets and patients are selected: seizure outcomes and adverse effects. Targets can be chosen with the idea to interfere with seizure propagation; this is the case of cerebellar, vagal, subthalamic, and thalamic stimulation. Currently, studies are being performed stimulating the epileptic focus. Even though many controversies regarding which is the best target and stimulating parameters still exist, there is no doubt neuromodulation reduces seizures and has the advantage of being reversible and safe.

Keywords Neuromodulation • Electrical brain stimulation • Epilepsy • Refractory seizures • Stimulation anatomical targets • Epilepsy surgery

17.1 Introduction

Neuromodulation is an alternative method to traditional ablative surgery. It emerged from the mandatory need to halt seizures and preserve neurological function in those patients who are rejected from ablative procedures due to several reasons, for example bilateral or multiple epileptic foci, focus involving primary functional areas of the brain, generalized seizures, or non-lesional imaging studies. Berg et al.

A.L. Velasco (✉) • F. Velasco
Department of Neurology and Neurosurgery, General Hospital of Mexico, CDA, Bosques de Moctezuma 55 La Herradura, Huixquilucan, Mexico State 52784, Mexico
e-mail: analuisav@yahoo.com

L. Rocha and E.A. Cavalheiro (eds.), *Pharmacoresistance in Epilepsy: From Genes and Molecules to Promising Therapies*, DOI 10.1007/978-1-4614-6464-8_17,

(2003) calculate that approximately 30 % of patients who need epilepsy surgery are rejected.

In 1973, Cooper et al. stimulated the cerebellum based on experimental observations indicating that low-frequency stimulation (10 Hz) of paravermian cerebellar cortex decreased paroxysmal electroencephalographic (EEG) discharges and seizures induced by electric shocks (Moruzzi 1941) or cobalt powder (Dow et al. 1962) applied on the motor cortex in cats. Furthermore Iawata and Snider (1959) stimulated the cerebellum to stop seizures and long after-discharges that were induced by hippocampal electrical stimulation. In normal conditions paravermian cortex inhibits deep brain cerebellar nuclei activity, which facilitates both cortical excitability and spinal cord monosynaptic reflex (Cooper 1978).

Since then several targets have been proposed to control seizures. Although there might be discrepancies about which target is the best, all authors agree that neuromodulation of all of them improves seizure control without deteriorating neurological functions. Many studies have been performed in different epilepsy surgery centers in the world proposing several seizure types that respond, different and stimulation modes.

17.2 Patient Selection

As with all surgical procedures that are used to treat refractory seizures, patient selection is the first step to ensure a good outcome. The neuromodulation procedure is designed for each patient. If we fail to recognize the appropriate candidate, even the best surgery is a failure; this principle applies to neuromodulation. Furthermore, this procedure is expensive. In the future, neuromodulation might become the first option when considering a surgical method for refractory epilepsy. This is due to its low surgical risk and reversible qualities. But for now ablative surgery is less expensive and shows good results. Criteria to select a patient are the following:

- Primary generalized seizures
- Multifocal or bilateral foci
- Seizures arising from eloquent areas (motor, memory, and language for example)

In all the above clinical settings, conventional surgery has proven to be risky due to the fact that it can be a major surgery with high probability of infection, bleeding, or loss of neural function. Since surgeries restrict the amount of tissue to be removed to avoid loss of function, residual seizures are frequent. Some of the patients have non-lesional magnetic resonance imaging (MRI), the risk and outcome are worse, and patients are discarded from surgical options.

17.3 Period of Time to Obtain Seizure Reduction

We must bear in mind some inherent features of electric neuromodulation of the brain. Seizures do not disappear as soon as the stimulator is turned on. There is a variable period of time to obtain seizure reduction. This period of time varies according to the stimulated target and stimulation mode. If the cerebellum or vagus nerve is chosen, the best effect will take years to be reached; if the thalamus is stimulated, seizure reduction will take from 3 to 6 months to be achieved; if the target is hippocampal focus, the time span is reduced to 2–6 weeks if the hippocampus shows no signs of sclerosis in the MRI. If we stimulate the cortical epileptic focus in a programmed cyclic mode, seizures diminish in a matter of days (Velasco et al. 2009) and if the mode is based on a closed-loop fashion seizures take months to years to decrease (Fountas and Smith 2007).

17.4 Nervous System Targets

Multiple targets that intend to achieve seizure reduction have been stimulated. The different targets work either by interfering with seizure propagation or seizure generation. The basis of interfering with seizure propagation seems natural in generalized seizures but it has also been used in cases of partial seizures when the focus cannot be determined with precision or in cases of multiple foci. Several targets have been proposed: cerebellum, vagus nerve, thalamus (anterior nucleus, centromedian nucleus), and others such as subthalamic nuclei.

Since Cooper suggested that low-frequency stimulation of the cerebellar cortex (dorsal paravermian area) decreased seizures in humans, a review of different studies with a total of 129 patients showed that 49 % had significant seizure reduction, 27 % being seizure free. This and other studies (Velasco et al. 2005) have shown that the seizure type that best responds is primary generalized tonic–clonic seizures and atypical absences and that even though there is an initial seizure reduction within the first 2 months of stimulation: the effect is maintained and further increased with time. Vagus nerve stimulation has been used in all types of refractory seizures. Its effects on seizure reduction are modest (~30 %). Even though the precise antiepileptic mechanism remains unclear, it appears that the thalamocortical relay neurons modulate cortical excitability, influencing seizure generation or propagation (Ben-Menachem 2002). It can produce dysphonia and headache and increases peptic ulcer and insulin-dependant diabetes mellitus. It is not recommended for children under 12 years old.

According to the centro-encephalic theory by Penfield and Jasper (1954) high-frequency stimulation of nonspecific thalamic nuclei (such as centro-median or anterior thalamic nuclei) interferes with propagation of cortically or subcortically initiated seizures. In 1984, Velasco et al. performed the first bilateral centro-median electrode implantation in a 12-year-old boy with severe generalized seizures of the Lennox–Gastaut syndrome. Five years later they published a report of children and adults with generalized seizures of the Lennox–Gastaut syndrome (Velasco et al. 1987). Best results are obtained in the parvocellular portion and that neurophysiologic definition based on electrocortical responses elicited by stimulation of the electrode contacts within different zones of the centro-median nucleus (Velasco et al. 2000a, b, 2006). When these anatomic and neurophysiologic criteria are met in patients with generalized seizures and epilepsia partialis continua, the results are

>80 % seizure reduction and some patients have become seizure free. An improvement in ability scales is also observed with no adverse effects.

As described above, the anterior nucleus is a nonspecific thalamic nucleus and as such, interferes with propagation of cortical or subcortical initiated seizures but it also blocks seizures initiated in mesial temporal structures and propagated through the fornix, mammillary body, and anterior nucleus of the thalamus (Mirski and Fisher 1994). The SANTE study Group has stimulated the anterior nucleus of the thalamus (Fisher et al 2010); best results have been obtained in complex partial and secondary generalized seizures, which were reduced by stimulation. By 2 years, there was a 56 % median percent reduction in seizure frequency.

The subthalamic nucleus has been stimulated for seizure control based on the suppressive effects of pharmacological or electrical inhibition seen on different types of seizures in animal models of epilepsy (Chabardes et al. 2002). It is considered that inhibition of the subthalamic nucleus causes activation of an endogenous system referred to as the nigral control of epilepsy system (Gale and Iadarola 1980). Patients with frontal lobe and myoclonic seizures are the best responders. Improvement varies from 30 to 80 % (Vesper et al. 2007). Secondary effects include mild facial twitching and paresthesias in legs and arms that responded to adjustment of the stimulation parameters.

Weiss et al. (1998) found that low-frequency stimulation (1 Hz for 15 min), applied after kindling stimulation of the amygdala, inhibited the development and expression of amygdala-kindled seizures. Velasco et al. (2000a, b) stimulated the hippocampal foci in patients with diagnostic intracranial electrodes who were undergoing temporal lobectomy, and seizures were diminished. Clinical studies using neurophysiologic testing and single positron emission tomography and benzodiazepine receptor binding studies show that an inhibitory mechanism could explain seizure control (Velasco et al. 2000a, b; Cuellar-Herrera et al. 2004).

Various authors (Boon et al. 2007; Velasco et al. 2007) have shown the beneficial effects in seizure reduction in patients with hippocampal foci stimulation; best responders are those patients whose epileptic focus can be pinpointed with hippocampal electrodes and thus stimulated directly and have non-lesional MRI. In these latter cases seizure reduction is >90 % with several patients being seizure free. Wyckhuys et al. (2007) found that high-frequency stimulation of the hippocampus in kindled rats increases after-discharge thresholds with the consequent seizure reduction.

There are studies that have shown evidence that neuromodulation works by inhibiting the stimulated area. Clinical studies using neurophysiologic testing and single positron emission tomography and benzodiazepine receptor binding studies show that an inhibitory mechanism could explain seizure control (Velasco et al. 2000a, b; Cuellar-Herrera et al. 2004).

Cortical stimulation for motor seizures has been performed in two modes: an open (Velasco et al. 2009) and closed loop (Sun et al. 2008). In case of the open loop mode, a significant (>90 %) seizure decrease takes place over several days and effect persists thereafter; the stimulation mode is preestablished in a 24-h cyclic 1 min ON, 4 min OFF. When the closed-loop mode is used, a seizure detection system is implanted too so that every time a seizure is detected, the stimulation therapy is delivered. In the latter mode, seizure reduction takes a longer period of time to produce a modest difference.

17.5 Rationale for Target Selection

No matter what target we choose we must consider that there should be a neurophysiologic rationale in our reasoning. First we have to ask ourselves if we are able to detect the precise epileptic focus to be able to interfere with seizure generation; if not, we have to go for the disruption of the epileptic activity propagation. Either way we need to make sure that we are in the correct location. From the anatomic point of view this should be easy, but several problems have to be faced. In case that we decide to go for seizure propagation we must target a precise anatomic region. The localization of the target is performed by the use of the current technology: stereotactic surgery, neuro-navigation, MRI, and neurophysiology. All expertise is needed to ensure the localization. Despite all these efforts, anatomy may be disrupted. This is particularly the case of reaching thalamic targets. We prefer patients whose thalamus and brain stem are intact and symmetric. MRI is used to verify position. Even so, the best-placed electrodes must have neurophysiologic confirmation. In the case of centro-median stimulation, detailed analysis of incremental response morphology, polarity, peak latency, and cortical distribution may aid in defining the relation of the stimulated area with specific anatomophysiologic systems within the centro-median nucleus. To perform the physiologic confirmation of the electrode position in the parvocellular portion, the three pairs of combinations of the four contacts in each deep brain stimulation electrode are stimulated (0–1, 1–2, and 2–3). Unilateral stimulation is performed at 6 Hz, 1.0 ms, and 320–800 μA with 10-s duration to induce recruiting responses, and unilateral high frequency is conducted as well at 60 Hz, 1.0 ms, and 320–800 μA to induce focalized desynchronization and negative DC shift of the EEG baseline. Scalp distribution analysis of electrocortical responses is performed. Within centro-median nucleus, suprathreshold stimulation in parvocellular subnucleus induces monophasic negative waxing and waning potentials, with peak latencies from 40 to 60 ms, recorded bilaterally in frontal and central regions, with emphasis on the stimulated side. Outside this subnucleus, incremental responses remain mainly biphasic positive–negative, with 16–20 ms latency, fixed amplitudes for the positive component, and distribution extending more toward the posterior leads. If the electrode is localized in the posterior and basal area of the centro-median nucleus within boundaries with the parafascicular nucleus induces only short-latency positive potentials at low frequency and occasionally painful sensation at high frequencies (Velasco et al. 1997). In the case of epileptic focus stimulation, localizing the precise site where it is located is mandatory; it could make the difference in seizure outcome. In our epilepsy clinic, patients are implanted with externalized diagnostic multicontact intracranial electrodes, and recorded outside the operating room to be able to detect spontaneous seizures. In case of hippocampal stimulation we implant bilateral hippocampal electrodes; if the focus is unilateral, the diagnostic electrodes are explanted and only a single therapeutic permanent electrode is implanted; if the patient has bilateral foci, two electrodes, one in each hippocampus, are implanted. The selected stimulation contacts are those that overlap with the epileptic focus. All electrode implantations are verified with MRI.

17.6 Stimulation Parameter Setup

One of the most controversial matters is regarding the stimulation parameters; several clinical and basic studies are required for the implementation of double-blinded protocols. Despite all this, there are some suggestions of the current parameters used for epilepsy:

- The electrical stimulation cycling mode of the nervous tissue was originally proposed to avoid electrical current overcharge in areas under or around electrodes, and therefore damaging neural tissue (Cooper et al. 1976).
- Discontinuous and cycling ES have been successfully used in treatment epilepsy (Ebner et al. 1980; Davis and Emmonds 1992; George et al. 2000). Although the main reason for using this mode of stimulation has been to save battery charge, its efficacy indicates that the beneficial effect outlasts each stimulation period.

Information derived from basic research has shown the importance of setting stimulation parameters that take into account principally the charge density-per-phase, which for safety's sake should not exceed 4 $\mu C/cm^2$/phase (Babb et al. 1977; Ebner et al. 1980). In all of our centro-median nucleus stimulation cases, the stimulating pulse amplitude remained between 2.0 and 3.0 V while in hippocampus and motor cortex stimulation up to 3.5 V and only rarely were they changed during follow-up. This voltage represents between 50 and 80 % of that which is necessary for inducing recruiting responses and DC shifts. It is important to mention that in cases with poor outcome, increasing the voltage two or three times the average did not improve efficacy.

Experience on neuromodulation studies in patients with movement disorders and those with pain shows that high-frequency stimulation is inhibitory. The same occurs in epilepsy; almost all studies use frequency in the range of 130 Hz. Velasco et al. (1997) demonstrated that low frequencies produced recruiting responses when stimulating the centro-median nucleus, and when bilateral stimulation at 3 Hz was performed in these nuclei, a typical absence seizure was reproduced. On the contrary, high-frequency stimulation produced cortical inhibition of epileptic activity. In the case of neuromodulation of the subthalamic nucleus, low frequency has been used for good results (Chabardes et al. 2002).

Recent instances of clinical application of closed-loop seizure control, which are limited to stimulation with pulse trains in response to epileptiform activity, have been reviewed (Osorio et al. 2001; Sun et al. 2008). This method requires the implementation of a seizure detection algorithm to control the delivery of therapy using a suitable device. Further studies are mandatory to improve this methodology and solve issues regarding efficacy of the closed-loop mode and cost of implanting a dual system.

17.7 Long-Term Assessment

Neuromodulation in epilepsy has certain difficulties for its long-term assessment due to several reasons:

- The inherent characteristics of the symptoms (seizures).
- Patients do not experience any sensations or secondary effects at all that indicate that stimulation is being delivered.

The time that neuromodulation takes to show a positive effect in seizure reduction is known as "carry-on" effect. Unlike movement disorders like tremor in Parkinson's disease, seizures appear once in a while and are not predictable, so it is not a matter of turning the pulse generator on or off and observing if seizures disappear to know if the stimulation system is working.

Except for the dysphonia that a few patients who undergo vagus nerve stimulation experiment when the stimulator is ON, other patients do not have sensations or secondary effects that could indicate if the stimulation is taking place. Two other important observations are that stimulation takes a variable time to show its effect; this period can take from several days to months; and that, when stimulation is stopped, there is a variable period of "carry-on" effect. This term refers to the observed phenomenon in which the seizure reduction is maintained for days to months after the stimulator is turned OFF, the battery depletes, or the stimulation is interrupted for any reason. Seizures reappear later in a progressive manner without reaching basal (before neuromodulation) level either in number or severity. Today, the neuromodulation community accepts the "carry-on effect." These inherent characteristics carry the need to check the system every 6–12 months or when the patient returns to consult us because seizures are increasing in intensity or number. We must check the following:

- Pulse generator battery current.
- Electrode impedance: If there is an increase, it could mean that either the system extension or the electrode is broken or disconnected. In this case simple X-rays are mandatory.
- Perform acute stimulation trial using the internalized stimulating system to generate recruiting responses. This will allow us to know that the system is working correctly and that the brain tissue is being stimulated; if not, either the system is broken or there is something in the tissue that is preventing a correct stimulation (blood, gliosis) (Velasco et al. 2006). Similar responses are found in hippocampal stimulation but are localized in ipsilateral temporal region and in motor cortex stimulation localized in ipsilateral frontal region.

17.8 Impact on Neural Functions

One of the main reasons to use neuromodulation is to preserve the functional areas of the brain. Neuromodulation in cases of abnormal movements or chronic pain has proven to be effective and to preserve function. Even when some undesirable effects are present, stimulation parameters and even the stimulated contacts can be changed and the adverse effects revert. When our group started stimulation of the centro-median thalamic nuclei for seizure control, we were dealing with patients with severe epilepsy, some of them Lennox–Gastaut patients with relentless psychomotor worsening due to the amount and severity of their seizures. The surgical options were not going to spare any function. So the functional implications of neuromodulation were not our main concern and we knew that the method was reversible. What we did not expect to find was an important improvement in the functions of these patients. We were surprised of how bedridden, totally dependent patients would start "learning" again. So we started evaluating their progress. Neuropsychological evaluation of this group was for the most part difficult in view of their deteriorated condition; several patients were in non-convulsive status, which made it impossible to apply a battery of standardized psychological tests in basal conditions. Nevertheless, the ability scales demonstrated that no patient had signs of neurologic or mental deterioration during electrical stimulation of the centro-median nuclei (Velasco et al. 2006); on the contrary, all patients improved their scales, some of them becoming independent and a couple of them seizure free and living a normal life.

Patients with normal development before Lennox–Gastaut syndrome onset tend to regain their abilities regardless of convulsive syndrome severity. Patients who had an early childhood onset had to learn everything from the start. The seizure and medication reduction added to the normalization of EEG background activity could explain this improvement (Velasco et al. 1993). Another explanation is that we are stimulating the reticular formation and thus improving the attention mechanisms of the brain; if a patient attends, he is able to learn new tasks. In patients with neuromodulation of the hippocampus focus, using pulse amplitudes higher than needed, not only are the clinical benefits not increased, but also speech problems such as anomia can be produced. The problem disappears when the amplitude is decreased again (Nuche-Bricaire et al. 2010).

In regard to stimulating the epileptic focus localized in the hippocampus, the groups mentioned above that have performed neuromodulation of the hippocampal foci have not reported a worsening of the memory function. Neuropsychological batteries for memory function have been applied and no deterioration has been found, and possibly a tendency to improve has occurred (Velasco et al. 2007). The same thing happens with patients with stimulation of the primary or supplementary motor cortices: no decrease in motor function has been observed (Velasco et al. 2009). Numbers or patients are small up to now and more studies need to be performed.

17.9 Possible Mechanisms for Neuromodulation Effect in Epilepsy

In 2000, Velasco et al. published the first results of subacute hippocampus foci stimulation in ten patients. These patients had undergone intracranial electrode implantation as part of their surgical protocol to localize the epileptic focus; once localized, a 2- to 3-week trial of subacute stimulation was delivered before performing temporal lobectomy. This study design allowed the performance of a number of neurophysiologic (after-discharges, paired pulse trials before and after stimulation), and SPECT studies comparing basal conditions with post-stimulation conditions. Since patients underwent lobectomy, stimulated tissue was recovered and analyzed using high-performance liquid chromatography techniques (Cuellar-Herrera et al. 2004). All studies suggested an inhibitory mechanism to explain seizure control. Wyckhuys et al. (2007) found that after-discharges were inhibited and seizures disappeared in rats that had been kindled to induce epileptic seizures. None of the rats had an increase in seizure number.

According to experimental observations, intralaminar and midline thalamic nuclei participate in the genesis and propagation of epileptic seizures (Pollen et al. 1963; Miller and Farandelli 1990; Velasco et al. 1990). These structures are also anatomically linked with brain stem once involved in seizure onset (Gloor et al. 1997). Although the controversy on the cortical vs. subcortical origin of epileptic attacks remains unsolved, there is a general consensus that thalamo-cortical interactions are essential in the development and propagation of most types of seizures (Avoli et al. 1983; Velasco et al. 1982). High-frequency stimulation in centromedian thalamic nucleus, which is part of intralaminar thalamic nuclei, intends to interfere with seizure propagation.

17.10 Conclusion

Neuromodulation is a remarkable surgical therapy that can be used safely in patients with epilepsy to reduce or even control seizures. A huge amount of information is available and the challenge remains in being able to "tailor" the best therapy for each patient.

References

Avoli M, Gloor P, Kostopoulus G, Gutman J. An analysis of penicillin-induced generalized spike and wave discharges using simultaneous recording of cortical and thalamic single neurons. J Neurophysiol. 1983;50:819–37.

Babb TL, Soper HV, Lieb JP, Brown WJ, Ottino CA, Crandall PH. Electrophysiological studies of long-term electrical stimulation of the cerebellum in monkeys. J Neurosurg. 1977;47:353–65.

Ben-Menachem E. Vagus-nerve stimulation for the treatment of epilepsy. Lancet Neurol. 2002;1: 477–82.

Berg AT, Vickrey BG, Langfitt JT, Sperling MR, Walczak TS, Shinnar S, et al. Multicenter study of epilepsy surgery. The multicenter study of epilepsy surgery: recruitment and selection for surgery. Epilepsia. 2003;44:1425–33.

Boon P, Vonck K, De Herdt V, Van Dycke A, Goethals M, Goossens L, et al. Deep brain stimulation in patients with refractory temporal lobe epilepsy. Epilepsia. 2007;48:1551–60.

Chabardes S, Kahane P, Minotti L, Koudsie A, Hirsch E, Benabid AL. Deep brain stimulation in epilepsy with particular reference to the subthalamic nucleus. Epileptic Disord. 2002; 4:S83–93.

Cooper IS. Cerebellar stimulation in man. New York: Raven; 1978. p. 3–265.

Cooper IS, Amin I, Gilman S. The effect of chronic cerebellar stimulation upon epilepsy in man. Trans Am Neurol Assoc. 1973;98:192–6.

Cooper IS, Amin I, Riklan M, Waltz JM, Poon TP. Chronic cerebellar stimulation in epilepsy. Clinical and anatomical studies. Arch Neurol. 1976;33:559–70.

Cuellar-Herrera M, Velasco M, Velasco F, Velasco AL, Jimenez F, Orozco S, et al. Evaluation of GABA system and cell damage in parahippocampus of patients with temporal lobe epilepsy showing antiepileptic effects after subacute electrical stimulation. Epilepsia. 2004;45(5):459–66.

Davis R, Emmonds SE. Cerebellar stimulation for seizure control: 17-year study. Stereotact Funct Neurosurg. 1992;58:200–8.

Dow RS, Fernandez-Guardiola A, Manni E. The influence of the cerebellum on experimental epilepsy. Electroencephalogr Clin Neurophysiol. 1962;14:383–98.

Ebner TJ, Bantli H, Bloedel JR. Effects of cerebellar stimulation on unitary activity within a chronic epileptic focus in a primate. Electroencephalogr Clin Neurophysiol. 1980;49:585–99.

Fisher R, Salanova V, Witt T, Worth R, Henry T, Gross R, et al. Electrical stimulation of the anterior nucleus of thalamus for treatment of refractory epilepsy Epilepsia. 2010;51:899–908.

Fountas KN, Smith JR. A novel closed-loop stimulation system in the control of focal, medically refractory epilepsy. Acta Neurochir Suppl. 2007;97:357–62.

Gale K, Iadarola MJ. Seizure protection and increased nerve-terminal GABA: delayed effects of GABA transaminase inhibition. Science. 1980;208:288–91.

George MS, Nahas Z, Bohning DE, Lomarev M, Denslow S, Osenbach R, et al. Vagus nerve stimulation: a new form of therapeutic brain stimulation. CNS Spectr. 2000;5:43–52.

Gloor P, Quesney LF, Zumstein H. Pathophysiology of generalized penicillin seizures in the cat. The role of cortical and subcortical structures II topical application of penicillin to the cerebral cortex and subcortical structures. Electroencephalogr Clin Neurophysiol. 1997;48:79–94.

Iatawa K, Snider RS. Cerebello-hippocampal influences on the electroencephalogram. Appl Neurophysiol. 1959;11:439–46.

Miller JW, Farandelli JA. The central medial nucleus: thalamic site of seizure regulation. Brain Res. 1990;508:297–300.

Mirski MA, Fisher RS. Electrical stimulation of the mammillary nuclei increases seizure threshold to pentylenetetrazol in rats. Epilepsia. 1994;35:1309–16.

Moruzzi G. Sui rapporti fra cervelleto e corteccia cerebrale: Azione d'impulse cerebellari sulle attivita motriciti provocate della stimulazione farandica o chimica del giro sigmoldeo nel gato. Arch Fisiol. 1941;41:157–82.

Nuche-Bricaire A, Montes De Oca M, Marcos-Ortega M, Trejo D, Núñez JM, Vazquez D, Velasco AL. Voltage-dependant verbal memory. Effects on the cognitive function through changing voltage parameters in deep brain stimulation. Proceedings of the 64th American epilepsy society meeting, San Antonio, USA, December 2010.

Osorio I, Frei MG, Manly BF, Sunderam S, Bhavaraju NC, Wilkinson SB. An introduction to contingent (closed-loop) brain electrical stimulation for seizure blockage, to ultra-short-term clinical trials, and to multidimensional statistical analysis of therapeutic efficacy. J Clin Neurophysiol. 2001;18:533–44.

Penfield W, Jasper H. Epilepsy and the functional anatomy of the human brain. Boston: Little Brown; 1954.

Pollen DA, Perot P, Reid KH. Experimental bilateral spike and wave from thalamic stimulation in relation to the level of arousal. Electroencephalogr Clin Neurophysiol. 1963;15:459–73.

Sun FT, Morrell MJ, Wharen REJ. Responsive cortical stimulation for the treatment of epilepsy. Neurotherapeutics. 2008;5:68–74.

Velasco F, Velasco M, Romo R. Specific and nonspecific multiple unit activities during pentylenetetrazol seizures in animal with mesencephalic transections. Electroencephalogr Clin Neurophysiol. 1982;53:289–97.

Velasco F, Velasco M, Ogarrio C, Fanghanel G. Electrical stimulation of the centromedian thalamic nucleus in the treatment of convulsive seizures: a preliminary report. Epilepsia. 1987;28:421–30.

Velasco F, Velasco M. Mesencephalic structures and tonic clonic generalized seizures. In: Avoli M, Gloor P, Kustopoulus G, Naquet R, editors. Generalized epilepsy. Neurobiological approaches. Boston: Birkhouser; 1990, p. 368–84.

Velasco M, Velasco F, Velasco AL, Velasco G, Jimenez F. Effect of chronic electrical stimulation of the centromedian thalamic nuclei on various intractable seizure patterns: II. Psychological performance and background EEG activity. Epilepsia. 1993;34:1065–74.

Velasco M, Velasco F, Velasco AL, Brito F, Jimenez F, Marquez I, et al. Electrocortical and behavioral responses produced by acute electrical stimulation of the human centromedian thalamic nucleus. Electroencephalogr Clin Neurophysiol. 1997;102:461–71.

Velasco AL, Velasco M, Velasco F, Menes D, Gordon F, Rocha L, et al. Subacute and chronic electrical stimulation of the hippocampus on intractable temporal lobe seizures: preliminary report. Arch Med Res. 2000a;31:316–28.

Velasco F, Velasco M, Jimenez F, Velasco AL, Brito F, Rise M, et al. Predictors in the treatment of difficult-to-control seizures by electrical stimulation of the centromedian thalamic nucleus. Neurosurgery. 2000b;47:295–304.

Velasco F, Carrillo-Ruiz JD, Brito F, Velasco M, Velasco AL, Marquez I, et al. Double-blind, randomized controlled pilot study of bilateral cerebellar stimulation for treatment of intractable motor seizures. Epilepsia. 2005;46:1071–81.

Velasco AL, Velasco F, Jimenez F, Velasco M, Castro G, Carrillo-Ruiz JD, et al. Neuromodulation of the centromedian thalamic nuclei in the treatment of generalized seizures and the improvement of the quality of life in patients with Lennox-Gastaut syndrome. Epilepsia. 2006;47:1203–12.

Velasco AL, Velasco F, Velasco M, Trejo D, Castro G, Carrillo-Ruiz JD. Electrical stimulation of the hippocampal epileptic foci for seizure control: a double-blind, long-term follow-up study. Epilepsia. 2007;48:1895–903.

Velasco AL, Velasco F, Velasco M, Nuñez JM, Trejo D, Garcia I. Neuromodulation of epileptic foci in patients with non-lesional refractory motor epilepsy. Int J Neural Syst. 2009;19:139–47.

Vesper J, Steinhoff B, Rona S, Wille C, Bilic S, Nikkhah G, et al. Chronic high-frequency deep brain stimulation of the STN/SNr for progressive myoclonic epilepsy. Epilepsia. 2007;48:1984–9.

Weiss SR, Eidsath A, Li XL, Heynen T, Post RM. Quenching revisited: low level direct current inhibits amygdala-kindled seizures. Exp Neurol. 1998;154:185–92.

Wyckhuys T, De Smedt T, Claeys P, Raedt R, Waterschoot L, Vonck K, et al. High frequency deep brain stimulation in the hippocampus modifies seizure characteristics in kindled rats. Epilepsia. 2007;48:1543–50.

Chapter 18
Transcranial Magnetic Stimulation and Refractory Partial Epilepsy

Lilia Maria Morales Chacón, Lázaro Gómez Fernández, Otto Trápaga Quincoses, Genco Marcio Estrada Vinajera, Lourdes Lorigados Pedre, Marilyn Zaldivar Bermudes, and Luisa Rocha

Abstract This chapter reviews the principles of transcranial magnetic stimulation (TMS) concerning its potential clinical use in diagnosis and therapy in medically intractable epilepsies. After introducing basic principles, stimulation protocols, and risks, TMS applications in epilepsies are summarized. Next, we discuss several clinical trials and animal studies, which show how low-frequency repetitive TMS (rTMS) may reduce seizure frequency and epileptiform discharges, mainly in focal epilepsy patients with neocortical epileptogenic zones such as malformations of cortical development. Lastly, we address some TMS effects on neurofunctional imaging. We conclude that rTMS should be considered one of the future noninvasive, relatively safe, and inexpensive therapeutic methods in patients with medically intractable epilepsies.

Keywords Epilepsy • Medically intractable epilepsies • Seizures • Transcranial magnetic stimulation • Repetitive transcranial magnetic stimulation • Electroencephalography

18.1 Introduction

According to the World Health Organization (WHO), 50 million people worldwide, representing about 2%, have epilepsy (Engel 2003). Though the availability of antiepileptic drugs (AEDs) has increased in recent decades, about 30% of the

L.M. Morales Chacón (✉) • L. Gómez Fernández • O. Trápaga Quincoses
• G.M. Estrada Vinajera • L. Lorigados Pedre • M. Zaldivar Bermudes
Clinical Neurophysiology Service, International Center for Neurological Restoration,
Ave 25 No 15805 e/158 y 160, Habana, Playa 11 300, Cuba
e-mail: lily@neuro.ciren.cu; genesvin@yahoo.es

L. Rocha
Department of Pharmacobiology, Center for Research and Advanced Studies,
Mexico City, Mexico

L. Rocha and E.A. Cavalheiro (eds.), *Pharmacoresistance in Epilepsy: From Genes and Molecules to Promising Therapies*, DOI 10.1007/978-1-4614-6464-8_18,

population who suffer from epilepsy are considered medically intractable or *pharmacoresistant*, and 5–10% of these may be candidates for resective surgery (Engel 2001; Uijl et al. 2012). There is no doubt that, for patients who develop intractable epilepsy, surgery is superior to medical treatment (Morales et al. 2009; Tellez-Zenteno and Wiebe 2008). Although surgery does better in temporal lobe epilepsy (TLE), it is also recommended for extratemporal epilepsy patients (Abou-Khalil 2012; Al-Otaibi et al. 2011; Alexopoulos et al. 2007; Bonilha et al. 2012; Nakken et al. 2012).

Electrical stimulation of both central and peripheral nervous systems has emerged as a possible alternative for patients who are not deemed to be good candidates for resective surgical procedures (Al-Otaibi and Al-Khairallah 2012). Apart from well-established treatments like vagus nerve stimulation, epilepsy centers are investigating the efficacy and safety of neurostimulation of different brain targets, such as the thalamus, hippocampus, and subthalamic nucleus (Fisher 2012; Velasco et al. 2001). Also exciting are the preliminary results of responsive neuromodulation studies, which involve the delivery of stimulation to the brain in response to detected epileptiform activity (Rolston et al. 2012). In addition to electrical stimulation, novel therapeutic methods that may open new horizons in the management of epilepsy include focal drug delivery, cellular transplantation, gene therapy, and transcranial magnetic stimulation (TMS) (Al-Otaibi et al. 2011). Repetitive TMS (rTMS) has been used with the aim of modifying brain activity over longer timescales in patients with specific neurological disorders with therapeutic intent (Fregni and Pascual-Leone 2007; Rossi et al. 2009; Rossini and Rossi 2007).

This review focuses on TMS, which—at least theoretically—fulfils some of the requirements of an optimal therapeutic method. Basic principles, stimulation protocols, and risks are discussed as well as current applications of TMS in epilepsies.

18.2 Transcranial Magnetic Stimulation: Basic Principles and Protocols

TMS is a noninvasive and painless method providing focal cortical stimulation that is emerging as a novel clinical tool (Barker and Cain 1985; Kobayashi and Pascual-Leone 2003). TMS is based on the principle of "electromagnetic induction," the process by which electrical energy is converted into magnetic fields, and vice versa. This principle was discovered by Faraday in 1831. Later, in 1896, D. Arsonval was the first to apply a magnetic field to the human brain. This was followed by several experiments and the construction of different magnetic stimulators by several researchers (Hallett 2007). The modern era of TMS began in 1985, when Barker et al. developed the first modern TMS device to investigate the human motor cortex (Barker and Cain 1985).

It has been suggested that TMS stimulates the brain through an electromagnetic field that penetrates the tissue with minimal resistance and produces synaptic excitation within the stimulated cortical neurons. A 0.1-ms stimulation has been shown to induce currents that can last the same amount of time and are confined to 1 cm^2 of cortex (Pascual-Leone and Pridmore 1995). The magnetic field is simply used to pass the high-intensity pulses through the skull without inducing pain and it can reach up to about 2 T and typically lasts for about 100 ms. An electric field is induced perpendicularly to the magnetic field. The voltage of the field itself may excite neurons, but the induced currents are likely more important (Hallett 2007).

For magnetic stimulation, a brief, high-current pulse is induced in a coil of wire, called the magnetic coil. These magnetic coils may have different shapes. Round coils are relatively powerful. Figure-eight-shaped coils are more focal, producing maximal current at the intersection of the two round components. Another configuration is called the H coil, with complex windings that permit a slower falloff of the magnetic field intensity with depth (Zangen et al. 2005). In another design, the windings of a coil are around an iron core rather than air. This focuses the field and allows greater strength and depth of penetration (Yang et al. 2008).

TMS can be applied as one stimulus at a time (single pulse), as trains of stimuli delivered at a fixed frequency (conventional repetitive TMS, usually in the range of 1–20 Hz), or in more complex trains combining different frequencies (Theodore 2002). Repetitive TMS is a special form of TMS made possible in the late 1980s thanks to the development of stimulators capable of delivering TMS pulses at frequencies up to 60 Hz. Recent developments have provided magnetic stimulators that allow for stimulation at even higher frequencies.

Repetitive TMS can produce powerful effects that outlast the period of stimulation, inhibition with stimulation at about 1 Hz, and excitation with stimulation at 5 Hz and higher. Low-frequency-rTMS (LF-rTMS) between 0.2 and 1 Hz reduces cortical excitability (Chen et al. 1997) as evidenced by increased cortical silent period duration (Cincotta et al. 2003), and reduced motor-evoked potential (MEP) amplitudes (Muellbacher et al. 1998). In contrast, higher frequencies, approximately 5 Hz or faster, enhance cortical excitability, particularly at high intensities (Thut et al. 2003a). The term "slow-frequency" rTMS is used to refer to stimulus rates of 1 Hz or less, in contrast to "rapid-rate" or "high-frequency" rTMS meaning stimulus rates higher than 1 Hz. This division is somewhat arbitrary, but it is based on the different physiological effects and degrees of risks associated with low- and high-frequency stimulation (Hallett 2007; Thut et al. 2003a, b).

TMS can also be used repetitively in a mode where very-short- and very-high-frequency trains of stimuli are delivered at theta frequency, about 5 Hz. This is called theta burst stimulation (TBS). A typical paradigm would be three stimuli at 50 Hz, repeated at 5 Hz (Di Lazarro et al. 2005).

It is also important to distinguish between online and offline rTMS, as these two rTMS protocols have different possible applications in clinical practice and research. In offline rTMS, the focus lies on the rTMS effects that outlast the rTMS train and can be demonstrated after the rTMS train has ceased (offline effects). In the online protocol, rTMS is used mainly with the aim to disrupt specific brain functions during the application of the rTMS train itself (online effects) (Pascual-Leone et al. 1991). In the clinical setting, this could help to identify the speech-dominant hemisphere, obviously important for presurgical evaluations as well as for establishing causal brain–behavior relations (Thut et al. 2003a).

Offline effects of rTMS have been probed mainly through assessment of a number of electromyography (EMG) responses to a single TMS pulse over the motor cortex and their changes due to rTMS. The magnitude of the evoked muscle contraction in a contralateral limb (typically a hand muscle) can be quantified by skin electrodes and the recording of an MEP (Kobayashi and Pascual-Leone 2003). These EMG responses can provide measures of various aspects of motor cortex excitability (Pascual-Leone et al. 1998). From MEPs, a number of measures can be derived to probe cortical excitability. One is the threshold to muscle activation, or motor threshold (MT). The MT appears to largely reflect neuronal membrane excitability and is increased by anticonvulsants, such as phenytoin and carbamazepine that inhibit voltage-gated sodium channels.

On the other hand, paired-pulse TMS-EMG provides measures of γ-aminobutyric acid (GABA)-mediated cortical inhibition and glutamate-dependent cortical excitability. In the most common paired-pulse TMS-EMG protocols, a subthreshold conditioning stimulus is delivered before each succeeding TMS pulse (Kobayashi and Pascual-Leone 2003; Theodore 2003). Short (1–5 ms) interstimulus intervals lead to reduction of the MEP, and likely reflect GABA(A)-receptor-mediated short-intervals. TMS can be used not only to investigate phenomena of intracortical inhibition (ICI) and facilitation (ICF) in the motor cortex but also to view interactions between motor cortices, such as interhemispheric inhibition (IHI) (Badawy et al. 2010; Hallett 2007).

18.3 Safety and Tolerability of rTMS

Early studies documented rTMS-induced epileptic seizures in healthy subjects that raised safety concerns (Pascual-Leone et al. 1993, 1994). Based on these studies, conditions for seizure induction have been evaluated and safety guidelines have been established. Since their initial publication, new but rare incidences of seizure induction have led to adaptations of these guidelines (Chen et al. 2008; Rossi et al. 2009).

Stimulus parameters, which increase the probability of adverse effects, include high TMS pulse intensities, high rTMS frequencies and high number of pulses for individual trains, as well as short inter-train intervals and high number of trains delivered in a single session. Safety guidelines for the use of rTMS have been formulated by the International Society for Transcranial Stimulation (ISTS) (Wassermann et al. 1999) and the International Federation for Clinical Neurophysiology (IFCN) (Benninger et al. 2009).

Seizure induction is a rare but serious adverse effect of the—otherwise very safe—method of TMS. There are only very few single case reports concerning seizures in single-pulse TMS. Most of them describe individuals with neurological disorders or anticonvulsant medication (Hufnagel et al. 1990a; Hufnagel and Elger 1991a). However, one study found evidence for subclinical, epileptiform activity induced by rTMS, applied within safety margins in a non-epileptic subject (Kanno et al. 2001). In 2011, Kratz et al. also reported a healthy subject who developed symptoms of a seizure after single-pulse TMS during motor threshold estimation (Kratz et al. 2011). This case report provides evidence that single-pulse TMS may cause seizures, even in the absence of neurological risk factors.

Electroencephalographic (EEG) monitoring of non-epileptic volunteers before, during, and after rTMS generally found no apparent EEG abnormalities that could be attributed to rTMS (Boutros et al. 2000; Graf et al. 2001; Loo et al. 2008). Furthermore, there is no conclusive evidence that rTMS can facilitate interictal epileptic EEG activity in epilepsy patients, even though in some of these studies, stimulus parameters fell outside the safety guidelines or patients were off antiepileptic medication (Davies et al. 1994; Schuler et al. 1993; Schulze-Bonhage et al. 1999).

We have recently described a 58-year-old chronic stroke patient with multiple risk factors, who developed focal motor seizures with secondary tonic–clonic generalization during his first 10 Hz rTMS session as an experimental subject of a placebo-controlled clinical trial. It is very interesting to remark that the stimulation at 10 Hz and subthreshold intensity of 90% induced the seizure just within the first 2-s TMS train. We concluded that the identification of epileptiform activity in the EEG from a stroke patient is a warning signal when proposing high-frequency rTMS as a therapy. In addition, high-frequency rTMS should not be used when any other systemic or chronic conditions, such as toxic addiction or withdrawal syndrome, are present (Gomez et al. 2011).

It is important to remember that pathophysiological conditions are completely different in patients than in healthy subjects, who have been the main source of data for establishing safety margins. The issue of safety and tolerability of rTMS in patients with epilepsy is obviously of pivotal importance for any further development of the method as a therapeutic tool.

In 2007, Bae et al. summarized the experience from 26 studies in a total of 280 subjects and concluded that in epilepsy patients, seizures may occur by chance during a TMS session (Bae et al. 2007). In order to minimize the risk of such rare adverse effects, existing and new suggestions are combined to provide reasonable precautions to be taken before and during TMS application. rTMS applied correctly and carefully might be used to safely modulate neuronal elements in a potentially meaningful manner for diagnosis or therapy of a wide range of neurological diseases (Thut et al. 2003a).

18.4 TMS as Diagnostic and Investigative Procedure in Epilepsies

According to the literature reviewed, single-pulse and paired-pulse TMS may be used as a diagnostic procedure to map cortical function and measure cortical excitability (Staudt 2010).

Various TMS measures of the motor cortex can evaluate different aspects of cortical excitability. Some of the common measures are threshold for producing an MEP, recruitment curve, short intracortical inhibition and facilitation, silent period, short and long afferent inhibition, and transcallosal inhibition (TCI) (Hallett 2007; Werhahn et al. 2000; Ziemann 2011). A number of TMS applications as diagnostic and investigative procedures in epilepsies are mentioned below.

18.4.1 TMS for Assessment of Cortical Excitability in Epileptic Syndrome

Changes in cortical excitability in patients with epilepsy vary depending on epilepsy type, time of testing (ictal vs. interictal), and AED intake (Tassinari et al. 2003). A reduced MT indicating cortical hyperexcitability was observed only in subsets of untreated patients with idiopathic generalized epilepsy (IGE) (Reutens et al. 1993; Reutens and Berkovic 1992). In contrast, Delvaux et al. reported that MT usually increased in treated patients with IGE or partial epilepsy, likely due to antiepileptic treatment. They also found an MT increase 48 h after a generalized seizure (Delvaux et al. 2001). On the other hand, Aguglia et al. (2000) described that interhemispherical divergences in MT can be exaggerated in patients with asymmetric motor seizures.

In 2001, Macdonell and collaborators found that the mean cortical silent period (CSP) duration increased at all stimulus intensities, indicating that ICI is increased in patients with untreated IGE (Macdonell et al. 2001). Other authors demonstrated specific differences in cortical excitability between progressive myoclonic epilepsy (PME) and juvenile myoclonic epilepsy (JME) using TMS, particularly at long latencies in the paired-pulse paradigm, implicating a role for GABA B-mediated networks (Badawy et al. 2010).

18.4.2 TMS for Assessment of Ictal–Interictal Cortical Excitability Changes

Recently, Richardson and Lopes da Silva (2011) described that motor responses to TMS differ between the interictal state remote from any seizure and a period of hours immediately prior to a seizure. These studies reveal that intracortical mechanisms responsible for paired-pulse inhibition and facilitation (probably involving synaptic processes and small networks) are impaired in the pre-ictal period, producing "increased excitability" or "reduced inhibition," or both (Richardson and Lopes da Silva 2011).

18.4.3 TMS for Functional Mapping of Eloquent Cortical Areas and Presurgical Localization of the Epileptogenic Zone

Using TMS, the brain can be briefly activated or inhibited. This effect can be used to localize brain functions in both space and time. Since the 1990s, TMS has been used for presurgical localization and evaluation of the epileptogenic zone (Dhuna et al. 1991; Hufnagel et al. 1990a; Schuler et al. 1993) and for mapping functionally eloquent cortical areas (Jennum and Winkel 1994; Pascual-Leone et al. 1991; Theodore 2003).

Applications were first directed at the motor system, but are now being used to map sensory processes and cognitive function. Mapping the motor cortex by moving the coil over the surface of the scalp and recording MEPs from different muscles has been fairly straightforward. MEP mapping is an example of mapping in space with activation, whereas TMS of the occipital cortex can also produce a transient scotoma, which provides mapping in time with inhibition.

rTMS is used to transiently modulate brain function in healthy people beyond TMS to probe for the implication of the stimulated area (or network) in perception and cognition (Robertson et al. 2003). It has been useful for evaluating memory processes. For example, several studies give evidence for a role of the left dorsolateral prefrontal cortex (DLPFC) in working memory. There are numerous examples of how this technique has helped localize a wide variety of other cognitive functions. For example, LF-rTMS over right or left prefrontal cortex impaired behavior on a task involving visuospatial planning (Basso et al. 2006; Knoch et al. 2006).

Although language lateralization through rTMS-induced speech arrest shows a fairly high concordance with the results of the intracarotid amytal (Wada) test in epilepsy patients (Jennum et al. 1994; Wassermann et al. 1999) there are some drawbacks to cortical mapping of linguistic functions using this approach. Online rTMS appears to lack sensitivity for determination of language dominance, as some studies report difficulties to obtain speech arrest in more than two-thirds of all tested patients (Jennum et al. 1994; Michelucci et al. 1994). Even when rTMS parameters are adjusted to reliably induce speech arrest, online rTMS shows a relatively poor prognostic value for postoperative language deficits (Epstein et al. 2000). Of special interest in this respect is a study on the susceptibility of Wernicke's area to rTMS-induced language disruption (in a picture–word matching task) and the relationship to language lateralization in the same, healthy subjects as assessed through functional magnetic resonance imaging (fMRI) (Knecht et al. 2002).

In future studies, rTMS protocols will have to be adapted to target other aspects of language than speech production, if online rTMS is to become a useful tool in epilepsy presurgical evaluation. A major intrinsic limitation of TMS to map the human brain lies in the unclear relationship between the position of the stimulating coil on the scalp and the underlying stimulated cortex. The relationship between structure and function as the major feature constituting a brain mapping modality can therefore not be established. Recent advances in image processing have allowed refinement of TMS by combining magnetic resonance imaging (MRI) modalities with TMS using a neuronavigation system to measure the position of the stimulating coil and map this position onto an MRI data set. In 2010, Saisanen et al. showed that navigated transcranial magnetic stimulation (nTMS) is a safe and feasible clinical tool for noninvasive preoperative localization of motor cortex in patients with intractable epilepsy due to focal lesions adjacent or within the presumed primary motor cortex in MRI (Saisanen et al. 2010).

A further conceivable application of rTMS in diagnosis and evaluation of epilepsy is its potential to increase cortical excitability and reduce seizure threshold, if applied at high frequencies. It has been argued that rTMS could be used as an epileptogenic activation procedure to endorse other approaches for seizure induction or for localization of seizure foci in epilepsy evaluation (Hufnagel et al. 1990b). However, studies so far have failed to induce epileptiform discharges in the EEG in most epilepsy patients by either high- or low-frequency rTMS. Altogether, these studies suggest that TMS has limited practical use in localization of the epileptogenic zone, and that high-frequency rTMS possibly has a greater anti- than proconvulsant effect in epilepsy patients when applied by conventional, commercially available magnetic stimulators (Hufnagel and Elger 1991b).

18.5 TMS as Therapeutic Procedure

In therapeutic applications, the capacity of rTMS to induce a lasting change in cortical excitability has been tested in several diseases (Pascual-Leone et al. 1999). The 2008 US Food and Drug Administration (FDA) clearance of rTMS for treatment of major depression is testament to its gain of acceptance in the clinical setting. The clinical potential of TMS and rTMS (TMS/rTMS) also drives translational research where these methods are tested in animal disease models. Translational work with TMS/rTMS includes tests of its antidepressant, anti-manic, and antiepileptic potential (Akamatsu et al. 2001; Anschel et al. 2003), as well as experiments aimed to evaluate the safety of TMS/rTMS (Nitsche et al. 2002).

The most promising characteristic of rTMS in relation to possible future clinical applications in epilepsy is its potential for seizure reduction at low frequencies. In comparison to healthy controls, patients with epilepsy show signs of cortical hyperexcitability (decreased motor threshold, decreased ICI, shortening of the silent period, increased ICF) (Brodtmann et al. 1999; Brown et al. 1996; Caramia et al. 1996; Cicinelli et al. 2000; Manganotti et al. 2001; Valzania et al. 1999; Werhahn et al. 2000), as indicated by the variety of single- and paired-pulse TMS protocols probing motor cortex excitability. In patients with epilepsy, there is an enhanced probability of neuronal networks to fire synchronously at high frequency, initiated by a paroxysmal depolarization shift. Reducing neuronal excitability is a common target of antiepileptic therapies. In addition to pharmacological interventions, excitability-reducing brain stimulation is pursued as an alternative therapeutic approach (Nitsche and Paulus 2009).

18.5.1 Rationale for Using TMS as a Therapeutic Procedure in Epilepsy

The reasoning for using TMS as a therapeutic tool is precisely based on the fact that the effects of each single pulse or single train can summate with repeated application, leading to effects outlasting a stimulation session (Kimiskidis 2010; Ridding and Rothwell 2007; Rossi et al. 2004). rTMS can produce effects that outlast the application of a train of stimuli for minutes or hours. It is assumed that these aftereffects can be used to modulate neuronal activity in a targeted area of dysfunctional cortex to induce a functional benefit. The exact nature of TMS-induced effects depends on the frequency, intensity, and length of time for which the stimulation is applied (Fregni and Pascual-Leone 2007). The duration of the antiepileptic effects is obviously of paramount importance if TMS is to become a clinically meaningful treatment against epilepsies.

At an experimental level, LF-rTMS (0.5 Hz) reduced the occurrence of status epilepticus and increased the onset latency of pentylenetetrazole-induced seizures in rats (Akamatsu et al. 2001).

It was also demonstrated that low-frequency (1 Hz) electrical stimulation is able to prevent interictal epileptic discharges and epilepsy-like events in an intensity-, frequency-, and distance-dependent manner in hippocampal and neocortical rat slices (Albensi et al. 2004; Schiller and Bankirer 2007). Moreover, these effects remain after the end of stimulation and are NMDA-receptor dependent, thus indicating that long-term depression (LTD)-inducing protocols might have antiepileptic properties. Consequently, the application of LF-rTMS for treating epilepsy in humans seems to be promising.

The effects induced by rTMS are reminiscent of LTD and long-term potentiation (LTP), two forms of synaptic plasticity elicited in animal models of cortical circuitry by low- and high-frequency electrical stimulation, respectively. It has been suggested that LF-rTMS may exert antiepileptic effects by inducing LTD whereas high-frequency stimulation may act in a proconvulsant manner (Ziemann 2011). Although this theoretical framework is appealing, it should be noted that there is—in fact—very little actual evidence that rTMS induces LTD in the human brain, and that other mechanisms, including enhancement of GABAergic inhibition (Pascual-Leone et al. 1994), may be involved in its antiepileptic action.

Moreover, other scientists reported the effect of LF-TMS on neuropeptide-Y (NPY) expression and apoptosis of hippocampal neurons in epileptic rats induced by pilocarpine. They found that LF-TMS alleviated neuron injury in the hippocampus, and concluded that LF-TMS might play an important role in resisting the progression of epilepsy. They also showed that NPY-positive cell numbers increased in all areas of the hippocampus, which indicated a close relation between NPY and epilepsy. These results also indicated that NPY might have some function in intractable epilepsy (Wang et al. 2007). All these reported effects in animal models suggest the possible therapeutic use of LF-rTMS in patients with intractable seizures.

18.5.2 Clinical Trials

The antiepileptic effects of TMS have been investigated in a series of open-label studies (Brasil-Neto et al. 2004; Brighina et al. 2006; Daniele et al. 2003; Fregni et al. 2005; Kinoshita et al. 2005; Rotenberg et al. 2009; Santiago-Rodriguez et al. 2008; Sun et al. 2011; Tergau et al. 1999), single-case reports (Graff-Guerrero et al. 2004; Menkes and Gruenthal 2000; Misawa et al. 2005; Rossi et al. 2004; Rotenberg et al. 2008), and controlled studies (Cantello et al. 2007; Fregni et al. 2006; Joo et al. 2007; Tergau et al. 2003; Theodore et al. 2002; Sun et al. 2011). Table 18.1 summarizes clinical trials of rTMS treatment of epilepsies.

Single-case reports as well as small-scale series have also been carried out (Brasil-Neto et al. 2004; Fregni et al. 2005; Graff-Guerrero et al. 2004; Kinoshita et al. 2005; Menkes and Gruenthal 2000; Misawa et al. 2005; Rossi et al. 2004; Rotenberg et al. 2008) describing the effects of TMS on various seizure types of diverse etiologies. Misawa et al. reported an illustrative case of a 31-year-old patient suffering from epilepsia partialis continua (EPC) for 15 years due to a motor cortical dysplasia. TMS resulted in a dramatic improvement of EPC in the right upper extremity, which lasted approximately 2 months. A second trial of rTMS produced similarly good effects (Misawa et al. 2005). In a single patient with epilepsy associated with a focal cortical dysplasia, Menkes et al. applied LF-rTMS (0.5 Hz) stimulation and found a decrease in seizure frequency and interictal spikes, by 70 and 77%, respectively (Menkes and Gruenthal 2000).

Overall, the available open-label studies show a reduction in seizure frequency and epileptic discharges, using TMS with stimulation frequencies of 1 Hz or lower (Brasil-Neto et al. 2004; Fregni and Pascual-Leone 2005; Joo et al. 2007; Kinoshita et al. 2005; Rotenberg and Pascual-Leone 2009; Santiago-Rodriguez et al. 2008) (Table 18.1). LF-rTMS was performed between 0.3 and 0.9 Hz, but the specific frequency had no impact on the efficacy of stimulation when comparing the different studies. The stimulation intensity was between 90 and 120% of motor threshold, and the number of stimuli applied was between 100 and 1,000. When comparing the efficacy of stimulation to reduce seizures there is slight indication in favor of stronger and longer stimulation. However, since other parameters were not identical among the various studies, this statement is also somewhat preliminary.

The enthusiasm created by open-label studies was subsequently tempered by the results of controlled rTMS studies (Cantello et al. 2007; Fregni et al. 2006; Theodore et al. 2002).

The results derived from controlled trials are mixed in relation to antiepileptic rTMS efficacy, and the field would benefit from further carefully controlled trials. The published placebo-controlled trials employed distinct rTMS protocols and subject selection, with inconsistent conclusions (Cantello et al. 2007; Fregni et al. 2006; Theodore et al. 2002). Definitive reasons for these heterogeneous results are difficult to assess because the studies differ in more than one aspect (Table 18.1). Fregni and Theodore included only patients with focal epilepsy, whereas patients with primary generalized epilepsies also participated in the study by Cantello et al. Thus, it

Table 18.1 Clinical trials and case reports of rTMS to treat intractable epilepsy

Authors (year)	No. patients/ mean age and/ or age range in years	Study protocol	Epilepsy syndrome/ underlying etiology	rTMS protocol: frequency (Hz) / Intensity stimuli / Schedule	Coil/position	Outcome seizures	Outcome epileptiform discharges	No. AEDs
Cantello et al. (2007)	43/36.9	Randomized, double blind, sham controlled	Focal (mTLE = 7, NE = 34) generalized = 2	0.3 Hz 100% MT ($n = 34$) 65% MSO ($n = 9$) 500/train 2 trains/day for 5 days	0/Vertex	No change	Decreasing	2–4
Fregni et al. (2006)	12/21.9	Randomized, double blind, sham controlled	Focal (MCD)	1 Hz 70% MSO 1,200/train 1 train/day for 5 days	8/Epileptogenic focus ($n = 9$), vertex ($n = 3$)	Decreasing	Decreasing	1–3
Theodore, et al. (2002)	24/26–54	Randomized, double blind, sham controlled	Focal (mTLE = 10, lTLE = 10, ETLE = 4)	1 Hz 120% MT 900/train 2 trains/day for 1 week	8/Epileptogenic focus	Trend for reduction	NR	≥2
Joo et al. (2007)	35/25 (18–46)	Randomized	Focal ($n = 18$), multifocal ($n = 8$), non-localized ($n = 9$)	0.5 Hz 100% MT 3,000/train ($n = 19$) 1,500/train ($n = 16$) 1 train/day for 5 days	0/Vertex ($n = 17$) temporal ($n = 12$)	Trend for reduction (correlation with no. of stimuli)	Decreasing	3.6 ± 1.4 (2–7)

(continued)

Table 18.1 (continued)

Authors (year)	No. patients/ mean age and/ or age range in years	Study protocol	Epilepsy syndrome/ underlying etiology	rTMS protocol: frequency (Hz) Intensity stimuli Schedule	Coil/position	Outcome seizures	Outcome epileptiform discharges	No. AEDs
Tergau et al. (2003)	17/29 ± 10	Crossover, placebo controlled	mTLE = 2, ETLE = 11, multifocal = 2, generalized = 2	0.33, 1 Hz Slightly below MT 1,000/train 1 train/day for 5 days	0/Vertex	Decreasing (at 0.33 Hz only)	NR	NR
Daniele et al. (2003)	4/27–33	Open label	Focal (frontal = 2, multifocal = 2, due to CD)	0.5 Hz 90% MT 100/train Biweekly, 4 weeks	8/Epileptogenic focus or vertex	Decreasing (in patients with a single focus)	NR	2–3
Fregni et al. (2005)	8/24.2 (14–38)	Open label	TLE = 3, multifocal = 4, ETLE = 1, all due to MCD	0.5 Hz 65% MSO 600 single session	8/Epileptogenic focus or vertex	Decreasing (for 1 month)	Decreasing (for 1 month)	2–4
Kinoshita et al. (2005)	7/23.3 (16–33)	Open label	Focal (frontal = 5, parietal = 1, hypothalamic hamartoma = 1)	0.9 Hz 90% rMT 810/train 2 trains/day for 5 days/week for 2 weeks	0/FCz, PCz	Decreasing	NR	2–4
Tergau et al. (1999)	9/19-47	Open label	TLE = 2, ETLE = 7	0.33 Hz 100% MT 500 ×2/train 2 train/day for 5 days	0/Vertex	Decreasing	NR	Various

Brasil-Neto et al. (2004)	5/27.4	Open label	Focal (TLE=2, FLE=3)	0.3 Hz 95% MT 20/train 5 trains/day biweekly for 3 months	0/Vertex	Decreasing	NR	1–3
Brighina et al. (2006)	6/37±6.3 (28–44)	Open label	Focal	5 Hz 90% MT 800 Biweekly for 4 weeks	8/Epileptogenic focus or Cz	Reduction only by stimulation over the epileptogenic region	Not recorded	2–5
Santiago-Rodriguez et al. (2008)	12/29.3	Open label	Focal neocortical	0.5 Hz 110% rMT 900 pulse/day 2 weeks	8/Epileptic focus	Reduction	No reduction	NR
Rotenberg et al. (2009)	7/(11–79)	Open label	Continuous partial seizures	1, 20–100 Hz 100% MT Diverse Different	8/Epileptogenic focus	Reduction, in most cases short lasting	NA	NR
Graff-Guerrero et al. (2004)	2/7–11	Case report	Continuous partial seizures	20 Hz 50% MD, 128% MT 40 15 days	8/Epileptogenic focus	Reduction in one of the two patients	Reduction	4
Sun et al. (2011)	17/18.12±7.40	Open label	Focal	0.5 Hz 90% RMT 3 sessions 500 pulses each session for 2 weeks	8/Epileptogenic focus	Decreasing and improved psychological conditions	Decreasing interictal epileptiform discharges per 30 min	1

(continued)

Table 18.1 (continued)

Authors (year)	No. patients/ mean age and/ or age range in years	Study protocol	Epilepsy syndrome/ underlying etiology	rTMS protocol: frequency (Hz) / Intensity stimuli / Schedule	Coil/position	Outcome seizures	Outcome epileptiform discharges	No. AEDs
Rotenberg et al. (2008)	1/14	Case report	Continuous partial seizures	1 Hz 100%MT 1,800 9 days	8/Epileptogenic focus	Reduction of seizure duration only during stimulation	Reduction	6
Misawa et al. (2005)	1/31	Case report	Continuous partial seizures due to CD	0.5 Hz 90% rMT 100 single session repeated at 3 months	8/Epileptogenic focus	Decreasing (for 2 months)	NR	2
Rossi et al. (2004)	1/34	Case report	Continuous partial seizures due to CD	1 Hz 90% rMT 900 single session	8/Epileptogenic focus	Decreasing	Decreasing	2
Menkes and Gruenthal (2000)	1/38	Case report	ETLE (parietal CD)	0.5 Hz 95% rMT 20/train 5 trains/day biweekly for 3 months	0/Epileptogenic focus	Decreasing	Decreasing	3

AEDs antiepileptic drug, *CD* malformations of cortical development, *ETLE* extratemporal lobe epilepsy, *FLE* frontal lobe epilepsy, *LTLE* lateral temporal lobe epilepsy, *MCD* cortical dysplasia, *mTLE* mesial temporal lobe epilepsy, *MSO*, maximum stimulator output, *MT* motor threshold, *NE* neocortical epilepsy, *NR* not reported, *rMT* resting motor threshold, *rTMS* repetitive transcranial magnetic stimulation, *0* circular, *8* figure of eight cannot be excluded that the type of epilepsy has an impact on the proneness to profit from rTMS. From a pathophysiological perspective, it would make sense that focal epilepsies with a cortical origin, which are more easily influenced by rTMS, might profit more from rTMS than primary generalized epilepsies.

In the studies conducted by Fregni and Theodore, intensity was stronger than in the study conducted by Cantello and more stimuli were applied. The focality of stimulation is determined by the position of the coil relative to the epileptogenic region and the focality of the stimulation coil. In the Fregni and Theodore studies, the epileptogenic zone was stimulated, whereas in the latter study, stimulation over the vertex was performed. As a result, it could be argued that more intense rTMS and rTMS over the epileptogenic zone might be preferable. Even less is known about the impact of the focality of the coil, current flow direction, and optimal suited frequency of stimulation. It might be that high-frequency stimulation has a disruptive effect on epileptic seizures, while LF-rTMS prevents seizure induction. However, this assumption is derived rather from presumed mechanisms than supported by controlled studies.

In general, it is not known whether optimum stimulation parameters differ in focal and primary generalized epilepsies or whether the specific antiepileptic medication has an effect on the efficacy of rTMS.

Hsu et al. conducted a meta-analysis to reevaluate the antiepileptic efficacy of LF-rTMS in medically intractable epilepsy. This review identified 11 articles, with a total of 164 participants. For outcome measures, effect size and 95% confidence intervals (CIs) were calculated for seizure frequency, spike number, duration of epileptiform abnormalities (EAs), and resting motor threshold (RMT) by using fixed and random effect models. They concluded that LF-rTMS has a favorable effect on seizure reduction, which suggests that rTMS is an alternative intervention, and that the antiepileptic effect lasts at least 2–4 weeks by using the 1–2-week stimulation paradigm. They also concluded that patients with neocortical epilepsy or cortical dysplasia compared with other epileptic disorders might benefit more from rTMS (Hsu et al. 2011)

As has been shown in recent years, several studies have demonstrated that LF-rTMS may reduce seizure frequency in patients with refractory epilepsy (Daniele et al. 2003; Fregni et al. 2005; Joo et al. 2007; Kinoshita et al. 2005; Menkes and Gruenthal 2000; Tergau et al. 1999).

On the other hand, inconsistent findings related to seizure suppression in controlled trials, as well as the discrepancy between open-label and controlled data, suggest that further placebo-controlled trials of rTMS in epilepsy are necessary to fully characterize its antiepileptic potential. Estimation of the placebo effect of rTMS is necessary in trial design, particularly for power analyses and sample size calculations.

In addition, because of the limitations of available rTMS sham methods, it is important to investigate whether there are differences in placebo effect among the sham methods used in published trials. Bae et al. conducted a meta-analysis of individual data from placebo-controlled rTMS trials to estimate the rTMS placebo effect. They measured the placebo effect at follow-up intervals of 2, 4, and 8 weeks after sham rTMS treatment. These authors employed three methods in the reviewed studies: (1) coil positioning orthogonal to the scalp, (2) spring-loaded sham coil, and (3) double active–sham coil. The placebo response overall was consistently low across follow-up intervals, both for median change in seizure frequency and for responder (defined as ≥50% seizure frequency reduction) rate. The aggregate effect of the placebo condition was a 0–2% median seizure reduction rate and a responder rate of 16–20%. Finally, the authors anticipated that these data will contribute to future power analysis as well as selection and design of rTMS sham methods for controlled rTMS trials (Bae et al. 2011).

18.6 Evaluation of TMS Effects on EEG

Functional imaging techniques such as positron emission tomography, fMRI, and EEG mapping enable assessment of TMS-related functional brain activation (Gomez et al. 2011; Thut and Pascual-Leone 2010).

A combination of TMS and functional imaging can be useful in three principal ways: (1) brain imaging before TMS is helpful in defining the accurate coil position over a distinct cortical area targeted by TMS; (2) imaging the brain during TMS is a promising approach for assessing cortical excitability and intracerebral functional connectivity; and (3) brain imaging after TMS can be employed to study the plasticity of the human cortex by evaluating lasting effects of TMS. Moreover, this approach will help to advance our understanding of the therapeutical effects related to TMS (Siebner et al. 2009).

TMS-EEG co-registration in human beings and in animals may enhance clinical and translational TMS/rTMS applications (Bonato et al. 2006; Boutros et al. 2000; Ilmoniemi et al. 1999; Rotenberg et al. 2008). TMS-EEG integration provides real-time information on cortical reactivity and connectivity such as interhemispheric connections, and on how functional activity is linked to behavior (Komssi and Kahkonen 2006; Thut et al. 2003a).

Although TMS-EEG has been largely applied in neurophysiology research, there are prospects for its use in clinical practice, particularly in epilepsy where EEG is widely used, and where TMS is emerging as a diagnostic, investigative, and therapeutic tool (Ferreri et al. 2011). Especially attractive in clinical epilepsy are prospects for TMS-EEG to detect an anticonvulsive effect or a proconvulsive side effect of repetitive stimulation. Brodbeck et al. indicated a consistent effect of rTMS stimulation on interictal spike discharges, but speak in favor of a rather weak and individually variable-immediate effect of rTMS on focal epileptic activity (Brodbeck et al. 2010). For therapeutic purposes, TMS-EEG may be used for the selection of appropriate TMS strength outside of the motor cortex where the threshold for cortical activation is more apparent with the aid of EEG. In other realistic clinical applications, TMS-EEG may be useful in real-time monitoring of epileptiform activity in vulnerable populations where TMS may trigger seizures, or as a component of a responsive neurostimulation setup in which TMS timing is determined by underlying EEG activity. Figure 18.1 shows a representative EEG of a patient with focal intractable epilepsy where the application of TMS was determined by underlying ictal EEG onset.

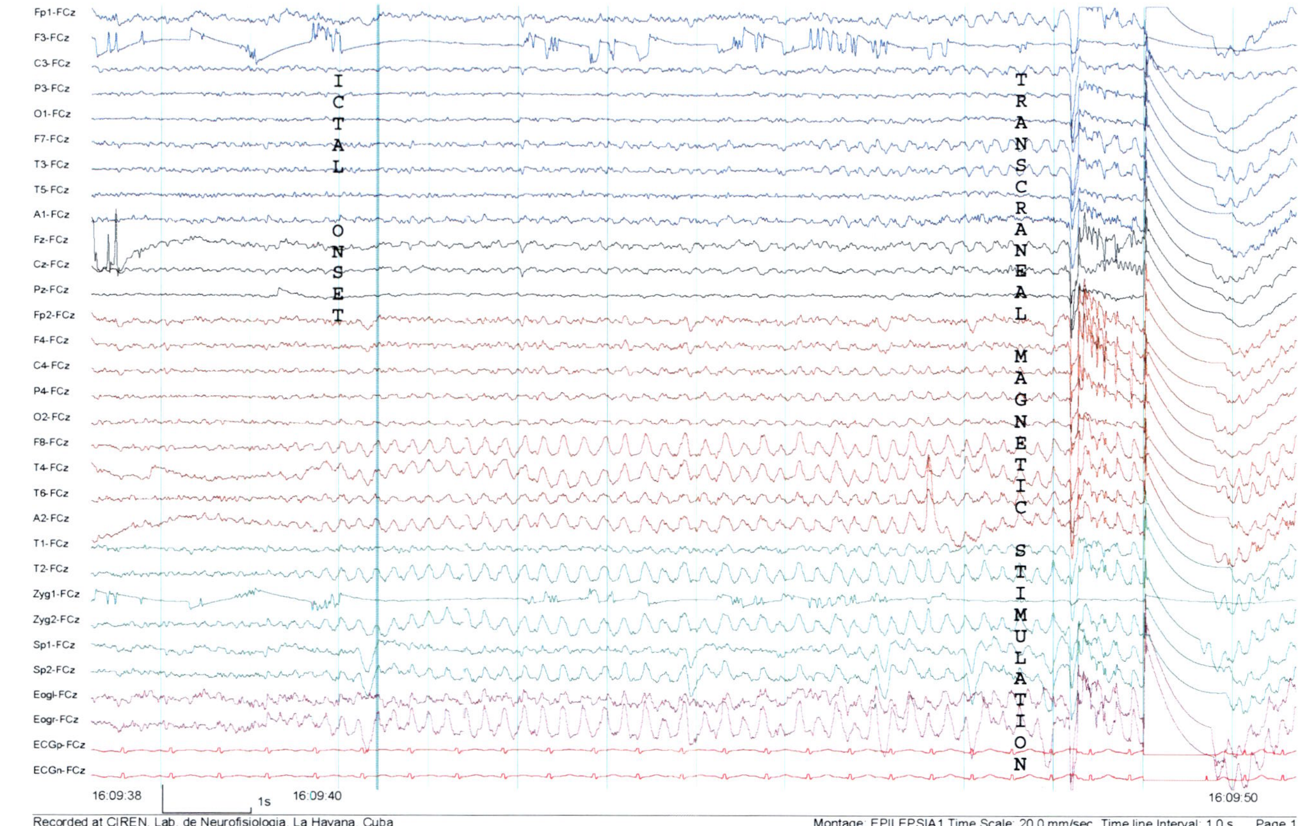

Fig. 18.1 Representative ictal EEG recording during a complex partial seizure in a patient with temporal lobe epilepsy (LF: 0.3, HF: 35 Notch on, sensibility: 30.00 μV/mm, timescale: 20 mm/s or 30 s/page). rTMS application was determined by ictal EEG onset. Notice the artifact induced as a consequence of TMS

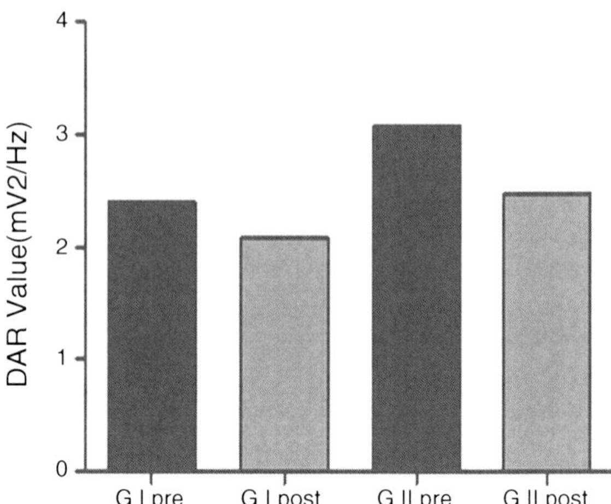

Fig. 18.2 Global delta/alpha ratio (DAR, mV^2/Hz) obtained from EEG recordings before (pre-) and after (post-) rTMS sessions in a patient with stroke submitted to sham (GI) and real 1 Hz rTMS (GII)

Thut and Pascual-Leone found the EEG aftereffects of rTMS to be robust with a mean effect-size of 30–35% change from baseline or sham and a mean duration of 35 min. Furthermore, there is evidence that the aftereffect direction (suppression vs. facilitation) depends on the protocol employed such as conventional low-frequency (1 Hz) and high-frequency TMS, differing in terms of their suppressive versus facilitative impact on brain activity (Thut and Pascual-Leone 2010).

Neuroimaging has also been applied to understand the process of clinical recovery after other neurological diseases such as stroke. The use of EEG and TMS helps to interpret these findings (Rossini and Rossi 2007) (Gerloff et al. 2006). EEG studies using coherence analysis showed that cortico-cortical connections were reduced in the stroke hemisphere but increased in the contralesional hemisphere.

We recently conducted a double-blind prospective and longitudinal study (unpublished data) in order to assess the electrical brain activity and to evaluate the clinical evolution in nine patients with chronic stroke after rehabilitation and the application of 1 Hz rTMS over the contralesional hemisphere. The sample evaluated was randomly divided into two groups: five patients received sham rTMS (group I) and four patients received real rTMS (1 Hz) (group II) both with daily sessions for 20 days. EEGs were recorded before and after rTMS sessions. The neurophysiological measures used were resting EEG-power spectrum (EEG-PS), delta/alpha ratio (DAR), spike-frequency, and spike-amplitude. Clinical characterization was assessed using Scandinavian (SS) and Barthel Index (BI) scales. Stroke patients who received 1 Hz rTMS sessions experienced modifications on resting EEG-PS and epileptiform activity, suggesting likely cortical activation in both brain hemispheres. In general, rTMS induced a better clinical and brain electrical activity recovery, both reflected in the modifications of the SS and in the DAR parameter (Figs. 18.2 and 18.3).

In summary, relatively little can be concluded about the effect of rTMS on EEG characteristics due to the limited data available. An advance in the understanding of these issues is imminent and promises to have a substantial impact on many areas of clinical and basic neuroscience.

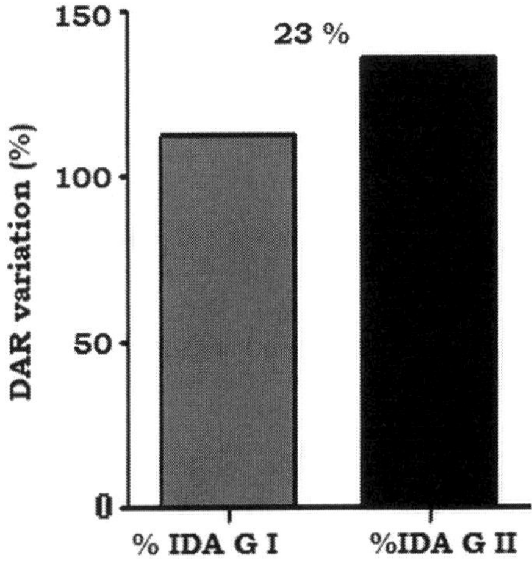

Fig. 18.3 Percentage of delta/alpha ratio (DAR) variation in patients with stroke receiving sham (GI) and rTMS (GII). Notice the higher delta/alpha ratio (DAR) parameter variation in GII after 1 Hz rTMs sessions, suggesting a better clinical and electrical brain activity recovery

18.7 Conclusions

rTMS should be considered one of the future noninvasive, relatively safe, and inexpensive therapeutic methods in patients with medically intractable epilepsies. In recent years, several studies have shown that LF-rTMS may reduce seizure frequency and epileptiform discharges in epilepsy patients, mainly in those with localized cortical epileptogenic zones such as malformations of cortical development (MCDs).

However, rTMS antiepileptic efficacy will have to be determined in future randomized placebo-controlled trials, which should use measurements of the rTMS-placebo effect for power analysis and trial design. Likewise, further clinical studies are required to clarify crucial methodological issues such as rTMS protocols (intervention duration, stimulus parameters, coil selection), inclusion criteria of patients, AED effects, and measures of outcome assessment.

Acknowledgments We thank Odalys Morales Chacón and Dr. Erika Brust-Mascher for English assistance and Maria Luisa Rodriguez, Abel Sanchez, Hector Vazquez, and Leticia Neri for their useful cooperation. This work was sponsored by CONACYT (Project 98386).

References

Abou-Khalil BW. Do we need EEGs after temporal lobe epilepsy surgery, and how many? Epilepsy Curr. 2012;12:29–31.

Aguglia U, Gambardella A, Quartarone A, Girlanda P, Le PE, Messina D, et al. Interhemispheric threshold differences in idiopathic generalized epilepsies with versive or circling seizures determined with focal magnetic transcranial stimulation. Epilepsy Res. 2000;40:1–6.

Akamatsu N, Fueta Y, Endo Y, Matsunaga K, Uozumi T, Tsuji S. Decreased susceptibility to pentylenetetrazol-induced seizures after low-frequency transcranial magnetic stimulation in rats. Neurosci Lett. 2001;310:153–6.

Albensi BC, Ata G, Schmidt E, Waterman JD, Janigro D. Activation of long-term synaptic plasticity causes suppression of epileptiform activity in rat hippocampal slices. Brain Res. 2004; 998:56–64.

Alexopoulos AV, Gonugunta V, Yang J, Boulis NM. Electrical stimulation and gene-based neuromodulation for control of medically-refractory epilepsy. Acta Neurochir Suppl. 2007; 97:293–309.

Al-Otaibi F, Al-Khairallah T. Functional neurosurgery. The modulation of neural and mind circuits. Neurosciences (Riyadh). 2012;17:16–31.

Al-Otaibi FA, Hamani C, Lozano AM. Neuromodulation in epilepsy. Neurosurgery. 2011;69: 957–79.

Anschel DJ, Pascual-Leone A, Holmes GL. Anti-kindling effect of slow repetitive transcranial magnetic stimulation in rats. Neurosci Lett. 2003;351:9–12.

Badawy RA, Macdonell RA, Jackson GD, Berkovic SF. Can changes in cortical excitability distinguish progressive from juvenile myoclonic epilepsy? Epilepsia. 2010;51:2084–8.

Bae EH, Theodore WH, Fregni F, Cantello R, Pascual-Leone A, Rotenberg A. An estimate of placebo effect of repetitive transcranial magnetic stimulation in epilepsy. Epilepsy Behav. 2011;20:355–9.

Bae EH, Schrader LM, Machii K, Alonso-Alonso M, Riviello Jr JJ, Pascual-Leone A, et al. Safety and tolerability of repetitive transcranial magnetic stimulation in patients with epilepsy: a review of the literature. Epilepsy Behav. 2007;10:521–8.

Barker AT, Cain MW. The claimed vasodilatory effect of a commercial permanent magnet foil: results of a double-blind trial. Clin Phys Physiol Meas. 1985;6:261–3.

Basso D, Lotze M, Vitale L, Ferreri F, Bisiacchi P, Olivetti BM, et al. The role of prefrontal cortex in visuo-spatial planning: A repetitive TMS study. Exp Brain Res. 2006;171:411–5.

Benninger DH, Lomarev M, Wassermann EM, Lopez G, Houdayer E, Fasano RE, et al. Safety study of 50 Hz repetitive transcranial magnetic stimulation in patients with Parkinson's disease. Clin Neurophysiol. 2009;120:809–15.

Bonato C, Miniussi C, Rossini PM. Transcranial magnetic stimulation and cortical evoked potentials: a TMS/EEG co-registration study. Clin Neurophysiol. 2006;117:1699–707.

Bonilha L, Martz GU, Glazier SS, Edwards JC. Subtypes of medial temporal lobe epilepsy: influence on temporal lobectomy outcomes? Epilepsia. 2012;53:1–6.

Boutros NN, Berman RM, Hoffman R, Miano AP, Campbell D, Ilmoniemi R. Electroencephalogram and repetitive transcranial magnetic stimulation. Depress Anxiety. 2000;12:166–9.

Brasil-Neto JP, de Araujo DP, Teixeira WA, Araujo VP, Boechat-Barros R. Experimental therapy of epilepsy with transcranial magnetic stimulation: lack of additional benefit with prolonged treatment. Arq Neuropsiquiatr. 2004;62:21–5.

Brighina F, Daniele O, Piazza A, Giglia G, Fierro B. Hemispheric cerebellar rTMS to treat drug-resistant epilepsy: case reports. Neurosci Lett. 2006;397:229–33.

Brodbeck V, Thut G, Spinelli L, Romei V, Tyrand R, Michel CM, et al. Effects of repetitive transcranial magnetic stimulation on spike pattern and topography in patients with focal epilepsy. Brain Topogr. 2010;22:267–80.

Brodtmann A, Macdonell RA, Gilligan AK, Curatolo J, Berkovic SF. Cortical excitability and recovery curve analysis in generalized epilepsy. Neurology. 1999;53:1347–9.

Brown P, Ridding MC, Werhahn KJ, Rothwell JC, Marsden CD. Abnormalities of the balance between inhibition and excitation in the motor cortex of patients with cortical myoclonus. Brain. 1996;119:309–17.

Cantello R, Rossi S, Varrasi C, Ulivelli M, Civardi C, Bartalini S, et al. Slow repetitive TMS for drug-resistant epilepsy: clinical and EEG findings of a placebo-controlled trial. Epilepsia. 2007;48:366–74.

Caramia MD, Gigli G, Iani C, Desiato MT, Diomedi M, Palmieri MG, et al. Distinguishing forms of generalized epilepsy using magnetic brain stimulation. Electroencephalogr Clin Neurophysiol. 1996;98:14–9.

Chen R, Gerloff C, Classen J, Wassermann EM, Hallett M, Cohen LG. Safety of different inter-train intervals for repetitive transcranial magnetic stimulation and recommendations for safe ranges of stimulation parameters. Electroencephalogr Clin Neurophysiol. 1997;105:415–21.

Chen R, Cros D, Curra A, Di Lazzaro V, Lefaucheur JP, Magistris MR, et al. The clinical diagnostic utility of transcranial magnetic stimulation: report of an IFCN committee. Clin Neurophysiol. 2008;119:504–32.

Cicinelli P, Mattia D, Spanedda F, Traversa R, Marciani MG, Pasqualetti P, et al. Transcranial magnetic stimulation reveals an interhemispheric asymmetry of cortical inhibition in focal epilepsy. Neuroreport. 2000;11:701–7.

Cincotta M, Borgheresi A, Gambetti C, Balestrieri F, Rossi L, Zaccara G, et al. Suprathreshold 0.3 Hz repetitive TMS prolongs the cortical silent period: potential implications for therapeutic trials in epilepsy. Clin Neurophysiol. 2003;114:1827–33.

Daniele O, Brighina F, Piazza A, Giglia G, Scalia S, Fierro B. Low-frequency transcranial magnetic stimulation in patients with cortical dysplasia – a preliminary study. J Neurol. 2003;250:761–2.

Davies KG, Maxwell RE, Jennum P, Dhuna A, Beniak TE, Destafney E, et al. Language function following subdural grid-directed temporal lobectomy. Acta Neurol Scand. 1994;90:201–6.

Delvaux V, Alagona G, Gerard P, De Pasqua V, Delwaide PJ, Maertens de Noordhout A. Reduced excitability of the motor cortex in untreated patients with de novo idiopathic "grand mal" seizures. J Neurol Neurosurg Psychiatry. 2001;71:772–6.

Dhuna A, Gates J, Pascual-Leone A. Transcranial magnetic stimulation in patients with epilepsy. Neurology. 1991;41:1067–71.

Di Lazarro V, Pilato F, Saturno E, Oliviero A, Dileone M, Mazzone P, et al. Theta-burst repetitive transcranial magnetic stimulation suppresses specific excitatory circuits in the human motor cortex. J Physiol. 2005;565:945–50.

Engel Jr J. A greater role for surgical treatment of epilepsy: why and when? Epilepsy Curr. 2003;3:37–40.

Engel J Jr. Intractable epilepsy: definition and neurobiology. Epilepsia. 2001;42 Suppl 6:3.

Epstein CM, Woodard JL, Stringer AY, Bakay RA, Henry TR, Pennell PB, et al. Repetitive transcranial magnetic stimulation does not replicate the Wada test. Neurology. 2000;55:1025–7.

Ferreri F, Pasqualetti P, Maatta S, Ponzo D, Ferrarelli F, Tononi G, et al. Human brain connectivity during single and paired pulse transcranial magnetic stimulation. Neuroimage. 2011;54:90–102.

Fisher RS. Therapeutic devices for epilepsy. Ann Neurol. 2012;71:157–68.

Fregni F, Pascual-Leone A. Transcranial magnetic stimulation for the treatment of depression in neurologic disorders. Curr Psychiatry Rep. 2005;7:381–90.

Fregni F, Pascual-Leone A. Technology insight: noninvasive brain stimulation in neurology-perspectives on the therapeutic potential of rTMS and tDCS. Nat Clin Pract Neurol. 2007;3:383–93.

Fregni F, Thome-Souza S, Bermpohl F, Marcolin MA, Herzog A, Pascual-Leone A, et al. Antiepileptic effects of repetitive transcranial magnetic stimulation in patients with cortical malformations: an EEG and clinical study. Stereotact Funct Neurosurg. 2005;83:57–62.

Fregni F, Otachi PT, Do VA, Boggio PS, Thut G, Rigonatti SP, et al. A randomized clinical trial of repetitive transcranial magnetic stimulation in patients with refractory epilepsy. Ann Neurol. 2006;60:447–55.

Gerloff C, Bushara K, Sailer A, Wassermann EM, Chen R, Matsuoka T, et al. Multimodal imaging of brain reorganization in motor areas of the contralesional hemisphere of well recovered patients after capsular stroke. Brain. 2006;129:791–808.

Gomez L, Morales L, Trapaga O, Zaldivar M, Sanchez A, Padilla E, et al. Seizure induced by subthreshold 10-Hz rTMS in a patient with multiple risk factors. Clin Neurophysiol. 2011;122:1057–8.

Graf T, Engeler J, Achermann P, Mosimann UP, Noss R, Fisch HU, et al. High frequency repetitive transcranial magnetic stimulation (rTMS) of the left dorsolateral cortex: EEG topography during waking and subsequent sleep. Psychiatry Res. 2001;107:1–9.

Graff-Guerrero A, Gonzales-Olvera J, Ruiz-Garcia M, Avila-Ordonez U, Vaugier V, Garcia-Reyna JC. rTMS reduces focal brain hyperperfusion in two patients with EPC. Acta Neurol Scand. 2004;109:290–6.

Hallett M. Transcranial magnetic stimulation: a primer. Neuron. 2007;55:187–99.

Hsu WY, Cheng CH, Lin MW, Shih YH, Liao KK, Lin YY. Antiepileptic effects of low frequency repetitive transcranial magnetic stimulation: a meta-analysis. Epilepsy Res. 2011;96: 231–40.

Hufnagel A, Elger CE. Induction of seizures by transcranial magnetic stimulation in epileptic patients. J Neurol. 1991a;238:109–10.
Hufnagel A, Elger CE. 1991b. Responses of the epileptic focus to transcranial magnetic stimulation. Electroencephalogr Clin Neurophysiol Suppl. 1991;43(86–99):86–99.
Hufnagel A, Elger CE, Durwen HF, Boker DK, Entzian W. Activation of the epileptic focus by transcranial magnetic stimulation of the human brain. Ann Neurol. 1990a;27:49–60.
Hufnagel A, Elger CE, Klingmuller D, Zierz S, Kramer R. Activation of epileptic foci by transcranial magnetic stimulation: effects on secretion of prolactin and luteinizing hormone. J Neurol. 1990b;237:242–6.
Ilmoniemi RJ, Ruohonen J, Virtanen J, Aronen HJ, Karhu J. EEG responses evoked by transcranial magnetic stimulation. Electroencephalogr Clin Neurophysiol Suppl. 1999;51(22–9):22–9.
Jennum P, Winkel H. Transcranial magnetic stimulation. Its role in the evaluation of patients with partial epilepsy. Acta Neurol Scand Suppl. 1994;152(93–6):93–6.
Jennum P, Friberg L, Fuglsang-Frederiksen A, Dam M. Speech localization using repetitive transcranial magnetic stimulation. Neurology. 1994;44:269–73.
Joo EY, Han SJ, Chung SH, Cho JW, Seo DW, Hong SB. Antiepileptic effects of low-frequency repetitive transcranial magnetic stimulation by different stimulation durations and locations. Clin Neurophysiol. 2007;118:702–8.
Kanno M, Chuma T, Mano Y. Monitoring an electroencephalogram for the safe application of therapeutic repetitive transcranial magnetic stimulation. J Neurol Neurosurg Psychiatry. 2001;71:559–60.
Kimiskidis VK. Transcranial magnetic stimulation for drug-resistant epilepsies: rationale and clinical experience. Eur Neurol. 2010;63:205–10.
Kinoshita M, Ikeda A, Begum T, Yamamoto J, Hitomi T, Shibasaki H. Low-frequency repetitive transcranial magnetic stimulation for seizure suppression in patients with extratemporal lobe epilepsy-a pilot study. Seizure. 2005;14:387–92.
Knecht S, Floel A, Drager B, Breitenstein C, Sommer J, Henningsen H, et al. Degree of language lateralization determines susceptibility to unilateral brain lesions. Nat Neurosci. 2002;5:695–9.
Knoch D, Gianotti LR, Pascual-Leone A, Treyer V, Regard M, Hohmann M, et al. Disruption of right prefrontal cortex by low-frequency repetitive transcranial magnetic stimulation induces risk-taking behavior. J Neurosci. 2006;26:6469–72.
Kobayashi M, Pascual-Leone A. Transcranial magnetic stimulation in neurology. Lancet Neurol. 2003;2:145–56.
Komssi S, Kahkonen S. The novelty value of the combined use of electroencephalography and transcranial magnetic stimulation for neuroscience research. Brain Res Rev. 2006;52:183–92.
Kratz O, Studer P, Barth W, Wangler S, Hoegl T, Heinrich H, et al. Seizure in a nonpredisposed individual induced by single-pulse transcranial magnetic stimulation. J ECT. 2011;27:48–50.
Loo CK, McFarquhar TF, Mitchell PB. A review of the safety of repetitive transcranial magnetic stimulation as a clinical treatment for depression. Int J Neuropsychopharmacol. 2008;11:131–47.
Macdonell RA, King MA, Newton MR, Curatolo JM, Reutens DC, Berkovic SF. Prolonged cortical silent period after transcranial magnetic stimulation in generalized epilepsy. Neurology. 2001;57:706–8.
Manganotti P, Tamburin S, Zanette G, Fiaschi A. Hyperexcitable cortical responses in progressive myoclonic epilepsy: a TMS study. Neurology. 2001;57:1793–9.
Menkes DL, Gruenthal M. Slow-frequency repetitive transcranial magnetic stimulation in a patient with focal cortical dysplasia. Epilepsia. 2000;41:240–2.
Michelucci R, Valzania F, Passarelli D, Santangelo M, Rizzi R, Buzzi AM, et al. Rapid-rate transcranial magnetic stimulation and hemispheric language dominance: usefulness and safety in epilepsy. Neurology. 1994;44:1697–700.
Misawa S, Kuwabara S, Shibuya K, Mamada K, Hattori T. Low-frequency transcranial magnetic stimulation for epilepsia partialis continua due to cortical dysplasia. J Neurol Sci. 2005; 234:37–9.

Morales LM, Sanchez C, Bender JE, Bosch J, Garcia ME, Garcia I, et al. A neurofunctional evaluation strategy for presurgical selection of temporal lobe epilepsy patients. MEDICC Rev. 2009;11:29–35.
Muellbacher W, Artner C, Mamoli B. Motor evoked potentials in unilateral lingual paralysis after monohemispheric ischaemia. J Neurol Neurosurg Psychiatry. 1998;65:755–61.
Nakken KO, Kostov H, Ramm-Pettersen A, Heminghyt E, Bakke SJ, Nedregaard B, et al. [Epilepsy surgery – assessment and patient selection]. Tidsskr Nor Laegeforen. 2012;132:1614–8.
Nitsche MA, Paulus W. Noninvasive brain stimulation protocols in the treatment of epilepsy: current state and perspectives. Neurotherapeutics. 2009;6:244–50.
Nitsche MA, Liebetanz D, Tergau F, Paulus W. [Modulation of cortical excitability by transcranial direct current stimulation]. Nervenarzt. 2002;73:332–5.
Pascual-Leone A, Pridmore H. Transcranial magnetic stimulation (TMS). Aust N Z J Psychiatry. 1995;29:698.
Pascual-Leone A, Gates JR, Dhuna A. Induction of speech arrest and counting errors with rapid-rate transcranial magnetic stimulation. Neurology. 1991;41:697–702.
Pascual-Leone A, Houser CM, Reese K, Shotland LI, Grafman J, Sato S, et al. Safety of rapid-rate transcranial magnetic stimulation in normal volunteers. Electroencephalogr Clin Neurophysiol. 1993;89:120–30.
Pascual-Leone A, Valls-Sole J, Wassermann EM, Hallett M. Responses to rapid-rate transcranial magnetic stimulation of the human motor cortex. Brain. 1994;117:847–58.
Pascual-Leone A, Tormos JM, Keenan J, Tarazona F, Canete C, Catala MD. Study and modulation of human cortical excitability with transcranial magnetic stimulation. J Clin Neurophysiol. 1998;15:333–43.
Pascual-Leone A, Tarazona F, Keenan J, Tormos JM, Hamilton R, Catala MD. Transcranial magnetic stimulation and neuroplasticity. Neuropsychologia. 1999;37:207–17.
Reutens DC, Berkovic SF. Increased cortical excitability in generalised epilepsy demonstrated with transcranial magnetic stimulation. Lancet. 1992;339:362–3.
Reutens DC, Berkovic SF, Macdonell RA, Bladin PF. Magnetic stimulation of the brain in generalized epilepsy: reversal of cortical hyperexcitability by anticonvulsants. Ann Neurol. 1993;34:351–5.
Richardson MP, Lopes da Silva FH. TMS studies of preictal cortical excitability change. Epilepsy Res. 2011;97:273–7.
Ridding MC, Rothwell JC. Is there a future for therapeutic use of transcranial magnetic stimulation? Nat Rev Neurosci. 2007;8:559–67.
Robertson EM, Theoret H, Pascual-Leone A. Studies in cognition: the problems solved and created by transcranial magnetic stimulation. J Cogn Neurosci. 2003;15:948–60.
Rolston JD, Englot DJ, Wang DD, Shih T, Chang EF. Comparison of seizure control outcomes and the safety of vagus nerve, thalamic deep brain, and responsive neurostimulation: evidence from randomized controlled trials. Neurosurg Focus. 2012;32:E14.
Rossi S, Ulivelli M, Bartalini S, Galli R, Passero S, Battistini N, et al. Reduction of cortical myoclonus-related epileptic activity following slow-frequency rTMS. Neuroreport. 2004;15:293–6.
Rossi S, Hallett M, Rossini PM, Pascual-Leone A. Safety, ethical considerations, and application guidelines for the use of transcranial magnetic stimulation in clinical practice and research. Clin Neurophysiol. 2009;120:2008–39.
Rossini PM, Rossi S. Transcranial magnetic stimulation: diagnostic, therapeutic, and research potential. Neurology. 2007;68:484–8.
Rotenberg A, Pascual-Leone A. Safety of 1 Hz repetitive transcranial magnetic stimulation (rTMS) in patients with titanium skull plates. Clin Neurophysiol. 2009;120:1417.
Rotenberg A, Depositario-Cabacar D, Bae EH, Harini C, Pascual-Leone A, Takeoka M. Transient suppression of seizures by repetitive transcranial magnetic stimulation in a case of Rasmussen's encephalitis. Epilepsy Behav. 2008;13:260–2.
Rotenberg A, Bae EH, Takeoka M, Tormos JM, Schachter SC, Pascual-Leone A. Repetitive transcranial magnetic stimulation in the treatment of epilepsia partialis continua. Epilepsy Behav. 2009;14:253–7.

Saisanen L, Kononen M, Julkunen P, Maatta S, Vanninen R, Immonen A, et al. Non-invasive preoperative localization of primary motor cortex in epilepsy surgery by navigated transcranial magnetic stimulation. Epilepsy Res. 2010;92:134–44.
Santiago-Rodriguez E, Cardenas-Morales L, Harmony T, Fernandez-Bouzas A, Porras-Kattz E, Hernandez A. Repetitive transcranial magnetic stimulation decreases the number of seizures in patients with focal neocortical epilepsy. Seizure. 2008;17:677–83.
Schiller Y, Bankirer Y. Cellular mechanisms underlying antiepileptic effects of low- and high-frequency electrical stimulation in acute epilepsy in neocortical brain slices in vitro. J Neurophysiol. 2007;97:1887–902.
Schuler P, Claus D, Stefan H. Hyperventilation and transcranial magnetic stimulation: two methods of activation of epileptiform EEG activity in comparison. J Clin Neurophysiol. 1993;10:111–5.
Schulze-Bonhage A, Scheufler K, Zentner J, Elger CE. Safety of single and repetitive focal transcranial magnetic stimuli as assessed by intracranial EEG recordings in patients with partial epilepsy. J Neurol. 1999;246:914–9.
Siebner HR, Bergmann TO, Bestmann S, Massimini M, Johansen-Berg H, Mochizuki H, et al. Consensus paper: combining transcranial stimulation with neuroimaging. Brain Stimul. 2009;2:58–80.
Staudt M. The role of transcranial magnetic stimulation in the characterization of congenital hemiparesis. Dev Med Child Neurol. 2010;52:113–4.
Sun W, Fu W, Mao W, Wang D, Wang Y. Low-frequency repetitive transcranial magnetic stimulation for the treatment of refractory partial epilepsy. Clin EEG Neurosci. 2011;42:40–4.
Tassinari CA, Cincotta M, Zaccara G, Michelucci R. Transcranial magnetic stimulation and epilepsy. Clin Neurophysiol. 2003;114:777–98.
Tellez-Zenteno JF, Wiebe S. Long-term seizure and psychosocial outcomes of epilepsy surgery. Curr Treat Options Neurol. 2008;10:253–9.
Tergau F, Naumann U, Paulus W, Steinhoff BJ. Low-frequency repetitive transcranial magnetic stimulation improves intractable epilepsy. Lancet. 1999;353:2209.
Tergau F, Neumann D, Rosenow F, Nitsche MA, Paulus W, Steinhoff B. Can epilepsies be improved by repetitive transcranial magnetic stimulation? Interim analysis of a controlled study. Suppl Clin Neurophysiol. 2003;56(400–5):400–5.
Theodore WH. Handbook of transcranial magnetic stimulation. Edited by A. Pascual-Leone, N.J. Davey, J. Rothwell, E.M. Wasseran, B.K. Puri. Epilepsy Behav. 2002;3:404.
Theodore WH. Transcranial magnetic stimulation in epilepsy. Epilepsy Curr. 2003;3:191–7.
Theodore WH, Hunter K, Chen R, Vega-Bermudez F, Boroojerdi B, Reeves-Tyer P, et al. Transcranial magnetic stimulation for the treatment of seizures: a controlled study. Neurology. 2002;59:560–2.
Thut G, Pascual-Leone A. A review of combined TMS-EEG studies to characterize lasting effects of repetitive TMS and assess their usefulness in cognitive and clinical neuroscience. Brain Topogr. 2010;22:219–32.
Thut G, Northoff G, Ives JR, Kamitani Y, Pfennig A, Kampmann F, et al. Effects of single-pulse transcranial magnetic stimulation (TMS) on functional brain activity: a combined event-related TMS and evoked potential study. Clin Neurophysiol. 2003a;114:2071–80.
Thut G, Theoret H, Pfennig A, Ives J, Kampmann F, Northoff G, et al. Differential effects of low-frequency rTMS at the occipital pole on visual-induced alpha desynchronization and visual-evoked potentials. Neuroimage. 2003b;18:334–47.
Uijl SG, Leijten FS, Moons KG, Veltman EP, Ferrier CH, van Donselaar CA. Epilepsy surgery can help many more adult patients with intractable seizures. Epilepsy Res. 2012;101(3):210–6.
Valzania F, Strafella AP, Tropeani A, Rubboli G, Nassetti SA, Tassinari CA. Facilitation of rhythmic events in progressive myoclonus epilepsy: a transcranial magnetic stimulation study. Clin Neurophysiol. 1999;110:152–7.
Velasco F, Velasco M, Velasco AL, Menez D, Rocha L. Electrical stimulation for epilepsy: stimulation of hippocampal foci. Stereotact Funct Neurosurg. 2001;77:223–7.

Wang YL, Zhai Y, Huo XL, Zhang JN. [The effect of low frequency transcranial magnetic stimulation on neuropeptide-Y expression and apoptosis of hippocampus neurons in epilepsy rats induced by pilocarpine]. Zhonghua Wai Ke Za Zhi. 2007;45:1685–7.

Wassermann EM, Blaxton TA, Hoffman EA, Berry CD, Oletsky H, Pascual-Leone A, et al. Repetitive transcranial magnetic stimulation of the dominant hemisphere can disrupt visual naming in temporal lobe epilepsy patients. Neuropsychologia. 1999;37:537–44.

Werhahn KJ, Lieber J, Classen J, Noachtar S. Motor cortex excitability in patients with focal epilepsy. Epilepsy Res. 2000;41:179–89.

Yang S, Xu G, Wang L, Zhang X. Effect of the different winding methods of coil on electromagnetic field during transcranial magnetic stimulation. Conf Proc IEEE Eng Med Biol Soc. 2008;4270–3:4270–3.

Zangen A, Roth Y, Voller B, Hallett M. Transcranial magnetic stimulation of deep brain regions: evidence for efficacy of the H-coil. Clin Neurophysiol. 2005;116:775–9.

Ziemann U. Transcranial magnetic stimulation at the interface with other techniques: a powerful tool for studying the human cortex. Neuroscientist. 2011;17:368–81.

Chapter 19
Effects of Transcranial Focal Electrical Stimulation via Concentric Ring Electrodes on Seizure Activity

Walter G. Besio

Abstract Epilepsy affects approximately one percent of the planets population. There does not appear to be any single therapy that works for all types of epilepsy. As an alternative we have been developing a noninvasive, or minimally invasive, transcranial focal electrical stimulation (TFS) based on the novel tripolar concentric ring electrode (TCRE). By applying biphasic, charge balanced, constant current, pulses noninvasively through the TCRE we have realized acute seizure attenuation in rats. We found that the TFS significantly reduced penicillin-induced myoclonic jerks. There was also a significant improvement in survival for the TFS-treated animals compared to those without application of TFS due to the pilocarpine-induced status epilepticus (SE). Long-lasting control of SE, without antiepileptic drugs, provided positive proof that TFS had antiseizure effects. We also found that TFS via TCREs significantly reduced Pentylenetetrazole (PTZ)-induced hypersynchrony at the beta and gamma frequencies as quantified from cross channel coherence performed on the electroencephalograms (EEGs) recorded from the TCREs. Further, we developed a noninvasive automated seizure control system utilizing TFS and EEG signals from the TCREs. The automatically triggered TFS significantly reduced the power of the EEG. We have also performed safety testing, applying TFS once or multiple times. The histological analysis on scalp, cortex, and hippocampal areas suggests there is no significant difference between the controls and the TFS-treated samples. In conclusion we have found TFS to be effective at attenuating acute seizures from three different rat models and safe. In the future we need to test if TFS is effective in models of pharmacoresistant epilepsy.

W.G. Besio (✉)
Department of Electrical, Computer, and Biomedical Engineering,
Rhode Island University, 4 East Alumni Ave., Kingston, RI 02881, USA
e-mail: besio@ele.uri.edu

L. Rocha and E.A. Cavalheiro (eds.), *Pharmacoresistance in Epilepsy: From Genes and Molecules to Promising Therapies*, DOI 10.1007/978-1-4614-6464-8_19,

Keywords Transcranial focal electrical stimulation (TFS) • Tripolar concentric ring electrode (TCRE) • Noninvasive • Seizure • Penicillin • Pilocarpine • Pentylenetetrazole (PTZ)

19.1 Introduction

Epilepsy is a significant life altering chronic disease in which cognitive control is spontaneous and recurrently "seized" from the subject. We are pursuing a novel, noninvasive approach for epilepsy: transcranial focal electrical stimulation (TFS) via unique tripolar concentric ring electrodes (TCREs) that provides focal electrical stimulation. We have demonstrated both transcutaneously and transcranially that TFS provides anticonvulsant effects in acute seizure models with minimal or no side effects. We have even shown that TFS can shut down status epilepticus (SE)—more than 30 min of continuous seizure activity without full recovery of consciousness from seizures.

19.1.1 Medically Intractable Epilepsy and Its Consequences

Presently, antiepileptic medication is the primary treatment for epilepsy. However, approximately half of new-onset seizure patients are not cured by medical therapy (Kwan and Brodie 2000). An estimated 425,000 Americans suffer from pharmacoresistant epilepsy that does not respond to anticonvulsant drugs (Kwan and Brodie 2000). Uncontrolled seizures have been related to increased morbidity and mortality, resulting in an increased incidence of progressive developmental delay and sudden accidental deaths (Krumholz et al. 1995). Approximately 1% of the world population (~67 million) suffers from epilepsy, of which 85% live in developing countries where medication may be too costly (WHO). Each year in the USA, approximately 152,000 SE cases occur (Sirven and Waterhouse 2003) causing 22,000–42,000 deaths, with the mortality rate of at least 20% (Shorvon et al. 2007), and when persisting beyond one hour mortality has been reported at 65% (Drislane et al. 2009). Many more deaths occur in developing countries.

19.1.2 Brain Stimulation for Pharmacoresistant Epilepsy

Brain stimulation is a promising technology for treating medically intractable epilepsy (Theodore and Fisher 2004). Electrical stimulation of the brain and its periphery has a long history (for reviews see Thomas and Young 1993; George et al. 2000). Over the past 30 years, applications have included cerebellar stimulation (Davis 2000), the vagus nerve stimulation (VNS) (George et al. 2000), and deep brain stimulation (DBS) targeting sites such as the subthalamic nucleus (Chabardes et al. 2002), mesial temporal structures (Vonck et al. 2002), and anterior thalamic nucleus.

19.1.2.1 Invasive Approaches

As of this writing the VNS by Cyberonics is the only FDA-approved stimulation therapy for intractable epilepsy. Several controlled trials have assessed the efficacy of VNS (VNS Study Group 1995; Handforth et al. 1995; Ben-Menachem et al. 1994). Generally, it is found to be as effective as antiepileptic drugs for select seizure populations and serious complications are uncommon (Cyberonics Inc 2012).

Deep brain stimulation (DBS) by Medtronic is approved by the FDA to deliver electrical stimulation to structures in the brain that control movement and muscle function for movement disorders. Preliminary animal and clinical studies on DBS have shown promise for seizure control. One study showed that DBS suppressed the secondary generalization of limbic seizures in rats (Usui et al. 2005). There is also preliminary evidence that DBS led to clinical improvement in seizure control of refractory epilepsy patients (Velasco et al. 2000; Vonck et al. 2002; Kerrigan et al. 2004). For invasive approaches complications such as hemorrhage are few, on average in about 5% of the patients (Fisher 2003; Bhatia et al. 2011), and infection rates are similar with a 4.7% average (Ben-Haim et al. 2009; Pouratian et al. 2011).

The responsive neurostimulator (RNS) by Neuropace delivers a short train of electrical pulses to the brain through implanted leads in response to detected abnormal electrical signals of the brain. Preliminary results on RNS have been encouraging. In a study on rats, RNS using low frequency stimulation was shown to decrease the incidence of kindled seizures (Goodman et al. 2005). Analysis of individual cases suggested that RNS may have suppressed seizures in some patients (Kossoff et al. 2004). Results from the RNS pivotal clinical trial suggest that there was a decrease in seizure frequency (Gigante and Goodman 2011). VNS, DBS, and RNS all require invasive surgeries for implantation of electronics. Though the associated complication rates are comparable to the norm in neurosurgical practice, they do represent risks.

19.1.2.2 Noninvasive Approaches

Efforts to interrupt epileptic seizures noninvasively include transcranial magnetic stimulation (TMS), transcranial direct current stimulation (tDCS), and electroconvulsive therapy (ECT).

TMS applies magnetic fields to the cranium, producing electric fields in the brain. TMS has been studied extensively over the past decade with mixed results for controlling seizures and remains an experimental device (Hallett 2002; Wassermann 1998; Theodore et al. 2002; Tassinari et al. 2003). TMS in one study showed effectiveness for malformations where the seizure focus could be localized in the neocortex (Fregni et al. 2006a). TMS can reach into the cortex up to 2–3 cm below the scalp (George 2003). In the future, coils may be developed that stimulate at greater depth; however, to increase depth, they will have less focus (Zangen et al. 2005).

Transcranial electrical stimulation (TES) was used safely back in 1980 to noninvasively stimulate the cortex (Merton and Morton 1980). Limited pilot studies showed that two forms of TES—tDCS and ECT—might have antiepileptic effects on selected patients. Unfortunately, for either case, the stimulation is difficult to focus. In a pilot study on patients with malformations of cortical development and refractory epilepsy, tDCS demonstrated a decrease of epileptic discharges but no significant reduction in the number of seizures (Fregni et al. 2006b). For tDCS to be effective, the cathodic electrode is placed over an identified seizure focus and the anodic electrode placed far away from it. Although tDCS is safe (Fregni et al. 2006b) the charge passage is not balanced. Electroconvulsive therapy is typically used for severe depression (Chanpattana and Sackeim 2010). It induces a controlled seizure by applying electrical pulses to an anesthetized patient's head. A case study reported that ECT acutely controlled seizures in two children (Griesemer et al. 1997). Present day ECT has limited spatial distribution of electrical current or dosage in the brain. Sackeim (2004) proposed a method to improve the focus of ECT. DeGiorgio (2003) also assessed the efficacy of stimulating the trigeminal nerve noninvasively in humans.

To summarize, brain stimulation for epilepsy has shown promise but requires further research. As Theodore and Fisher (2004) concluded, the best structures to stimulate and the most effective stimuli to use are still unknown.

19.2 TCREs and TFS

We have developed a unique, noninvasive method of stimulation: TFS via novel TCREs (referred to as TFS for short). TFS delivers focal stimulation, providing the opportunity to target specific brain regions at depths of a few centimeters. Reciprocally, the TCREs also allow high fidelity focal recordings of neural activity. We have demonstrated that TFS via unique TCREs (transcutaneously and transcranially) successfully abolished or reduced experimentally induced acute seizures and SE in rats, with minimal or no side effects (Besio et al. 2007, 2009, 2010a, 2011a). For example, TFS via TCREs abolished pilocarpine-induced SE seizures and prevented them from returning even hours after the stimulation was stopped without using any anticonvulsant such as diazepam (Besio et al. 2007).

19.2.1 Innovation

The innovative nature of TFS via TCREs hinges on three core distinctions from existing technologies and methods: (a) an innovative electrode design (TCRE),

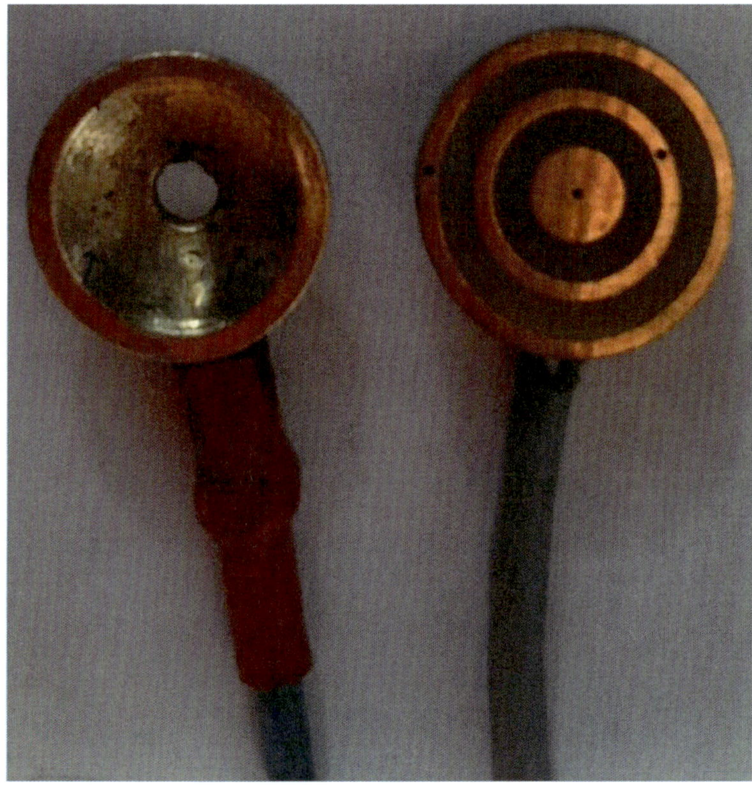

Fig. 19.1 (*Left*) Disk electrode. (*Right*) TCRE (Besio et al. 2006)

(b) providing noninvasive focal stimulation modality that has been demonstrated to have anticonvulsant effects in acute seizure models, and (c) allowing for both focal stimulation and recording from the same electrodes.

19.2.1.1 Innovative Electrode Design

The invention of the novel TCRE is a key to this new noninvasive stimulation modality. The TCRE consists of three electrode elements-outer ring, middle ring, and the center disk (Fig. 19.1). The invention of the TCRE is a significant improvement over the conventional disk electrode. Its details have been vetted in the peer reviewed scientific literature (Besio and Fasiuddin 2005; Besio et al. 2006, 2008, 2010b; Koka and Besio 2007; Besio and Chen 2007). TCREs have unique capabilities as they perform the second spatial derivative, i.e., the Laplacian, on the surface potentials (Fig. 19.1).

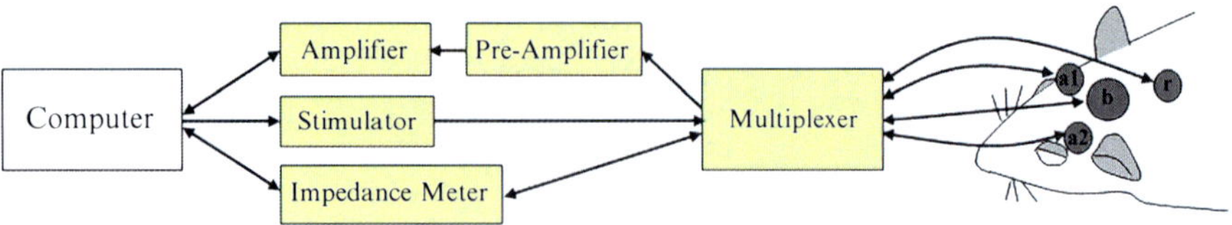

Fig. 19.2 Block diagram of the TFS system via tripolar concentric ring electrodes (TCREs) on the rat scalp: (a1 and a2) dia = 6 mm, (b) dia = 10 mm, (r) reference electrode, dia = 6 mm

19.2.1.2 Focal Stimulation

When used for stimulation, by reciprocity, the current density achieved by driving current through these electrodes yields a similar focused stimulation in the tissue below (Wiley and Webster 1982a, b; Van Oosterom and Strackee 1983). With particular balance of current among the three electrodes in the TCRE, we achieve focused stimulation into the tissue even through the skull, which is advantageous over the diffuse stimulation achieved by disk electrical stimulation applied across the head (Wiley and Webster 1982a, b; Van Oosterom and Strackee 1983).

19.2.1.3 Common Instrumentation for Focal Stimulation and Focal Transcranial Recordings from the Same Electrodes

We have developed custom instrumentation that can deliver TFS, and record Laplacian EEG and conventional EEG, all from the same TCRE. A block diagram of our custom designed TFS instrumentation system is shown in Fig. 19.2. The TCREs were placed on the scalp with conductive paste. One TCRE (b) (diameter = 10 mm), used to record from and stimulate, was centered on the top of the rat head, behind the eyes. Two other recording electrodes (a1, a2) (diameter = 6 mm) were placed bilaterally behind the eyes, closer to the subcortical structures such as the hippocampus. A reference electrode (r) was attached on the top of the neck behind the ears. The electrodes were fixed in place using dental cement (Fig. 19.2).

19.3 Results from Animal Models

TFS successfully abolished seizures or reduced seizure severity in three different acute seizures models (Besio et al. 2007, 2009, 2010a, 2011a).

19.3.1 Penicillin

When TFS was triggered manually after severe penicillin-induced myoclonic jerks, there was a significant reduction in the number and length of myoclonic jerks (Besio et al. 2009, 2010a). A small amount (approximately 0.2 cc) of cerebrospinal fluid was removed and replaced with penicillin G (2.5 MU/kg) (Besio et al. 2009, 2010a). Within 1 min of the penicillin injection, on average, myoclonic jerks began. Once the myoclonic jerks reached the rate of 30/min, TFS was applied to the electrode (b) Fig. 19.2. In the control group ($n=8$), not receiving TFS, the average maximal myoclonic jerk rate was 70/min with an average duration of 90 min. In the experimental group ($n=17$), various pulse widths and frequencies were examined. There was a significant decrease in the mean myoclonic jerk rate from 41/min to 21/min ($P<0.0001$, two-sample t-test) after the first application of TFS. After TFS was applied, myoclonic jerks stopped in all instances for a few minutes and then returned with a smaller amplitude and a lower frequency. In 13 cases, repeated stimulation led to complete cessation of myoclonic jerks. These results gave us hope that TFS had antiseizure effects. However, this seizure model is not a commonly used model and so we began work with the pilocarpine SE model.

19.3.2 Pilocarpine

To test the antiseizure effects of TFS in a more common model we decided to use pilocarpine, a muscarinic receptor agonist model of SE. TFS via TCREs led to a significant reduction in the intensity of pilocarpine-induced SE (an extreme form of seizures that is estimated to take 22,000–40,000 lives in the USA annually) with the effects lasting hours (Besio et al. 2007). Thirty minutes after the administration of scopolamine methylnitrate, pilocarpine HCl (310 mg/kg, i.p., Sigma) was administered. Rats were randomly assigned to one of two groups: control ($n=8$) and experimental ($n=8$). Symmetrical, biphasic, charge-balanced, constant current TFS pulses were applied to experimental rats via our custom-made stimulator. TFS was delivered via the outer ring and disk (with the middle ring floating) of the electrode at location (b) shown in Fig. 19.2. The range of TFS parameters used was 200, 300, 500, or 750 Hz, 200 or 300 μs pulse duration, and 50 or 60 mA intensity, applied for 1 min. TFS was started with the least intense parameter set (200 Hz, 200 μs pulse width, 50 mA) and progressively increased if there was no obvious change in electrographic and/or behavioral activity. Control rats did not receive TFS. Example traces from this study are shown in Fig. 19.3. Note that, without additional pharmacological intervention, the electrographic and behavioral activity did not return for hours. There was a significant improvement in survival for the TFS-treated animals compared to those without application of TFS due to the pilocarpine-induced status epilepticus. Long-lasting control of SE, without antiepileptic drugs, provided positive proof that TFS had antiseizure effects. However, the pilocarpine SE model is

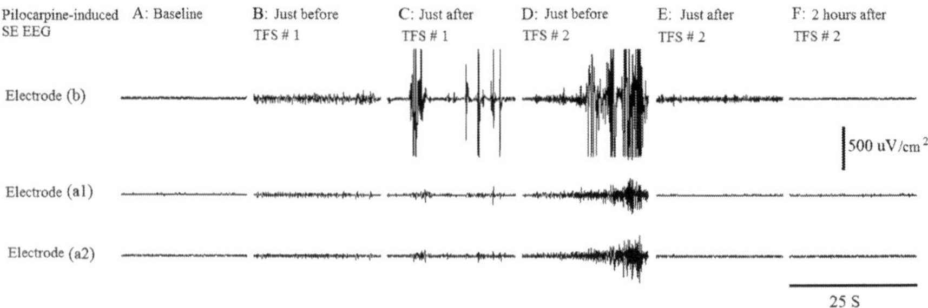

Fig. 19.3 Laplacian EEG recorded from three tripolar concentric ring electrodes (TCREs) at locations (b, a1, and a2) on the scalp of an experimental rat. A: baseline, B: 4 m 35 s after SE onset and before first TFS treatment, C: 6 m after SE onset and immediately after first TFS treatment (200 Hz, 200 μs pulse duration, 50 mA for 1 min), D: 10 m 35 s after SE onset and before second TFS treatment, E: 12 m after SE onset and immediately after second TFS treatment (300 Hz, 200 μs pulse duration, 50 mA for 1 min), and F: 2 h 12 m after SE onset and 2 h after second TFS treatment. The times refer to the starting time of each of the 25 s segments shown. The seizure electrographic activity is present in B, C, and D. During severe behavioral activity in C and D, the signals from location (b) were clipped. In E, the electrographic activity immediately after second TFS treatment resembles the baseline recording. In F, the baseline activity still persists 2 h after second TFS treatment without administering any AED. Electrode (b) is used for applying TFS and recording Laplacian EG

quite severe and not an efficient acute seizure model for testing stimulation parameters. Therefore, we began work with the pentylenetetrazole (PTZ) acute seizure rat model which is a widely used model for testing the effects of anticonvulsants (Fig. 19.3).

19.3.3 Pentylenetetrazole

19.3.3.1 TSF Reduced PTZ-Induced Hypersynchrony

TFS via TCREs significantly reduced PTZ-induced hypersynchrony at the beta and gamma frequencies (Besio et al. 2011a), as quantified from cross-channel coherence (CCC), which is similar to correlation however it is performed in the frequency domain rather than the time domain. Rat behavior was scored for seizure related phenomena (Mirski et al. 1997), and TFS was administered immediately after the first myoclonic jerk was observed. In each of the three electrode combinations the pre-TFS CCC, which was calculated from the signals recorded after administering the PTZ and just prior to applying the TFS, was consistently high over the full frequency range tested 1–50 Hz. The baseline (prior to administration of PTZ) and post-TFS (just after the TFS was terminated) CCC values were similar and lower than during the Pre-TFS stage. As shown in Fig. 19.4, for electrodes (a1) and (b) the CCC values after the application of TFS (blue/solid) return to pre-PTZ measured baseline values (green/dashed), in contrast to those prior to treatment (red/dotted).

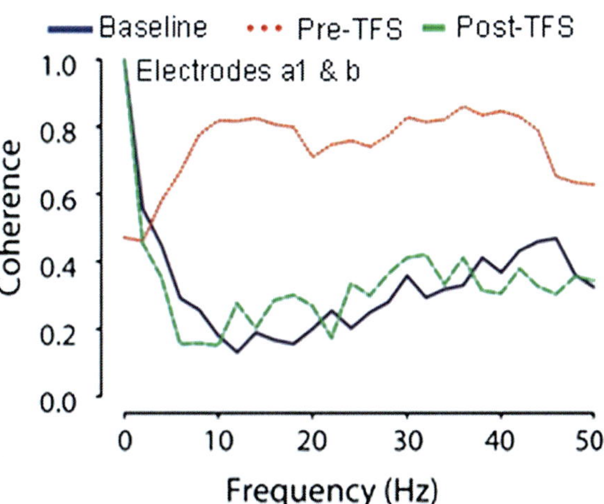

Fig. 19.4 Smoothed CCC for a TFS-treated rat between TCREs a1 and b. The pre-TFS CCC is distinctively high over a broad spectrum. The baseline and post-TFS values are similar and less than the pre-TFS value. Other rats had similar results

This was indicative for all electrode combinations and all rats. The high coherence suggests that there was a synchronization of brain electrographic activity over a wide area of the brain during the seizure. In contrast after the application of TFS the CCC was reduced suggesting that the synchronized activity was reduced by TFS.

For recording signals we have previously shown that TCREs, compared to conventional disk electrodes, provide less than one-tenth (8.27%) the mutual information (Koka and Besio 2007) and have strong attenuation of distant sources, −100 dB one radius from the electrode (Besio et al. 2006). The reduced mutual information and strong attenuation of distant sources infer that during the PTZ-induced seizures, since there was a high CCC between all electrodes, there is highly synchronized activity between major areas of the brain (Fig. 19.4).

19.3.3.2 TSF Reduced Two-Dose PTZ-Induced Behavioral Activity

In this study we expanded our analysis of the effect of TFS on behavioral seizure activity in two ways. First, four different metrics were used: (1) time of the first behavioral change, (2) seizure onset latency, (3) seizure duration, and (4) maximal seizure severity score. This allowed for a better description of the effect of TFS. Second, in our preliminary PTZ study two independent groups of animals were used (Besio et al. 2010a). The PTZ was administered to animals in both groups only once with only the TFS-treated group receiving TFS but not the control group. This previous approach did not account for variability (resistance to PTZ, etc.) among the animals of the two groups potentially obscuring the effect of TFS. To account for this variability, in this study, we used a different experimental design administering PTZ to the animals in both groups twice and giving TFS to the animals in the TFS-treated group after the second PTZ administration only. This approach allowed us to compare the results after the first PTZ administration in the TFS-treated and control groups confirming that there was no significant difference between controls and TFS-treated groups.

The results from the first application of PTZ and the resulting first seizure was considered the baseline to study the difference between the first and the second PTZ-induced seizures in each group separately. Finally, we compared the changes caused by recurrent PTZ administrations in control and TFS-treated groups to evaluate the effect of TFS.

The effect of recurrent administrations of PTZ producing a gradual increase in the seizure intensity is well established and used for the development of PTZ-induced kindling in rats (Ito et al. 1977; Corda et al. 1991; Han et al. 2000; Szyndler et al. 2002). Recurrent intraperitoneal administration of doses equal to 30 mg/kg (Corda et al. 1991), 35 mg/kg (Szyndler et al. 2002) and 40 mg/kg (Han et al. 2000; Ito et al. 1977), comparable to the dose used for our study (45 mg/kg), were shown to produce progressive sensitization to the convulsive effect of PTZ. Due to this sensitization effect of PTZ it would be difficult to reliably evaluate the effect of TFS using the same animals first as a part of the TFS-treated group and then as a control or vice versa. Even though including the animals in both legs of the study, as controls and then again in the treated group or vice versa, allows for a within-subject comparison it also convolutes the effect of TFS with the increased sensitivity to PTZ. This sensitization along with the possible obscuring/masking of PTZ tolerance when using a single PTZ administration on two separate groups of animals was why we administered two doses of PTZ in both groups. We compared the effect of TFS between the first and the second PTZ administrations in control and TFS-treated groups separately to overcome these limitations.

We found no significant differences in behavioral activity from the first PTZ treatment between the two groups (Makeyev et al. 2012b). Therefore, both groups had similar behavioral activity induced by the first administration of PTZ. It should also be noted that after the second administration of PTZ the TFS would not have had any effect on the time of the first behavioral change since the TFS was not turned on until the first behavioral change was observed. Therefore, until the time of the first behavioral change both groups are treated the same and were not found to be statistically different. We then compared the difference between the first and the second PTZ-induced seizures in each group separately. The same behavioral seizure activity metrics (seizure onset latency, time of the first behavioral change, duration of seizure and maximal seizure severity score) were used in both cases. There was a significant difference in all four metrics between the first and second PTZ-induced seizures for the control group. While the general trend was the same in the TFS-treated group (mean/median decrease in time of the first behavioral change, decrease in seizure onset latency, increase in seizure duration, and increase in maximal seizure severity score) the difference was statistically significant only for time of first behavioral change, that could not have been affected by TFS in the TFS-treated group (Makeyev et al. 2012b).

The fact that there was no statistically significant change in three behavioral seizure activity metrics that could have been affected by TFS clearly suggests that TFS may have an anticonvulsant effect. If this difference between two groups was due to some factor other than TFS all four behavioral seizure activity metrics affected or not affected by TFS would have been likely to exhibit similar behavior.

19.3.3.3 Automated Seizure Detection Triggers TSF and Reduces PTZ-Induced Electrographic Activity

After having previously shown that TFS was effective in altering convulsant-induced seizures we decided to determine if it was feasible to noninvasively and automatically control PTZ-induced seizures. We developed real-time seizure detectors using noninvasive electrographic seizure activity from TCREs based on a disjunctive combination of the cumulative sum (CUSUM) algorithm and generalized likelihood ratio test (GLRT). The seizure detectors automatically triggered TFS. The CUSUM is a signal change detector traditionally used in quality control, intrusion detection, spam filtering and medical systems to identify changes in probability distribution of a stochastic random process. Although there is no optimality associated with the GLRT it has been shown to work well in practice. We performed experiments following the methodology proposed in Makeyev et al. (2011) and Besio et al. (2011b) to confirm the effect of automatically triggered TFS on PTZ-induced electrographic seizure activity in rats. We applied the CUSUM and GLRT to verify the change in power between two data segments.

The performance of the two detectors, CUSUM and GLRT, was comparable in terms of all the performance metrics. The GLRT performed slightly better specially on sham seizure (specificity of 97.66% compared with 91.9% for CUSUM). The improved specificity is important since in real life applications a false positive detection may mean an extra dose of electrical stimulation or a dose of anticonvulsant drug. As a result of a tradeoff, higher specificities mean lower sensitivities, however even with the sensitivity of 33.73% for a disjunctive combination (logical OR) of all three detectors the seizure onset was detected prior to the first PTZ-induced myoclonic jerk in 76.92% of rats of the test set ($n=13$). According to the GLRT analysis comparing segments of comparable time between the control rats and TFS-treated rats the automatically triggered TFS significantly ($P=0.001$) reduced the electrographic seizure activity power, in the single dose TFS treated group ($n=5$) compared to controls ($n=4$), in 70% of the paired segments further suggesting its anticonvulsant effect. It was also observed that the second automated dose of TFS reduced the electrographic activity even further towards the baseline.

19.4 Tissue Safety

19.4.1 Scalp

Besides being effective at abolishing or diminishing seizures TFS must be safe for translation to clinical practice. We applied TFS to rat scalp and performed tissue histomorphological analysis to determine if the tissue was significantly damaged after TFS. We studied six different sets of stimulation parameters: 50 mA, 250 Hz, 200 μs ($J^2t=0.3$) ($A^2/cm^4/s$), 50 mA, 200 Hz, 300 μs ($J^2t=0.7$) ($A^2/cm^4/s$), 50 mA,

200 Hz, 500 μs ($J^2t=1.2$) ($A^2/cm^4/s$), 100 mA, 250 Hz, 200 μs ($J^2t=1.2$) ($A^2/cm^4/s$), 50 mA, 500 Hz, 300 μs ($J^2t=2.7$) ($A^2/cm^4/s$), 50 mA, 500 Hz, 300 μs, and 100 mA, 300 Hz, 500 μs ($J^2t=10.8$) ($A^2/cm^4/s$) each for 60 s. Immediately after the end of TFS we acquired a thermal image of the scalp. The maximum temperature measured from the rat experiments using ($J^2t=0.7$) ($A^2/cm^4/s$) low energy density stimulations was 38 °C. The maximum temperature measured from the experiments using ($J^2t=2.7$) ($A^2/cm^4/s$) high energy density stimulations was 47 °C. Stimulation at the energy density factor ($J^2t<0.92$) ($A^2/cm^4/s$) showed little or no damage. Some of the basal nuclei of the epidermis were more darkly stained than controls. The energy density factor ($J^2t=0.92$–1.5) ($A^2/cm^4/s$) showed some moderate changes. The epidermal cells were less distinct at most of the stimulation sites. The nuclei were shrunken darkly stained and sometimes indistinct. The thickness of the epidermis appeared thinner than in the controls. We also observed damage to the hair follicles and sebaceous glands. Energy density factor stimulation ($J^2t>1.5$) ($A^2/cm^4/s$) showed more pronounced damage to the epidermis. The epidermis was compact and homogenously stained and no nuclei were present. The cells in the deeper epidermis were indistinct with darkly stained elongated nuclei. Collagen fibers in the dermis were clumped and appeared to be different in orientation compared with the control tissue. From this study we concluded that as long as the specified energy density applied through the CRE was kept below ($J^2t<0.92$) ($A^2/cm^4/s$), the maximum temperature remained within the safe limits and also within the limits of the melting point of conductive paste and provide a safe current density distribution (Besio et al. 2010b).

19.4.2 *Cortex and Hippocampus*

Recently we conducted more safety experiments on adult male Sprague Dawley rats ($n=60$; two groups of 30). We applied TFS (50 mA, 200 μs, 300 Hz, 2 min, biphasic, charge-balanced pulses) via a TCRE. Group #1 received a single TFS application (9 controls, 21 TFS-treated). Group #2 received the same TFS on five consecutive days (9 controls, 21 TFS-treated). Cortical areas below the TFS site and hippocampal areas were assessed for neuronal damage. Following TFS application, rats were allowed to recover for 24 h, 1 week, and 1 month, respectively. Then the rats were anesthetized and transcardially perfused with 4% paraformaldehyde. The brains were removed, post-fixed, sliced (30 μm), stained (Nissl), and imaged (10×). No statistically significant difference was found in integrated optical density (IOD) values between the controls and TFS-treated rat brains for the three different latencies (t-test) (Mucio-Ramirez et al. 2011). Morphological analysis did not show any pyknotic neurons or gliosis that might confirm any neuronal damage. Cell counts in the CA1, CA3, and dentate gyrus hippocampal areas also showed no significant difference. This suggests that TFS, under these conditions, is innocuous to rat cortex and hippocampus.

19.5 Concluding Remarks

In summary we have shown the efficacy and safety of TFS in rats. In three different acute rat seizure models we have shown that TFS is effective. We first showed that TFS significantly reduced penicillin-induced myoclonic jerks in rats (Besio et al. 2009, 2010a). We then showed that TFS significantly reduced the risk of death due to pilocarpine induced status epilepticus and had a long-lasting effect (Besio et al. 2007). We also showed that TFS reduced the brain electrographic synchronization caused by PTZ (Besio et al. 2011a). Further, we found that TFS significantly reduced the PTZ-induced brain electrographic power and duration of myoclonic jerks (Besio et al. 2010a; Makeyev et al. 2011). We have also shown that an automated noninvasive seizure control system was possible utilizing TFS (Makeyev et al. 2012a). Though all of the models we have utilized to show the effectiveness of TFS have been acute seizure animal models, we believe that TFS will also be effective in the epileptic brain. Beyond seizure control we have also shown the safety of single and multiple doses of TFS. We initially showed that TFS was safe to rat scalp if the energy density factor was kept below 0.92 $A^2/cm^4/s$ (Besio et al. 2010b). Since brain tissue may be more sensitive than the scalp we then analyzed TFS-treated brain tissue. Our preliminary results show that TFS, in a single dose or in multiple doses, does not cause any significant difference in the rat cortex or hippocampus (Mucio-Ramirez et al. 2011). These findings all suggest that TFS is efficacious for controlling acute seizures in rats and does not cause significant safety concerns. Future studies have to be designed to evaluate if this strategy is able to reduce seizure activity in pharmacoresistant epilepsy.

References

Ben-Haim S, Asaad WF, Gale JT, Eskandar EN. Risk factors for hemorrhage during microelectrode-guided deep brain stimulation and the introduction of an improved microelectrode design. Neurosurgery. 2009;64:754–62.
Ben-Menachem E, Manon-Espaillat R, Ristanovic R, Wilder BJ, Stefan H, Mirza W, et al. Vagus nerve stimulation therapy for treatment of partial seizures, 1: a controlled study of effect on seizures. Epilepsia. 1994;35:616–26.
Besio WG, Chen T. Tripolar Laplacian electrocardiogram and moment of activation isochronal mapping. Physiol Meas. 2007;28:515–29.
Besio WG, Fasiuddin M. Quantizing the depth of bioelectrical sources for non-invasive 3D imaging. J Bioelectromagn. 2005;7:90–3.
Besio WG, Koka K, Aakula R, Dai W. Tri-polar concentric electrode development for high resolution EEG Laplacian electroencephalography using tri-polar concentric ring electrodes. IEEE Trans Biomed Eng. 2006;53:926–33.
Besio WG, Koka K, Cole A. Feasibility of non-invasive transcutaneous electrical stimulation for modulating pilocarpine-induced status epilepticus seizures in rats. Epilepsia. 2007;48:2273–9.
Besio WG, Cao H, Zhou P. Application of tripolar concentric electrodes and pre-feature selection algorithm for brain–computer interface. IEEE Trans Neural Syst Rehabil Eng. 2008;16:191–4.

Besio WG, Koka K, Gale KS, Medvedev AV. Preliminary data on anticonvulsant efficacy of transcutaneous electrical stimulation via novel concentric ring electrodes. In: Schachter SC, Guttag JV, Schiff SJ, Schomer DL, Summit Contributors. Advances in the application of technology to epilepsy: the CIMIT/NIO Epilepsy Innovation Summit, Boston, May 2008. Epilepsy Behav. 2009;16:3–46.

Besio WG, Gale KS, Medvedev A. Possible therapeutic effects of transcutaneous electrical stimulation via concentric ring electrodes. Epilepsia. 2010a;51:85–7.

Besio WG, Sharma V, Spaulding J. The effects of concentric ring electrode electrical stimulation on rat skin. Ann Biomed Eng. 2010b;38:1111–8.

Besio WG, Liu X, Wang L, Medvedev A, Koka K. Transcutaneous focal electrical stimulation via concentric ring electrodes reduces synchrony induced by pentylenetetrazole in beta and gamma bands in rats. IJ Neural Syst Spec Iss Neuromodulat Epilepsy. 2011a;21:1–11.

Besio WG, Liu X, Liu Y, Sun YL, Medvedev AV, Koka K. Algorithm for automatic detection of pentylenetetrazole-induced deizures in rats. Proceedings of 33rd annual international conference of the IEEE EMBS, Boston, USA, 30 August to 3 September; 2011b. p. 8283–6.

Bhatia R, Dalton A, Richards M, Hopkins C, Aziz T, Nandi D. The incidence of deep brain stimulator hardware infection: the effect of change in antibiotic prophylaxis regimen and review of the literature. Br J Neurosurg. 2011;25:625–31.

Chabardes S, Kahane P, Minotti L, Koudsie A, Hirsch E, Benabid AL. Deep brain stimulation in epilepsy with particular reference to the subthalamic nucleus. Epileptic Disord. 2002;4:83–93.

Chanpattana W, Sackeim HA. Electroconvulsive therapy in treatment-resistant schizophrenia: prediction of response and the nature of symptomatic improvement. J ECT. 2010;26:289–98.

Corda MG, Orlandi M, Lecca D, Carboni G, Frau V, Giorgi O. Pentylenetetrazol-induced kindling in rats: effect of GABA function inhibitors. Pharmacol Biochem Behav. 1991;40:329–33.

Cyberonics Inc. 2012. Press release obtained from http://www.cyberonics.com/en/press-room/Overview-to-Cyberonics.pdf. Accessed 13 Sept 2012.

Davis R. Cerebellar stimulation for cerebral palsy spasticity, function, and seizures. Arch Med Res. 2000;31:290–9.

DeGiorgio CM, Shewmon DA, Whitehurst T. Trigeminal nerve stimulation for epilepsy. Neurology. 2003;12:421–2.

Drislane FW, Blum AS, Lopez MR, Gautam S, Schomer DL. Duration of refractory status epilepticus and outcome: loss of prognostic utility after several hours. Epilepsia. 2009;50:1566–71.

Fisher R. Anterior thalamic nucleus stimulation: issues in study design. In: Luders H, editor. Deep brain stimulation and epilepsy. London: Martin Dunitz; 2003. p. 307–22.

Fregni F, Otachi P, do Valle A, Boggio P, Thut G, Rigonatti S, et al. A randomized clinical trial of repetitive transcranial magnetic stimulation in patients with refractory epilepsy. Ann Neurol. 2006a;60:447–55.

Fregni F, Thome-Souza S, Nitsche MA, Freedman SD, Valente KD, Pascual-Leone A. A controlled clinical trial of cathodal DC polarization in patients with refractory epilepsy. Epilepsia. 2006b;47:335–42.

George MS. Stimulating the brain. Sci Am. 2003;289:66–73.

George MS, Sackeim HA, Rush AJ, Marangell LB, Nahas Z, Husain MM, et al. Vagus nerve stimulation: a new tool for brain research and therapy. Biol Psychiatry. 2000;47:287–95.

Gigante PR, Goodman RR. Alternative surgical approaches in epilepsy. Curr Neurol Neurosci Rep. 2011;11:404–8.

Goodman J, Berger R, Theng T. Preemptive low-frequency stimulation decreases the incidence of amygdale-kindled seizures. Epilepsia. 2005;46:1–7.

Griesemer DA, Kellner CH, Beale MD, Smith GM. Electroconvulsive therapy for treatment of intractable seizures. Initial findings in two children. Neurology. 1997;49:1389–92.

Hallett M. Transcranial magnetic stimulation: a revolution in clinical neurophysiology. J Clin Neurophysiol. 2002;19:253–4.

Han D, Yamada K, Senzaki K, Xiong H, Nawa H, Nabeshima T. Involvement of nitric oxide in pentylenetetrazole-induced kindling in rats. J Neurochem. 2000;74:792–8.

Handforth A, DeGiorgio C, Schachter S, Uthman B, Naritoku D, Tecoma E, et al. Vagus nerve stimulation therapy for partial-onset seizures: a randomized active-control trial. Neurology. 1995;51:48–55.

Ito T, Hori M, Yoshida K, Shimizu M. Effect of anticonvulsants on seizures developing in the course of daily administration of pentetrazol to rats. Eur J Pharmacol. 1977;45:165–72.

Kerrigan J, Litt B, Fisher R, Cranstoun S, Frence J, Blum D, et al. Electrical stimulation of the anterior nucleus of the thalamus for the treatment of intractable epilepsy. Epilepsia. 2004;45:346–54.

Koka K, Besio WG. Improvement of spatial selectivity and decrease of mutual information of tripolar concentric ring electrodes. J Neurosci Methods. 2007;165:216–22.

Kossoff E, Ritzl E, Politsky J, Murro A, Smith J, Duckrow R, et al. Effect of an external responsive neurostimulator on seizures and electrographic discharges during subdural electrode monitoring. Epilepsia. 2004;45:1560–7.

Krumholz A, Sung GY, Fisher RS, Barry E, Bergey GK, Grattan LM. Complex partial status epilepticus accompanied by serious morbidity and mortality. Neurology. 1995;45:1499–504.

Kwan P, Brodie MJ. Early identification of refractory epilepsy. N Engl J Med. 2000;342:314–9.

Makeyev O, Liu X, Koka K, Kay SM, Besio WG. Transcranial focal stimulation via concentric ring electrodes reduced power of pentylenetetrazole-induced seizure activity in rat electroencephalogram. 33rd Annual international IEEE EMBS conference, Boston, USA, 30 August to 3 September; 1991. p. 7560–3.

Makeyev O, Liu X, Luna-Munguia H, Rogel-Salazar G, Mucio-Ramirez S, Liu Y, et al. Toward a noninvasive automatic seizure control system in rats with transcranial focal stimulations via tripolar concentric ring electrodes. IEEE TNSRE. 2012a;20:422–31.

Makeyev O, Luna-Munguía H, Rogel-Salazar G, Liu X, Besio WG. Noninvasive transcranial focal stimulation via tripolar concentric ring electrodes lessens behavioral seizure activity of recurrent pentylenetetrazole administrations in rats. IEEE TNSRE. 2012b. doi:10.1109/TNSRE.2012.2198244.

Merton PA, Morton HB. Stimulation of the cereberal cortex in the intact human subject. Nature. 1980;285:227.

Mirski M, Rossell L, Terry J, Fisher R. Anticonvulsant effect of anterior thalamic high frequency electrical stimulation in the rat. Epilepsy Res. 1997;28:89–100.

Mucio-Ramirez S, Makeyev O, Liu X, Leon-Olea M, Besio WG. Cortical integrity after transcutaneous focal electrical stimulation via concentric ring electrodes. Society for neuroscience 41st annual meeting, abs. 672.20/Y19, Washington, DC, 12–16 November; 2011.

Pouratian N, Reames DL, Frysinger R, Elias WJ. Comprehensive analysis of risk factors for seizures after deep brain stimulation surgery. J Neurosurg. 2011;115(2):310–5.

Sackeim HA. Convulsant and anticonvulsant properties of electroconvulsive therapy: towards a focal form of brain stimulation. Clin Neurosci Res. 2004;4:39–57.

Shorvon SD, Trinka E, Walker MC. The proceedings of the first London colloquium on status epilepticus. Epilepsia. 2007;48:1–3.

Sirven J, Waterhouse E. Management of status epilepticus. Am Fam Physician. 2003;68:469–76.

Szyndler J, Rok P, Maciejak P, Walkowiak J, Czlonkowska A. Effects of pentylenetetrazol-induced kindling of seizures on rat emotional behavior and brain monoaminergic systems. Pharmacol Biochem Behav. 2002;73:851–61.

Tassinari CA, Cincotta M, Zaccara G, Michelucci R. Transcranial magnetic stimulation and epilepsy. Clin Neurophysiol. 2003;114:777–98.

The Vagus Nerve Stimulation Study Group. A randomized controlled trial of chronic vagus nerve stimulation for treatment of medically intractable seizures. Neurology. 1995;45:224–30.

Theodore W, Fisher R. Brain stimulation for epilepsy. Lancet. 2004;3:111–8.

Theodore WH, Hunter K, Chen R, Vega-Bermudez F, Boroojerdi B, Reeves-Tyer P, et al. Transcranial magnetic stimulation for the treatment of seizures. A controlled study. Neurology. 2002;59:560–2.

Thomas RK, Young CD. A note on the early history of electrical stimulation of the human brain. J Gen Psychol. 1993;120:73–81.

Usui N, Maesawa S, Kajita Y, Endo O, Takebayashi S, Yoshida J. Suppression of secondary generalization of limbic seizures by stimulation of subthalamic nucleus in rats. J Neurosurg. 2005;102:1122–9.

Van Oosterom A, Strackee J. Computing the lead field of electrodes with axial symmetry. Med Biol Eng Comput. 1983;21:473–81.

Velasco AL, Velasco M, Velasco F, Menes D, Gordon F, Rocha L, et al. Subacute and chronic electrical stimulation of hippocampus on intractable temporal lobe seizures: preliminary report. Arch Med Res. 2000;31:16–328.

Vonck K, Boon P, Achten E, De Reuck J, Caemaert J. Long-term amygdalohippocampal stimulation for refractory temporal lobe epilepsy. Ann Neurol. 2002;52:556–65.

Wassermann E. Risk and safety of repetitive transcranial magnetic stimulation: report and suggested guidelines from the International Workshop on the Safety of Repetitive Transcranial Magnetic Stimulation. Electroencephalogr Clin Neurophysiol. 1998;108:1–16.

Wiley JD, Webster JG. Analysis and control of the current distribution under circular dispersive electrodes. IEEE Trans Biomed Eng. 1982a;29:381–5.

Wiley JD, Webster JG. Distributed equivalent-circuit model for circular dispersive electrodes. IEEE Trans Biomed Eng. 1982b;29:385–9.

Zangen A, Roth Y, Voller B, Hallett M. Transcranial magnetic stimulation of deep brain regions: evidence for efficacy of the H-Coil. Clin Neurophysiol. 2005;116:775–9.

Chapter 20
Physical Exercise as a Strategy to Reduce Seizure Susceptibility

Ricardo Mario Arida and Fulvio Alexandre Scorza

Abstract Effective strategies for preventing or treating epilepsy have been extensively used. Exercise has gained substantial attention to stimulate brain plasticity as well as noninvasive therapeutic strategy for achieving rehabilitation after brain damage. This chapter focuses on the beneficial effects of exercise programs observed in clinical studies and animal models of epilepsy, and their importance as complementary therapy for epilepsy. Information about the antiepileptogenic and neuroprotective effects of physical exercise is emphasized. Considering that exercise can promote beneficial actions such as reduction of seizure susceptibility, reduction of anxiety and depression, and improvement of quality of life of people with epilepsy, it can be suggested to be integrated with conventional therapy for epilepsy.

Keywords Epilepsy • Physical exercise • Seizure • Quality of life • Complementary therapy

20.1 Overview of Impact of Exercise on Functional Plasticity in the Intact and Injured Brain

Extensive literature review suggests that following injury the central nervous system has the capacity for self-repair and that this can be promoted through a diversity of experiences such as physical exercise programs (Griesbach 2011; Archer 2012).

R.M. Arida (✉)
Department of Physiology, Universadade Federal de Sao Paulo, Rua Botucatu, 862 Vila Clementino E. Ciencias Bioomedicas 5 Andar, Sao Paulo, Brazil
e-mail: arida.nexp@epm.br

F.A. Scorza
Department of Neurology/Neurosurgery, Escola Paulista de Medicina/Universidade Federal de Sao Paulo, Rua Botacatu, Rua Botucatu 862, Sao Paulo 04023-900, Brazil
e-mail: scorza.nexp@epm.br

L. Rocha and E.A. Cavalheiro (eds.), *Pharmacoresistance in Epilepsy: From Genes and Molecules to Promising Therapies*, DOI 10.1007/978-1-4614-6464-8_20,

In this sense, the major focus of researches has been the attempt to define the potential therapeutic capacity of exercise in brain injury. Regular physical exercise has been associated with changes in neurotransmitter levels (Bland et al. 1999), glial cell volume (Anderson et al. 1994), expression of endogenous neurotrophic factors (Neeper et al. 1995; Gomez-Pinilla et al. 1998), and growth of neuronal processes and neurogenesis (Kempermann et al. 1998; Gould et al. 1999). Considering these neurobiological effects of exercise, it is reasonable to suggest that such activity would have beneficial effects on neurodegenerative diseases.

In view of the above information, some questions are commonly raised: What time period should implementation of exercise as rehabilitative intervention is applied to produce its restorative effects on structural and functional brain damage? Which physical exercise stimulus, such as training length (acute vs. chronic), intensity and duration of the exercise are more adequate? How long do the consequences of physical exercise last in the damaged brain? In animal studies, performing exercise prior to brain lesion has been found to produce prophylactic effects such as limiting or preventing brain damage (Wang et al. 2001; Arida et al. 2011). Alternatively, exercise therapy may be beneficial for certain patient populations such as those who have sustained a transient ischemic attack and therefore have a high disposition to experience a secondary insult (Kleim et al. 2003). Nevertheless, we have bear in mind that as physical exercise has been shown to increase the energy demand in different parts of the brain (Vissing et al. 1996), it is conceivable that implementing physical activity during this compromised period may further accelerate cellular dysfunction. Thus, although positive outcomes in brain plasticity have been extensively observed with aerobic exercise, other types of exercise, such as strength exercise have demonstrated promising results (Cassilhas et al. 2010, 2012). Overall, exercise can provide a therapeutic tool for brain injury by managing its time of application, type, duration, and intensity of exercise (Arida et al. 2011).

While a considerable amount of literature is available on several positive effects of physical exercise for brain recovery in different conditions such as stroke, Alzheimer's and Parkinson's diseases, knowledge on their effects in epilepsy are limited. The efficacy of physical exercise for preventing or treating chronic epilepsy has been demonstrated in human and animal models of epilepsy (for review see Arida et al. 2008, 2009a). In this line, our primary concern in this chapter is to highlight the potential contribution of exercise in epilepsy.

20.2 Epilepsy: General Aspects

Epilepsy occurs in about 1 % of the world population is the most common acquired chronic neurological disorder (Hauser 1997). Epidemiological studies suggest that between 70 and 80 % of people developing epilepsy will go into remission, while the remaining patients continue to have seizures and are refractory to treatment with the currently available therapies (Kwan and Sander 2004). The most common risk factors for epilepsy are cerebrovascular diseases, brain tumors, alcohol, traumatic head injuries, malformations of cortical development, genetic inheritance, and infections of the central nervous system (Halatchev 2000). Thus, from the new patients that presented epilepsy, approximately 30 % have seizures originating from the temporal lobe (Manford et al. 1992). Individuals affected with temporal lobe epilepsy (TLE) usually have analogous clinical description, including an initial precipitating injury such as the status epilepticus (SE), head trauma, encephalitis, or childhood febrile seizures (Fisher et al. 1998; Cendes 2004).

Although the management of some antiepileptic drugs is effective for primary neuroprotection such as reduced neurodegeneration after SE, their efficacy for preventing the development of chronic epilepsy is not promising. Alternative strategies such as hormones or antioxidants seem useful for preventing and treating chronic TLE (Acharya et al. 2008). In addition, nonpharmacological therapies, including complementary and alternative medicine are often used by patients with epilepsy (Peebles et al. 2000; Schachter 2008). Considering the beneficial actions of exercise, both for seizure control and improvement of quality of life of individuals with epilepsy, physical exercise programs have been recently suggested as an effective complementary therapy for people with epilepsy (Arida et al. 2010a, b, 2012a). This chapter presents data of effects of physical exercise programs from human and animal studies and considerations of the potential application of exercise strategy for preventing or treating epilepsy.

20.3 Epilepsy and Physical Exercise: General Aspects in Human Studies

Many studies have demonstrated that as a population, those with epilepsy are usually less fit and less active than their non-affected peers. A low degree of participation in physical activities is found in several studies on this subject (Denio et al. 1989; Bjorholt et al. 1990, Jalava and Sillanpaa 1997; Arida et al. 2003a). These findings are also observed in pediatric population. Wong and Wirrell (2006) demonstrated that teens with epilepsy were less physically active than their sibling controls. Consequently, this considerable lack of physical fitness may have an impact on their general health and quality of life. Overprotection, loneliness, low self-esteem, depression, anxiety, and behavioral problems are considerable barriers to an active life (McEwan et al. 2004). Indeed, people with epilepsy present significant deficits in aerobic endurance, muscle strength endurance and physical flexibility (Steinhoff et al. 1996; Nakken et al. 1990; Wong and Wirrell 2006). This topic is explored elsewhere.

Psychiatric comorbidities frequently occur in patients with epilepsy (Devinsky 2003). Cognitive, emotional and behavioral conditions and adjustment to seizures seem to be especially crucial to the quality of life of people with epilepsy (Devinsky 1996; Kellett et al. 1997). Depression and anxiety are frequent comorbidities of epilepsy (Kobau et al. 2006; Tellez-Zenteno et al. 2007; Thapar et al. 2009) with a negative impact on quality of life. These conditions share common pathogenic mechanisms such as abnormalities of neurotransmitter systems (serotonergic, dopaminergic, and noradrenergic). Exercise has an important contribution in regulating these neurotransmitter systems involved in some mood disorders (Dunn et al. 2001, 2005). Along these lines, we have hypothesized that regular program of exercise might regulate depression associated with epilepsy (Arida et al. 2012b).

Fortunately, the above scenario is changing. In the last decade, some promising findings and decisions about this issue have occurred. Attitudes towards restriction and protection of the patient with epilepsy have been changing and extensive evidence regarding the beneficial effect of exercise on seizure frequency and severity has been reported (Elliott et al. 2008; Ablah et al. 2009; Arida et al. 2008, 2009a, 2010a). For instance, a study conducted by Arida et al. (2003a) analyzed the degree of participation in physical activities among Brazilian patients with epilepsy. Although only 15 % of patients were qualified as active, that is, exercised regularly, more than half of the patients participated in physical activities once or twice per week or on the weekends. In this sense, campaigns for more physical activity have been launched in mass media from several countries. The ILAE has formed a task force (Task Force on Sports and Epilepsy—http://www.ilae.org/Visitors/About_ILAE/TaskForces.cfm) to evaluate and establish new strategies (research directions, social, cultural, and educational efforts) to propagate information about physical exercise or sports participation in people with epilepsy (Arida et al. 2012c).

20.3.1 Epilepsy and Physical Exercise: Human Findings

For a long time it had been thought that exercise might exacerbate seizures either directly through hyperventilation, or indirectly through modifying levels of antiepileptic drugs. Hyperventilation is a significant activator of absence seizures and indeed this is routinely used as a provocative test during EEG. It causes a decrease in pCO_2 and cerebral vasoconstriction, decreased cerebral blood flow and hypoxia. Consequently a respiratory alkalosis is induced and all these factors may result in the triggering of epileptic discharges (McLaurin 1973; van Linschoten et al. 1990). However, during physical activity (involuntary hyperventilation) there is a compensatory mechanism, with greater metabolic and respiratory demand, different from the process of nonphysiological hyperventilation and therefore, in this condition, exercise does not exacerbate seizures (Esquivel et al. 1991).

The literature demonstrates that epileptiform discharges on EEG decrease during exercise (Gotze et al. 1967; Horyd et al. 1981; Nakken et al. 1997). A classic study of Gotze et al. (1967) reported that seizure discharges disappeared in most patients during exercise. Similarly, Horyd et al. (1981) had 43 patients with epilepsy exercise on a cycle ergometer and found that EEG discharges decreased during exercise. Nakken et al. (1997) noted that the majority of their patients had a decrease in the occurrence of epileptiform discharges in EEG during exercise on a cycle ergometer. Recent investigations reinforces that exercise have a normalizing effect on EEG. For instance, in Vancini and collaborators (2010) study, although no statistical difference in epileptiform discharges was detected during the periods analyzed, i.e., rest, exercise, and recovery, a decrease in the number of epileptiform discharges was observed between the rest state and exercise and between the rest state and recovery period. In a more recent study, the same parameters in subjects with juvenile myoclonic epilepsy were evaluated (de Lima et al. 2011). The number of epileptiform discharges was significantly reduced during the recovery period compared with the resting state. Indeed, the analysis of physiological variables during exercise may exhibit important physiological characteristics of people with epilepsy that could be of value in setting up efficient and safer physical exercise programs for this population. To this point, cardiovascular responses of people with TLE during an ergometric test demonstrated that neither seizures nor significant cardiovascular changes were observed during physical effort (Camilo et al. 2009). Overall, these findings support previous observations that, in general, physical exercise is not a seizure-inducing factor (Gotze et al. 1967; Denio et al. 1989; Howard et al. 2004; Sahoo and Fountain 2004).

With reference to the cited reports showing lower levels of physical fitness among people with epilepsy, studies have described reduced physical fitness in people with epilepsy as expressed by lower maximal oxygen uptake (VO_2max) and lower strength and flexibility (Nakken et al. 1990; Eriksen et al. 1994; McAuley et al. 2001). For instance, Nakken et al. (1990) found significant lower maximum oxygen uptake than average population. Others studies that explored the physiological responses to exercise have also shown lower VO_2max in people with epilepsy (Bjorholt et al. 1990; Vancini et al. 2010; de Lima et al. 2011). Another point to be considered is the association of antiepileptic drug and exercise. Although exercise may affect drug metabolism, absorption and serum drug concentration, some investigations report that physical training does not change their serum antiepileptic drug levels to a clinically important degree (Nakken et al. 1990; Eriksen et al. 1994).

20.3.2 Epilepsy and Physical Exercise: Experimental Findings

The effect of physical exercise in animal models of epilepsy can be investigated before or after brain insults. Researchers have only recently begun to explore the issue in experimental models of epilepsy at the end of the 1990s decade. The first animal study on this topic used the kindling model (Arida et al. 1998). Kindling can be induced by repeated administration of a subconvulsive stimulus administered into a limbic structure such as the amygdala, hippocampus, entorhinal cortex or other brain areas. Over a period of several stimulation days, the animal exhibits both behavioral and electrographic seizures that spread to become secondarily generalized. The initial stimulus elicits focal paroxysmal activity (afterdischarges) without apparent clinical seizure activity. Subsequent stimulations induce the progressive development of seizures, generally evolving through the following stages according to Racine (1972): 1—immobility, facial clonus, eye closure, twitching of the vibrissae, 2—head-nodding, 3—unilateral forelimb clonus, 4—rearing, 5—rearing and falling accompanied by secondary generalized clonic seizure. The effect of acute (bout) and chronic (training) physical exercise was tested on amygdala kindling development in rats (Arida et al. 1998). In Arida et al. (1998) study, animals submitted to physical training presented a higher number of stimulations to reach stage 5 when compared with sedentary animals. These findings suggest that physical exercise retards the amygdala kindling development in rats. Studies using the enriched environment also demonstrated lower susceptibility during kindling development than rats housed in isolated conditions (Auvergne et al. 2002).

The influence of exercise in epilepsy was evaluated using the pilocarpine model. The pilocarpine model of epilepsy reproduces the main features of human TLE in rats and mice. The systemic administration of pilocarpine in rats promotes sequential behavioral and electrographic changes that can be divided into three distinct periods: (a) an acute period that built up progressively into a limbic SE and that lasts 24 h, (b) a silent period with a progressive normalization of EEG and behavior which varies from 4 to 44 days, and (c) a chronic period with spontaneous recurrent seizures (SRSs). The main features of the SRSs observed during the long-term period resemble those of human complex partial seizures and recurs 2–3 times per week per animal (Cavalheiro 1995; Arida et al. 1999). In the pilocarpine model, chronic animals with epilepsy presented a significant reduction in seizure frequency (ca. 50 %) during the aerobic training period. As in the kindling model, Setkowicz and Mazur (2006) assessed the susceptibility to evoked seizures in the pilocarpine model of epilepsy after a physical training program. During the acute period of SE, all the behavioral parameters (the latency of the first motor sign, the intensity of seizures, the time when it occurred within the 6-h observation period, and the time when the acute period ended) were significantly better in trained animals compared to sedentary ones. Thus, in a seizure model, physical training, creatine supplementation, or a combination of both was able to attenuate pentylenetetrazol-induced seizures and oxidative damage in vivo (Rambo et al. 2009). One study that reviewed data from experimental studies of animals with epilepsy submitted to physical exercise observed that in all studies the physical training was able to reduce the number of SRSs and the seizure occurrence during exercise was relatively absent in the majority of studies (Arida et al. 2009b).

20.4 Mechanism by Which Physical Exercise Might Reduce Seizure Susceptibility

To understand the basic mechanisms by which exercise exerts positive influence in epilepsy, Arida et al. (2003b) evaluated whether physical training modifies the functional activity in brain areas in rats with epilepsy. An increase in local cerebral metabolic rates for glucose were observed in inferior colliculus and auditory cortex in trained rats with epilepsy compared to non-trained rats with epilepsy during the interictal phase of the pilocarpine model. In an electrophysiological study, it was observed a reduction in population spikes in different concentrations of extracellular potassium or bicuculline and enhanced the late phase of long term potentiation

(LTP) in trained rats with epilepsy (Arida et al. 2004). In another investigation, the number of parvalbumin-positive cells and staining intensity of parvalbumin-fibers in the hilus was significantly higher after acute voluntary (wheel running) and forced (treadmill running) physical exercise (Arida et al. 2007).

There are several factors which might be involved in this protective process. One mechanism by which exercise could reduce seizure susceptibility is related to neurotransmitters. Several lines of evidence show that brain neurotransmission is influenced by exercise and alterations in neurotransmitter systems could be mediating the inhibitory/excitatory balance to reduce the seizure frequency. Early studies have demonstrated increased levels of norepinephrine in the rat brain (Brown and Van Huss 1973; Brown et al. 1979; De Castro and Duncan 1985; Dunn et al. 1996). Noradrenaline has a tonic inhibitory effect on kindling development but not on kindling state (Westerberg et al. 2004). In accordance, depletion of noradrenaline induced by DSP4 facilitated the rate of hippocampal kindling (Bortolotto and Cavalheiro 1986). Therefore, the inhibition of amygdala kindling development in rats after exercise could partially attributed to alterations of brain noradrenaline (Arida et al. 1998). These findings reinforce not only the activation of the neurotransmitter systems but also possible circuitry alterations involved in this inhibitory effect. For example, exercise induced to prominent changes in the staining of the parvalbumin in the dentate gyrus from rats with epilepsy (Arida et al. 2007). Parvalbumin represents effective and sensitive marker of hippocampal cells (Celio 1990) and particularly it is co-expressed with GABAergic neurons (Freund and Buzsáki 1996). This possible inhibitory effect could also be related to the significant reduction in seizure frequency observed during exercise training period in other works utilizing the pilocarpine model of epilepsy (Arida et al. 1999, 2003b, 2004).

Among other hypothesis the increased sensory input from several organs during exercise, perhaps proprioceptive impulses, may contribute in the inhibition of seizures (Bennett 1981). We have to take in account that during exercise there are the involvements not only the motor function and proprioception but also parts of the brain responsible for attention, vigilance, and motivation. It has been suggested that increased vigilance and attention during exercise could reduce the number of seizures (Kuijer 1980), that is, some researches indicate a reduced likelihood of seizures during exercise (Howard et al. 2004; Sahoo and Fountain 2004; Arida et al. 2008, 2009a). The increased metabolic rate in structures related to vigilance and attention (inferior colliculus and auditory cortex) (Arida et al. 2003b) could possible explain a lower frequency of seizures in exercised rats with epilepsy in previous works (Arida et al. 1999, 2004, 2007).

The opioid system has an important involvement in seizure control (Hammers et al. 2007). Depending of exercise intensity, the release of circulating beta-endorphin will correspondingly increase. Although there are limited data in literature demonstrating the exercise influence on central opioids in epilepsy, it has been suggested that beta-endorphins released during exercise may participate in the inhibition of epileptic discharges (Albrecht 1986).

Among the several factors to be considered when prescribing physical activities to people with epilepsy, intensity of effort is a subject not well explored in epilepsy.

There are several sports activities which include anaerobic and aerobic components such as soccer, basketball, or volleyball. Concerning anaerobic exercise, short, intensive physical activity increases serum lactate content and causes metabolic acidosis. Seizures can markedly reduce extracellular pH, and acidosis in turn can terminate or prevent seizures in human and animal models of epilepsy (Ziemann et al. 2008). Enzymes controlling brain GABA concentrations seem to be influenced by pH changes, i.e., acidosis increases and alkalosis decreases GABA concentration (Velisek et al. 1994). In this regard, anaerobic, exhaustive exercise may decrease the pH of the blood, altering the enzymes involved in GABA metabolism which could produces a natural anticonvulsant effect. Thus, a proposition not yet explored in this context is activation of the adenosinergic system induced by exercise. During exhaustive exercise, extracellular adenosine (from AMP) concentrations rise promptly, which can activate all types of adenosine receptors (Pedata et al. 2001). Indeed, a significant increase in adenosine concentration after intense exercise has been observed (Dworak et al. 2007). As adenosine is a by-product of energy metabolism and ATP utilization, it has been suggested that it can be effective in preventing seizures.

20.5 Final Considerations

While there are several evidences addressing the effectiveness of physical exercise in epilepsy, there has been incomplete information about the mechanics by which exercise can reduce seizure susceptibility. In addition, there are still deficiencies in our current knowledge about questions mentioned in the introduction of this chapter.

Pertaining epilepsy, the first question cannot be fully clarified. What time period should implementation of exercise as rehabilitative intervention is applied to produce its restorative effects on structural and functional brain damage induced by "SE"? An initial precipitating injury induced by SE leads to neurodegeneration, abnormal reorganization of the brain circuitry and a significant imbalance of functional excitation/inhibition. All of these changes contribute to the development of chronic epilepsy. It is believed that epileptogenic changes occur during this latent period. Whether exercise intervention during this latent period can provides a beneficial impact in preventing or minimizing the progression of disease is not known. In experimental models, following SE, animals are unresponsive to their environment and behavior restore to normal over a 3- to 5-day period. Our experience shows inadequate performance to an exercise program for a period of 5–10 days. Although in some animal models of TLE (pilocarpine of kainate) the latent period may last 4–44 days, most animals can present a short silent period and in this regard, it becomes quite impossible to implement an adequate exercise program in these animals. In humans, physical exercise programs or sport activities should be introduced to attest possible beneficial outcomes.

Which physical exercise stimulus, such as training length (acute vs. chronic), intensity and duration of the exercise are more adequate "for people with epilepsy"? According to the scientific literature, aerobic exercise undoubtedly benefits

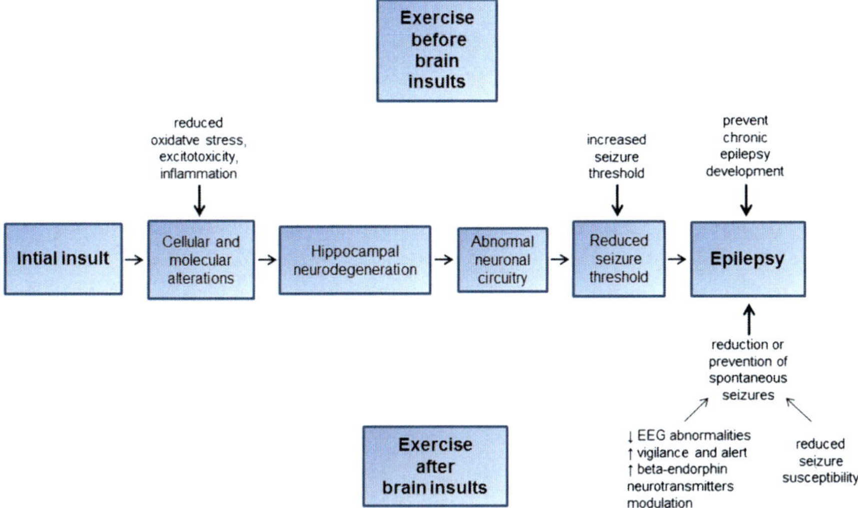

Fig. 20.1 Exercise strategy for preventing or treating epilepsy. Initial insult leads to abnormal structural and functional reorganization of the brain circuitry, which develops into epilepsy. The neuroprotective interventions such as exercise before brain insult or during the latent period can reduce seizure susceptibility and epileptogenesis. Exercise after chronic epilepsy can reduce or suppress spontaneous seizures

people with epilepsy due to the fact that it often reduces seizure frequency, reduces depression, anxiety, and social isolation, and promotes general health (Arida et al. 2012b). Although it is not well clarified whether other types of exercise can provide similar benefits for epilepsy, a recent study demonstrated that strength exercise program reduced the seizure frequency in animals with epilepsy (Peixinho-Pena et al. 2012). Scientific research has shown that strength training improves muscle strength and increases muscle and bone mass, flexibility, mood, self-confidence, and self-esteem (Kohrt et al. 2004; Garber et al. 2011). Therefore, it should be worthy to combine both aerobic and strength training into patient exercise program routine.

How long do the consequences of physical exercise last in the damaged "epileptic" brain? Information about this issue in humans is lacking in literature. One animal study reported reduced seizure frequency after 45 days of detraining compared to epileptic control animals.

Overall, the effects of exercise on epilepsy go beyond simply reducing the frequency of seizure or seizure susceptibility (see Fig. 20.1). Besides the physiologic benefits of physical exercise, improvements in psychosocial functioning and quality of life are of extreme importance. Several components such as cognitive, emotional and behavioral conditions, social functioning, family stability, self-esteem and stigma seem to be especially crucial to the quality of life of patients with epilepsy (Devinsky 1996). People with epilepsy have a considerable lack of physical fitness that might have an impact on their general health and quality of life. Epilepsy is more likely to be associated with psychiatric comorbidities compared to the general population.

These comorbidities are common and frequently more disabling than the seizures themselves (Duncan et al. 2006; Ottman et al. 2011). Studies have demonstrated reduction of depression in people with epilepsy after regular exercise programs. People with epilepsy participating in physical exercise programs have shown an improvement in behavioral outcomes (quality of life, mood, self-concept, self-esteem) (Nakken et al. 1990; Roth et al. 1994; Eriksen et al. 1994; McAuley et al. 2001). Although the knowledge about the impact of exercise in pharmacoresistant epilepsy is still lacking, we have to bear in mind that the psychosocial complications of epilepsy can be attenuated in patients who are involved in physical exercise programs. In view of the above information, exercise should be added to the pharmacological treatment for epilepsy and their associated comorbidities which may have a great impact on their quality of life.

References

Ablah E, Haug A, Konda K, Tinius AM, Ram S, Sadler T, et al. Exercise and epilepsy: a survey of midwest epilepsy patients. Epilepsy Behav. 2009;14:162–6.

Acharya MM, Hattiangady B, Shetty AK. Progress in neuroprotective strategies for preventing epilepsy. Prog Neurobiol. 2008;84:363–404.

Albrecht H. Endorphins, sport, and epilepsy: getting fit or having one. N Z Med J. 1986;99:915.

Arida RM, Vieira AJ, Cavalheiro EA. Effect of physical exercise on kindling development. Epilepsy Res. 1998;30:127–32.

Arida RM, Scorza FA, Peres CA, Cavalheiro EA. The course of untreated seizures in the pilocarpine model of epilepsy. Epilepsy Res. 1999;34:99–107.

Arida RM, Scorza FA, de Albuquerque M, Cysneiros RM, de Oliveira RJ, Cavalheiro EA. Evaluation of physical exercise habits in Brazilian patients with epilepsy. Epilepsy Behav. 2003a;4(5):507–10.

Arida RM, Fernandes MJS, Scorza FA, Preti SC, Cavalheiro EA. Physical training does not influence interictal LCMRglu in pilocarpine-treated rats with epilepsy. Physiol Behav. 2003b;200379:789–94.

Arida RM, Sanabria ERG, Silva AC, Faria LC, Scorza FA, Cavalheiro EA. Physical training reverts hippocampal electrophysiological changes in rats submitted to the pilocarpine model of epilepsy. Physiol Behav. 2004;83:165–71.

Arida RM, Scorza CA, Scorza FA, Silva SG, Naffah-Mazzacoratti MG, Cavalheiro EA. Effects of different types of physical exercise on the staining of parvalbumin-positive neurons in the hippocampal formation of rats with epilepsy. Prog Neuro-Psychopharmacol Biol Psychiatry. 2007;31:814–22.

Arida RM, Cavalheiro EA, da Silva AC, Scorza FA. Physical activity and epilepsy: proven and predicted benefits. Sports Med. 2008;38:607–15.

Arida RM, Scorza FA, Scorza CA, Cavalheiro EA. Is physical activity beneficial for recovery in temporal lobe epilepsy? Evidences from animal studies. Neurosci Biobehav. 2009a;33:422–31.

Arida RM, Scorza FA, Terra VC, Cysneiros RM, Cavalheiro EA. Physical exercise in rats with epilepsy is protective against seizures: evidence of animal studies. Arq Neuropsiquiatr. 2009b;67:1013–6.

Arida RM, Scorza FA, Gomes da Silva S, Schachter SC, Cavalheiro EA. The potential role of physical exercise in the treatment of epilepsy. Epilepsy Behav. 2010a;17:432–5.

Arida RM, Scorza FA, Cavalheiro EA. Favorable effects of physical activity for recovery in temporal lobe epilepsy. Epilepsia Suppl. 2010b;3:76–9.

Arida RM, Scorza FA, Gomes da Silva S, Cysneiros RM, Cavalheiro EA. Exercise paradigms to study brain injury recovery in rodents. Am J Phys Med Rehabil. 2011;90:452–65.
Arida RM, Peixinho-Pena LF, Scorza FA, Cavalheiro EA. Physical exercise: potential candidate as complementary therapy for epilepsy. Ann Indian Acad Neurol. 2012a;15:167.
Arida RM, Cavalheiro EA, Scorza FA. From depressive symptoms to depression in people with epilepsy: contribution of physical exercise to improve this picture. Epilepsy Res. 2012b;99:1–13.
Arida RM, Scorza FA, Cavalheiro EA, Perucca E, Moshé SL. Can people with epilepsy enjoy sports? Epilepsy Res. 2012c;98:94–5.
Anderson BJ, Li X, Alcantara AA, Isaacs KR, Black JE, Greenough WT. Glial hypertrophy is associated with synaptogenesis following motor-skill learning, but not with angiogenesis following exercise. Glia. 1994;11:73–80.
Archer T. Influence of physical exercise on traumatic brain injury deficits: scaffolding effect. Neurotox Res. 2012;21:418–34.
Auvergne R, Leré C, El Bahh B, Arthaud S, Lespinet V, Rougier A, et al. Delayed kindling epileptogenesis and increased neurogenesis in adult rats housed in an enriched environment. Brain Res. 2002;954:277–85.
Bjorholt PG, Nakken KO, Rohme K, Hansen H. Leisure time habits and physical fitness in adults with epilepsy. Epilepsia. 1990;31:83–7.
Bland ST, Gonzale RA, Schallert T. Movement-related glutamate levels in rat hippocampus, striatum, and sensorimotor cortex. Neurosci Lett. 1999;277:119–22.
Bennett DR. Sports and epilepsy: to play or not to play. Semin Neurol. 1981;1:345–57.
Bortolotto ZA, Cavalheiro EA. Effect of DSP4 on hippocampal kindling in rats. Pharmacol Biochem Behav. 1986;24:777–9.
Brown B, Van Huss C. Exercise and rat brain catecholamines. J Appl Physiol. 1973;34:664–9.
Brown B, Payne T, Kim C, Moore G, Krebs P, Martin W. Chronic response of rat brain norepinephrine and serotonin levels to endurance training. J Appl Physiol. 1979;46:19–23.
Camilo F, Scorza FA, de Albuquerque M, Vancini RL, Cavalheiro EA, Arida RM. Evaluation of intense physical effort in subjects with temporal lobe epilepsy. Arq Neuropsiquiatr. 2009;67:1007–12.
Cassilhas RC, Antunes HK, Tufik S, de Mello MT. Mood, anxiety, and serum IGF-1 in elderly men given 24 weeks of high resistance exercise. Percept Mot Skills. 2010;110:265–76.
Cassilhas RC, Lee KS, Fernandes J, Oliveira MG, Tufik S, Meeusen R, et al. Spatial memory is improved by aerobic and resistance exercise through divergent molecular mechanisms. Neuroscience. 2012;202:309–17.
Cavalheiro EA. The pilocarpine model of epilepsy. Ital J Neurol Sci. 1995;16:33–7.
Celio MR. Calbindin D28k and parvalbumin in the rat nervous system. Neuroscience. 1990;35:375–475.
Cendes F. Febrile seizures and mesial temporal sclerosis. Curr Opin Neurol. 2004;17:161–4.
De Castro J, Duncan G. Operantly conditioned running: effects on brain catecholamine concentrations and receptor densities in the rat. Pharmacol Biochem Behav. 1985;23:495–500.
de Lima C, Vancini RL, Arida RM, Guilhoto LM, de Mello MT, Barreto AT, et al. Physiological and electroencephalographic responses to acute exhaustive physical exercise in people with juvenile myoclonic epilepsy. Epilepsy Behav. 2011;22:718–22.
Denio LS, Drake ME, Pakalnis A. The effect of exercise on seizure frequency. J Med. 1989;20:171–6.
Devinsky O. Pychiatric comorbidity in patients with epilepsy: implications for diagnosis and treatment. Epilepsy Behav Suppl. 2003;4:S2–10.
Devinsky O. Quality of life in epilepsy. In: Wyllie E, editor. The treatment of epilepsy: principles and practice. 3rd ed. Baltimore: Williams & Wilkins; 1996. p. 1243–50.
Duncan JS, Sander JW, Sisodiya SM, Walker MC. Adult epilepsy. Lancet. 2006;367(9516): 1087–100.
Dunn AL, Reigle TG, Youngstedt SD, Armstrong RB, Dishman RK. Brain norepinephrine and metabolites after treadmill training and wheel running in rats. Med Sci Sports Exerc. 1996; 28:204–9.

Dunn AL, Trivedi MH, O'Neal HA. Physical activity dose–response effects on outcomes of depression and anxiety. Med Sci Sports Exerc. 2001;33:S587–97.
Dunn AL, Trivedi MH, Kampert JB, Clark CG, Chambliss HO. Exercise treatment for depression: efficacy and dose response. Am J Prev Med. 2005;28:1–8.
Dworak M, Diel P, Voss S, Hollmann W, Strüder HK. Intense exercise increases adenosine concentrations in rat brain: implications for a homeostatic sleep drive. Neuroscience. 2007;150:789–95.
Elliott JO, Lu B, Moore JL, McAuley JW, Long L. Exercise, diet, health behaviors, and risk factors among persons with epilepsy based on the California Health Interview Survey, 2005. Epilepsy Behav. 2008;13:307–15.
Esquivel E, Chaussain M, Plouin P, Ponsot G, Arthuis M. Physical exercise and voluntary hyperventilation in childhood absence epilepsy. Electroenceph Clin Neurophysiol. 1991;79:127–32.
Eriksen HR, Ellertsen B, Gronningaeter H, Nakken KO, Loyning Y, Ursin H. Physical exercise in women with intractable epilepsy. Epilepsia. 1994;35:1256–64.
Fisher PD, Sperber EF, Moshe SL. Hippocampal sclerosis revisited. Brain Dev. 1998;20:563–73.
Freund TF, Buzsáki G. Interneurons of the hippocampus. Hippocampus. 1996;6:345–470.
Garber CE, Blissmer B, Deschenes MR, Franklin BA, Lamonte MJ, Lee IM, et al. American College of Sports Medicine. American College of Sports Medicine position stand. Quantity and quality of exercise for developing and maintaining cardiorespiratory, musculoskeletal, and neuromotor fitness in apparently healthy adults: guidance for prescribing exercise. Med Sci Sports Exerc. 2011;43:1334–59.
Gomez-Pinilla F, So V, Kesslak JP. Spatial learning and physical activity contribute to the induction of fibroblast growth factor: neural substrates for increased cognition associated with exercise. Neuroscience. 1998;85:53–61.
Gotze W, Kubicki S, Munter M, Teichmann J. Effect of physical exercise on seizure threshold (investigated by electroencephalographic telemetry). Dis Nerv Syst. 1967;28:664–7.
Gould E, Beylin A, Tanapat P, Reeves A, Shors TJ. Learning enhances adult neurogenesis in the hippocampal formation. Nat Neurosci. 1999;2:260–5.
Griesbach GS. Exercise after traumatic brain injury: is it a double-edged sword? PM R. 2011;3(6 Suppl 1):S64–72.
Hauser WA. Incidence and prevalence. In: Engel Jr J, Pedley TA, editors. Epilepsy: a comprehensive textbook. Philadelphia: Lippincott-Raven; 1997. p. 47–57.
Halatchev VN. Epidemiology of epilepsy – recent achievements and future. Folia Med. 2000;42:17–22.
Hammers A, Asselin MC, Hinz R, Kitchen I, Brooks DJ, Duncan JS, et al. Upregulation of opioid receptor binding following spontaneous epileptic seizures. Brain. 2007;130:1009–16.
Horyd W, Gryziak J, Niedzielska K, Zielinski JJ. Exercise effect on seizure discharges in epileptics. Neurol Neurochir Pol. 1981;6:545–52.
Howard GM, Radloff M, Sevier TL. Epilepsy and sports participation. Curr Sports Med Rep. 2004;3:15–9.
Jalava M, Sillanpaa M. Physical activity, health-related fitness, and health experience in adults with childhood-onset epilepsy: a controlled study. Epilepsia. 1997;38:424–9.
Kellett MW, Smith DF, Chadwick DW. Quality of life after epilepsy surgery. J Neurol Neurosurg Psychiatry. 1997;63:52–8.
Kempermann G, Brandon EP, Gage FH. Environmental stimulation of 129/SvJ mice causes increased cell proliferation and neurogenesis in the adult dentate gyrus. Curr Biol. 1998;8:939–42.
Kleim JA, Jones TA, Schallert T. Motor enrichment and the induction of plasticity before and after brain injury. Neurochem Res. 2003;28:1757–69.
Kobau R, Gilliam F, Thurman DJ. Prevalence of self-reported epilepsy or seizure disorder and its associations with self-reported depression and anxiety: results from the 2004 HealthStyles Survey. Epilepsia. 2006;47:1915–21.
Kohrt WM, Bloomfield SA, Little KD, Nelson ME, Yingling VR. American College of Sports Medicine. American College of Sports Medicine Position Stand: physical activity and bone health. Med Sci Sports Exerc. 2004;36:1985–96.

Kuijer A. Epilepsy and exercise, electroencephalographical and biochemical studies. In: Wada JA, Penry JK, editors. Advances in epileptology: the 10th epilepsy international symposium. New York: Raven; 1980.

Kwan P, Sander JW. The natural history of epilepsy: an epidemiological view. J Neurol Neurosurg Psychiatry. 2004;75:1376–81.

Manford M, Hart YM, Sander JW, Shorvon SD. National general practice study of epilepsy (NGPSE): partial seizure patterns in a general population. Neurology. 1992;42:1911–7.

McAuley JW, Long L, Heise J, Kirby T, Buckworth J, Pitt C, et al. A prospective evaluation of the effects of a 12-week outpatient exercise program on clinical and behavioral outcomes in patients with epilepsy. Epilepsy Behav. 2001;2:592–600.

McEwan MJ, Espie CA, Metcalfe J, Brodie MJ, Wilson MT. Quality of life and psychosocial development in adolescents with epilepsy: a qualitative investigation using focus group methods. Seizure. 2004;13:15–31.

McLaurin RL. Epilepsy and contact sports. JAMA. 1973;225:285–7.

Nakken KO, Bjorholt PG, Johannessen SI, Løyning T, Lind E. Effect of physical training on aerobic capacity, seizure occurrence, and serum level of antiepileptic drugs in adults with epilepsy. Epilepsia. 1990;31:88–94.

Nakken KO, Loyning A, Loyning T, Gløersen G, Larsson PG. Does physical exercise influence the occurrence of epileptiform EEG discharges in children? Epilepsia. 1997;38:279–84.

Neeper SA, Gomez-Pinilla F, Choi J, Cotman C. Exercise and brain neurotrophins. Nature. 1995;373:109.

Ottman R, Lipton RB, Ettinger AB, Cramer JA, Reed ML, Morrison A, et al. Comorbidities of epilepsy: results from the Epilepsy Comorbidities and Health (EPIC) Survey. Epilepsia. 2011;52:308–15.

Pedata F, Corsi C, Melani A, Bordoni F, Latini S. Adenosine extracellular brain concentrations and role of A2A receptors in ischemia. Ann N Y Acad Sci. 2001;939:74–84.

Peebles CT, McAuley JW, Roach J, Moore JL, Reeves AL. Alternative medicine use by patients with epilepsy. Epilepsy Behav. 2000;1:74–7.

Peixinho-Pena LF, Fernandes J, de Almeida AA, Gomes FGN, Cassilhas R, Venancio DP, et al. A strength exercise program in rats with epilepsy is protective against seizures. Epilepsy Behav. 2012. In press 2012;25:323–8.

Racine RJ. Modification of seizure activity by electrical stimulation: II, motor seizure. Electroenceph Clin Neurophysiol. 1972;32:281–94.

Rambo LM, Ribeiro LR, Oliveira MS, Furian AF, Lima FD, Souza MA, et al. Additive anticonvulsant effects of creatine supplementation and physical exercise against pentylenetetrazol-induced seizures. Neurochem Int. 2009;55:333–40.

Roth DL, Goode KT, Williams VL, Faught E. Physical exercise, stressful life experience, and depression in adults with epilepsy. Epilepsia. 1994;35:1248–55.

Sahoo SK, Fountain NB. Epilepsy in football players and other land-based contact or collision sport athletes: when can they participate, and is there an increased risk? Curr Sports Med Rep. 2004;3:284–8.

Schachter SC. Complementary and alternative medical therapies. Curr Opin Neurol. 2008; 21:184–9.

Setkowicz Z, Mazur A. Physical training decreases susceptibility to subsequent pilocarpine-induced seizures in the rat. Epilepsy Res. 2006;71:142–8.

Steinhoff BJ, Neususs K, Thegeder H, Reimers CD. Leisure time activity and physical fitness in patients with epilepsy. Epilepsia. 1996;37:1221–7.

Tellez-Zenteno JF, Patten SB, Jette N, Williams J, Wiebe S. Psychiatric comorbidity in epilepsy: a population-based analysis. Epilepsia. 2007;48:2336–44.

Thapar A, Kerr M, Harold G. Stress, anxiety, depression, and epilepsy: investigating the relationship between psychological factors and seizures. Epilepsy Behav. 2009;14:134–40.

van Linschoten R, Backx FJ, Mulder OG, Meinardi H. Epilepsy and sports. Sports Med. 1990;10:9–19.

Vancini RL, de Lira CA, Scorza FA, de Albuquerque M, Sousa BS, de Lima C, et al. Cardiorespiratory and electroencephalographic responses to exhaustive acute physical exercise in people with temporal lobe epilepsy. Epilepsy Behav. 2010;19:504–8.

Velisek L, Dreier JP, Stanton PK, Heinemann U, Moshe SL. Lowering of extracellular pH suppresses low-Mg(2+)-induces seizures in combined entorhinal cortex-hippocampal slices. Exp Brain Res. 1994;101:44–52.

Vissing J, Andersen M, Diemer NH. Exercise-induced changes in local cerebral glucose utilization in the rat. J Cereb Blood Flow Metab. 1996;16:729–36.

Wang RY, Yang YR, Yu SM. Protective effects of treadmill training on infarction in rats. Brain Res. 2001;922:140–3.

Westerberg V, Lewis J, Corcoran ME. Depletion of noradrenaline fails to affect kindling seizures. Exp Neurol. 2004;84:237–40.

Wong J, Wirrell E. Physical activity in children/teens with epilepsy compared with that in their siblings without epilepsy. Epilepsia. 2006;47:631–9.

Ziemann AE, Schnizler MK, Albert GW, Severson MA, Howard III MA, Welsh MJ, et al. Seizure termination by acidosis depends on ASIC1a. Nat Neurosci. 2008;11:816–22.

Index

L. Rocha and E.A. Cavalheiro (eds.), *Pharmacoresistance in Epilepsy: From Genes and Molecules to Promising Therapies*, DOI 10.1007/978-1-4614-6464-8,

Printed by Publishers' Graphics LLC
FMRO140214.15.17.22